1 MONTH OF
FREE
READING

at

www.ForgottenBooks.com

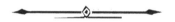

By purchasing this book you are eligible for one month membership to ForgottenBooks.com, giving you unlimited access to our entire collection of over 1,000,000 titles via our web site and mobile apps.

To claim your free month visit:

www.forgottenbooks.com/free922091

ISBN 978-0-260-01146-6
PIBN 10922091

This book is a reproduction of an important historical work. Forgotten Books uses state-of-the-art technology to digitally reconstruct the work, preserving the original format whilst repairing imperfections present in the aged copy. In rare cases, an imperfection in the original, such as a blemish or missing page, may be replicated in our edition. We do, however, repair the vast majority of imperfections successfully; any imperfections that remain are intentionally left to preserve the state of such historical works.

TRANSACTIONS

OF THE

SOUTHERN SURGICAL AND GYNECOLOGICAL ASSOCIATION
' ' '

VOLUME XXII

TWENTY-SECOND SESSION

HELD AT HOT SPRINGS, VA.

DECEMBER 14, 15 AND 16, 1909

EDITED BY W. D. HAGGARD, M.D.

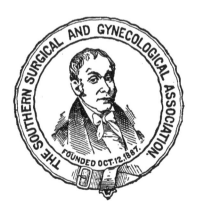

PUBLISHED BY THE ASSOCIATION

1910

DORNAN, PRINTER
PHILADELPHIA

CONTENTS.

CONTENTS

The Association does not hold itself responsible for the views enunciated in the papers and discussions published in this volume.

W. D. HAGGARD, M.D., *Secretary,*
NASHVILLE, TENN

OFFICERS FOR 1909–1910.

PRESIDENT.

W. O. ROBERTS, Louisville, Ky.

VICE-PRESIDENTS.

JOSEPH C. BLOODGOOD, Baltimore, Md.

LEWIS C. MORRIS, Birmingham, Ala.

SECRETARY.

WILLIAM D. HAGGARD, Nashville, Tenn.

TREASURER.

WM. S. GOLDSMITH, Atlanta, Ga.

COUNCIL.

HOWARD A. KELLY, Baltimore, Md.

STUART McGUIRE, Richmond, Va.

GEORGE H. NOBLE, Atlanta, Ga.

GEORGE BEN JOHNSTON, Richmond, Va.

BACON SAUNDERS, Fort Worth, Texas

CHAIRMAN COMMITTEE OF ARRANGEMENTS.

RUFUS E. FORT, Nashville, Tenn.

LIST OF OFFICERS

FROM THE ORGANIZATION TO THE PRESENT TIME

President.	Vice-Presidents.	Secretary.	Treasurer.
1888. *W. D. Haggard.	R. D. Webb. J. W. Sears.	*W. E. B. Davis.	Hardin P. Cochrane.
1889. *Hunter M. McGuire.	W. O. Roberts. *Bedford Brown.	*W. E. B. Davis.	Hardin P. Cochrane.
1890. *George J. Engelmann.	*Berthold E. Hadra. Duncan Eve.	*W. E. B. Davis.	Hardin P. Cochrane.
1891. Lewis S. McMurtry.	*J. McFadden Gaston. J. T. Wilson.	*W. E. B. Davis.	Hardin P. Cochrane.
1892. *J. McFadden Gaston.	*Cornelius Kollock. George Ben Johnston.	*W. E. B. Davis.	Hardin P. Cochrane.
1893. *Bedford Brown.	Joseph Price. George A. Baxter.	*W. E. B. Davis.	Hardin P. Cochrane.
1894. *Cornelius Kollock.	A. B. Miles. J. B. S. Holmes.	*W. E. B. Davis.	Hardin P. Cochrane.
1895. Lewis McLane Tiffany.	Ernest S. Lewis. Manning Simons.	*W. E. B. Davis.	*Richard Douglas.
1896. Ernest S. Lewis.	Joseph Taber Johnson. *Richard Douglas.	*W. E. B. Davis.	*A. M. Cartledge.
1897. George Ben Johnston.	W. E. Parker. Floyd W. McRae.	*W. E. B. Davis.	*A. M. Cartledge.
1898. *Richard Douglas.	*H. H. Mudd. James A. Goggans.	*W. E. B. Davis.	*A. M. Cartledge.
1899. Joseph Taber Johnson.	F. W. Parham. W. L. Robinson.	*W. E. B. Davis.	*A. M. Cartledge.
1900. *A. M. Cartledge.	Manning Simons. W. P. Nicolson.	*W. E. B. Davis.	W. D. Haggard.
1901. Manning Simons.	George H. Noble. L. C. Bosher.	W. D. Haggard.	Floyd W. McRae.
1902. *W. E. B. Davis.	J. Wesley Bovée. J. W. Long.	W. D. Haggard.	Floyd W. McRae.
1903. J. Wesley Bovée.	Christopher Tompkins. Bacon Saunders.	W. D. Haggard.	Floyd W. McRae.
1904. Floyd W. McRae.	George S. Brown. J. Shelton Horsley.	W. D. Haggard.	Charles M. Rosser.
1905. Lewis C. Bosher.	J. D. S. Davis. I. S. Stone.	W. D. Haggard.	Charles M. Rosser.
1906. George H. Noble.	Stuart McGuire. E. Denegre Martin.	W. D. Haggard.	Charles M. Rosser.
1907. Howard A. Kelly.	Rufus E. Fort. Hubert A. Royster.	W. D. Haggard.	Charles M. Rosser.
1908. F. W. Parham.	Henry D. Fry. W. F. Westmoreland.	W. D. Haggard.	Stuart McGuire.
1909. Stuart McGuire.	John Young Brown. R. S. Cathcart.	W. D. Haggard.	Wm. S. Goldsmith.
1910. W. O. Roberts.	Joseph C. Bloodgood. Lewis C Morris.	W. D. Haggard.	Wm. S. Goldsmith.

* Deceased.

HONORARY MEMBERS.

1894.—Foy, George   Dublin.

1894.—Jacobs, Charles   Brussels.

1894.—Martin, A.   Berlin.

1902.—Maury, Richard B.   Memphis, Tenn.

1894.—Morisani, O.   Naples.

1894.—Pozzi, S.   Paris.

1902.—*Reamy, Thaddeus   Cincinnati, Ohio.

1907.—Tiffany, L. M.   Baltimore, Md.

* Deceased.

MEMBERS.

1908.—ABELL, IRVIN, M.D. Professor of Principles and Practice of Surgery and Clinical Surgery, Medical Department, University of Louisville; Visiting Surgeon, University Hospital, Louisville City Hospital, and St. Mary and Elizabeth Hospital. 1228 Second St., Louisville, Ky.

1905.—BAKER, JAMES NORMENT, M.D. Visiting Surgeon, St. Margaret's Hospital; Secretary of the Medical Association of the State of Alabama. 719 Madison Avenue, Montgomery, Ala.

1894.—BALDRIDGE, FELIX E., M.D. Huntsville, Ala.

1900.—BALDY, JOHN MONTGOMERY, M.D. Professor of Gynecology, Philadelphia Polyclinic; Surgeon to Gynecean Hospital; Consulting Surgeon to Frederick Douglass Free Hospital and to the Jewish Hospital. 2219 De Lancey Place, Philadelphia, Pa.

1903.—BALLOCH, EDWARD A., M.D. Professor of Surgery, Medical Department of Howard University; Surgeon to Freedmen's Hospital; Member American Academy of Medicine. 1511 Rhode Island Avenue, N. W., Washington, D. C.

1908.—BARR, RICHARD ALEXANDER, M.D. Professor of Abdominal Surgery, Medical Department of Vanderbilt University; late Major of First Tennessee Infantry, U. S. A. First National Bank Building, N. Nashville, Tenn.

1905.—BARROW, DAVID, M.D. Ex-President Kentucky State Medical Society. 148 Market Street, Lexington, Ky.

1905.—BARTLETT, WILLARD, M.D. 4257 Washington Boulevard, St. Louis, Mo.

1904.—BATCHELOR, JAMES M., M.D. House Surgeon of Charity Hospital; Associate Professor of Surgery, Tulane University. New Orleans, La.

1901.—BAUGHMAN, GREER D., M.D. Lecturer on Hygiene; Demonstrator of Pathology; Demonstrator of Physiology; in charge of Gynecological Dispensary at Medical College of Virginia. 12 North Second Street, Richmond Virginia.

1907.—BEVAN, ARTHUR DEAN, M.D. Professor Surgery Rush Medical College, University of Chicago. 100 State Street, Chicago, Ill.

1908.—BLAIR, VILRAY PAPIN, A.M., M.D. Metropolitan Building, St. Louis, Mo.

1906.—BLOODGOOD, JOSEPH COLT, M.D. Associate Professor of Surgery, Johns Hopkins University; Associate Surgeon, Johns Hopkins Hospital; Surgeon to the Union Protestant Infirmary; Chief Surgeon to St. Agnes' Hospital. *Vice-President.* 904 North Charles Street, Baltimore Md.

1893.—BLOOM, J. D., M.D. Consulting Surgeon, Touro Infirmary; Lecturer on Diseases of Children, Tulane University. New Orleans, La.

1901.—BOLDT, HERMANN J., M.D. Gynecologist to Post-Graduate Hospital, St. Mark's Hospital, German Polyclinic; Consulting Gynecologist to the Beth Israel Hospital and to St. Vincent's Hospital; Professor of Gynecology, Post-Graduate Medical School; Member of the Gynecological Society of Germany; Fellow of the American Gynecological Society; Fellow of the Royal Society of Medicine (London); ex-President of the New York Obstetrical Society; of the German Medical Society of New York; of the Section of Obstetrics of the New York Academy of Medicine. 29 East Sixty-first Street, New York, N. Y.

1902.—BONIFIELD, CHARLES LYBRAND, M.D. Professor of Clinical Gynecology, Medical College of Ohio (Medical Department University of Cincinnati); Member American Association of Obstetricians and Gynecologists; ex-President Cincinnati Academy of Medicine; ex-President Cincinnati Obstetrical Society. 409 Broadway, Cincinnati, Ohio.

1890.—BOSHER, LEWIS CRENSHAW, M.D. Professor of Practice of Surgery and Clinical Surgery in the Medical College of Virginia; Visiting Surgeon to the Memorial Hospital; Member of American Surgical Association; Member of the American Association of Obstetricians and Gynecologists; Member of Association of American Anatomists; Member of American Urological Association; ex-President of Richmond Academy of Medicine and Surgery. *Vice-President,* 1901 *President,* 1905. 422 East Franklin Street, Richmond, Va.

1895.—BOVÉE, J. WESLEY, M.D. Fellow of American Gynecological Society; President of Washington Obstetrical and Gynecological Society; ex-President Medical and Surgical Society of the District of Columbia; Honorary Fellow Medical Society of Virginia; Professor of Gynecology of George Washington University, Washington, D. C.; Gynecologist to Providence, Columbia, and George Washington University Hospitals; Consulting Physician to St. Ann's Infant Asylum, and Attending Gynecologist to St. Elizabeth's Hospital for the Insane, Washington, D. C. *Vice-President*, 1902; *President*, 1903; Member of *Council*, 1903-1906. The Rochambeau, Washington, D. C.

1902.—BROOME, G. WILEY, M.D. Consulting Surgeon, St. Louis City and Female Hospitals; Member St. Louis Medical Society. 612 N. Taylor Avenue, St. Louis, Mo.

1898.—BROWN, GEORGE S., M.D. Ex-President Jefferson County Medical Society. *Vice-President*, 1804. Birmingham, Ala.

1905.—BROWN, JOHN YOUNG, M.D. Formerly Surgeon-in-Charge, St. Louis City Hospital; President of the American Association of Obstetricians and Gynecologists, 1906. *Vice-President*. Metropolitan Building, St. Louis, Mo.

1908.—BRYAN, ROBERT C., M.D. Professor of Descriptive Anatomy, University of Medicine, Visiting Surgeon to the Virginia Hospital. Fifth and Main Streets, Richmond, Va.

1907.—BURCH, LUCIUS E., M.D. Professor of Gynecology, Vanderbilt University, Medical Department; Gynecologist, St. Thomas' Hospital, Nashville; Gynecologist, Nashville City Hospital; Captain and Surgeon, N. G. S. T. 150 Eighth Avenue, N., Nashville, Tenn.

1899.—BURTHE, L., M.D. 124 Baronne Street, New Orleans, La.

1900.—BYFORD, HENRY T., M.D. Professor of Gynecology and Clinical Gynecology, College of Physicians and Surgeons (University of Illinois); Professor of Gynecology, Post-Graduate Medical School of Chicago; Surgeon to Woman's Hospital, etc. 100 State Street, Chicago, Ill.

1902.—CALDWELL, C. E., A.M., M.D. Professor of Principles of Surgery, Miami Medical College; Visiting Orthopedic Surgeon, Cincinnati Hospital; Member Cincinnati Academy of Medicine. 110 Cross Lane, Walnut Hills, Cincinnati, Ohio.

1906.—CANNADY, JOHN EGERTON, M.D. Former Surgeon-in-Charge to Sheltering Arms Hospital, Hansford, W. Va.; Fellow of the American Association of Obstetricians and Gynecologists; Non-resident Honorary Fellow of the Kentucky State Medical Society; Fellow of the West Virginia Medical Association, Virginia Medical Society, Tri-State Society of Virginia and the Carolinas, American Association of Railway Surgeons. Coyle and Richardson Building, Charleston, W. Va.

1904.—CAROTHERS, ROBERT, M.D. Professor of Clinical Surgery, Medical College of Ohio, Medical Department Cincinnati University; Surgeon to the Good Samaritan Hospital; 413 Broadway, Cincinnati, Ohio.

1903.—CARR, WILLIAM P. M.D. Professor of Physiology and Professor of Clinical Surgery, Columbian University; Surgeon to the Emergency Hospital and University Hospital; Consulting Surgeon to the Washington Asylum Hospital and the Government Hospital for the Insane, Washington, D. C. 1418 L Street, N. W., Washington, D. C.

*1891.—CARTLEDGE, ABIAH MORGAN, M.D.

1899.—CATHCART, R. S., M.D. Assistant to Chair of Clinical Surgery in the Medical College of the State of South Carolina. *Vice-President.* 66 Hasell Street, Charleston, South Carolina.

1904.—CHAMBERS, P. F., M.D. Attending Surgeon, Woman's Hospital; Consulting Surgeon, French Hospital. 49 West Fifty-seventh Street, New York, N. Y.

1907.—CLARK, JOHN G., M.D. Professor of Gynecology, University of Pennsylvania; Gynecologist-in-Chief, University Hospital. 2017 Walnut Street, Philadelphia Penna.

1907.—CLARK, S. M. D., M.D. Associate Professor Gynecology, Tulane Medical Department; Visiting Surgeon, Charity Hospital. 1435 Harmony Street, New Orleans, La.

1893.—COCRAM, HENRY S., M.D. 124 Baronne Street, New Orleans, La.

1908.—COFFEY, ROBERT C., M.D. Secretary Oregon State Board of Medical Examiners; Councellor Oregon State Medical Association. Portland, Oregon.

1909.—COLE, HERBERT PHALON, M.D. Instructor in Gynecology and Clinical Diagnosis, Medical Department of the University of Alabama; Gynecologist to City Hospital of Mobile. 202 Conti Street, Mobile Ala.

1893.—COLEY, ANDREW JACKSON, M.D. Councillor of the Medical Association of the State of Alabama. Alexander City, Ala.

1902.—COLEY, WILLIAM B., M.D. Clinical Lecturer on Surgery, College of Physicians and Surgeons; Assistant Surgeon in Hospital for Ruptured and Crippled; Attending Surgeon to General Memorial Hospital; Fellow of the American Surgical Association, New York Surgical Society, and New York Academy of Medicine. 5 Park Avenue, New York, N. Y.

1908.—CONNELL, F. GREGORY, M.D. Associate Surgeon St. Mary's Hospital. Oshkosh, Wis.

1907.—CRAWFORD, WALTER W., M.D. Ex-President Perry County Medical Society; Ex-president Mississippi State Medical Association; Surgeon to South Mississippi Infirmary. Hattiesburg, Miss.

1902.—CRILE, GEORGE W., M.D. Professor of Clinical Surgery, Medical College of Western Reserve University; Surgeon to St. Alexis' Hospital; Surgeon to Lakeside Hospital. 275 Prospect Street, Cleveland, Ohio.

1908.—CRISLER, JOSEPH AUGUSTUS, M.D. Professor of Anatomy and Operative Surgery, College of Physicians and Surgeons, Memphis, Tennessee; Lecturer on Minor Surgery, Medical Department, University of Mississippi; ex-Member Mississippi State Board of Health and Medical Examiners; ex-Vice-President Mississippi State Medical Association and Tri-State Medical Association; Member Mississippi Medical Association. Memphis Trust Building, Memphis, Tenn.

1893.—CROFFORD, T. J., M.D. Professor of Physiology and Clinical Lecturer on Gynecology in the Memphis Hospital Medical College. 155 Third Street, Memphis, Tenn.

1906.—CULLEN, THOMAS STEPHEN, M.D. Associate Professor of Gynecology, Johns Hopkins University; Associate in Gynecology, Johns Hopkins Hospital; Consultant in Abdominal Surgery, Church Home and Infirmary. Fellow of the American Gynecological Society; Honorary Member to La Societa Italiana Ostettricia Ginecologia, Rome; Corresponding Member of the Gesellschaft f. Geburtshülfe, Leipzig. 3 West Preston Street, Baltimore, Md.

Founder.—CUNNINGHAM, RUSSELL M., M.D. Professor of Practice of Medicine and Clinical Medicine, Birmingham

Medical College; Surgeon to the Pratt Mines Hospital. Ensley, Ala.

1906.—CUSHING, HARVEY, M.D. Associate Professor of Surgery in the Johns Hopkins University. 3 West Franklin Street, Baltimore, Md.

1907.—DANNA, JOSEPH A., M.D. First Assistant House Surgeon, Charity Hospital. Charity Hospital, New Orleans, La.

Founder.—DAVIS, JOHN D. S., M.D. Professor of Surgery, Birmingham Medical College; Surgeon to Hillman Hospital; ex-President of the Jefferson County Medical Society and of the Board of Health of Jefferson County. *Vice-President,* 1905. Avenue G and Twenty-first Street, Birmingham, Ala.

1891.—DEAN, G. R., M.D. Fellow of the American Association of Obstetricians and Gynecologists; ex-President of South Carolina State Medical Association; ex-President Association of Surgeons of Southern Railroad. Spartanburg, S. C.

1900.—DEAVER, JOHN B., M.D. Surgeon-in-Chief to the German Hospital. 1634 Walnut Street, Philadelphia.

1897.—DORSETT, WALTER B., M.D. Professor of Obstetrics and Clinical Gynecology, St. Louis University; Gynecologist to the Missouri Baptist Sanitarium and to Evangelical Deaconess' Hospital. 5070 Washington Boulevard, St. Louis, Mo.

1896.—DOUGHTY, W. H., M.D. Professor of Special Surgery and Surgical Pathology, Medical Department, University of Georgia; Chief Surgeon to Charleston and Western Carolina Railroad. 822 Greene Street, Augusta, Ga.

1890.—EARNEST, JOHN G., M.D. Professor of Clinical Gynecology, College of Physicians and Surgeons; formerly Professor of Gynecology, Southern Medical College; Visiting Gynecologist to the Grady Hospital. 828 Candler Building, Atlanta, Ga.

1907.—ELBRECHT, OSCAR HERMAN, M.D. Superintendent and Surgeon-in-Charge of St. Louis Female Hospital; Vice-President, St. Louis Obstetrical and Gynecological Society. 5600 Arsenal Street, St. Louis, Mo.

1891.—ELKIN, WILLIAM SIMPSON, M.D. Professor of Operative and Clinical Surgery, Atlanta College of Physicians and Surgeons; ex-President of the Atlanta Society of Medicine; Surgeon to Grady Hospital. 27 Luckie Street, Atlanta, Ga.

1900.—FERGUSON, ALEXANDER HUGH, M.D. Professor of Surgery, Chicago Post-Graduate; Professor of Surgery, Medical Department (College of Physicians and Surgeons), University of Illinois. 10 Drexel Square, Chicago, Ill.

1904.—FINNEY, J. M. T., M.D. Associate Professor of Surgery, Johns Hopkins University; Surgeon to Outpatients, Johns Hopkins Hospital. 1300 Eutaw Place Baltimore, Md.

1901.—FORT, RUFUS E., M.D. Chief Surgeon, Nashville Terminal Company; Surgeon to Southern and Illinois Central Railroads; Surgeon to Nashville Hospital; *Vice-President* 1907. 209 Seventh Avenue, N., Nashville, Tenn.

1895.—FORTIER, S. M., M.D. Visiting Surgeon to Charity Hospital. 4422 St. Charles Avenue, New Orleans, La.

1905.—FRANK, LOUIS, M.D. Professor of Abdominal and Pelvic Surgery, University of Louisville; Visiting Surgeon to the Louisville City Hospital. 400 Atherton Building, Louisville, Ky.

1902.—FREIBERG, ALBERT H., M.D. Professor of Orthopedic Surgery in the Medical College of Ohio, Medical Department of the University of Cincinnati; Orthopedic Surgeon to the Cincinnati Hospital and to the Jewish Hospital of Cincinnati. 19 West Seventh Street, Cincinnati, Ohio.

1895.—FRY, HENRY D., M.D. Professor of Obstetrics, Georgetown University; *Vice-President.* 1601 Connecticut Avenue, N. W., Washington, D. C.

1903.—GALE, JOSEPH A., M.D. Surgeon-General Norfolk and Western R. R.; ex-President of Medical Society of Virginia. Roanoke, Va.

1901.—GAVIN, GEORGE EDWIN, M.D. 11 South Conception Street, Mobile, Ala.

1902.—GILLESPIE, REESE B., M.D. Surgeon to Tazewell Sanitarium. Tazewell, Va.

1897.—GLASGOW, FRANK A., M.D. Professor of Clinical Gynecology of St. Louis Medical College; Gynecologist to St. Louis Mullanphy Hospital; on staff of Martha Parsons Free Hospital; Consulting Surgeon to St. Louis Female Hospital. 3894 Washington Boulevard, St. Louis, Mo.

Founder.—GOGGANS, JAMES A., M.D. Ex-President of the Tri-State Medical Society of Alabama, Georgia, and Tennessee; Senior Councillor of the Medical Association of the State of Alabama; Fellow of the British Gynecological Society. *Vice-President*, 1898. Alexander City, Ala.

1900.—GOLDSMITH, W. S., M.D. *Treasurer.* 262 Jackson Street, Atlanta, Ga.

1909.—GRAHAM, JOSEPH, M.D. Visiting Surgeon to Watts Hospital; Visiting Surgeon to the Lincoln Hospital. 410 Mangum Street Durham, N. C.

1892.—GRANT, HORACE H., M.D. Professor of Surgery in the Hospital College of Medicine; Surgeon to the Louisville City Hospital. 321 Equitable Building, Louisville, Ky.

1905.—GUERRY, LE GRAND, M.D. Surgeon, Columbia Hospital. Columbia, S. C.

1896.—GWATHMEY, LOMAX, M.D. Attending Gynecologist to St. Vincent Hospital and Dispensary. Norfolk, Va.

1896.—HAGGARD, WILLIAM DAVID, M.D. Professor of Clinical and Abdominal Surgery, Medical Department, University of Nashville, Tennessee; Gynecologist to St. Thomas' Hospital; Surgeon to Nashville City Hospital; Member Alumni Association of Woman's Hospital, of New York. *Treasurer*, 1900; *Secretary.* 148 Eighth Avenue, N., Nashville, Tenn.

1892.—HALL, RUFUS BARTLETT, A.M., M.D. Professor of Clinical Gynecology in the Miami Medical College; Gynecologist to the Presbyterian Hospital; ex-President of the Cincinnati Obstetrical Society; ex-President of the American Association of Obstetricians and Gynecologists; Fellow of British Gynecological Society. 628 Elm Street, Cincinnati, Ohio.

1901.—HAZEN, CHARLES M., M.D. Professor of Physiology, Medical College of Virginia. Bon Air (Richmond), Va.

1896.—HEFLIN, WYATT, M.D. Ex-President of the Jefferson County Medical Society. Birmingham, Ala.

1905.—HENDON, GEORGE A., M.D. Professor of Principles and Practice of Surgery and Surgical Pathology, Hospital College of Medicine. 1826 Baxter Avenue, Louisville, Ky.

Founder.—HERPF, FERDINAND, M.D. 308 East Houston Street, San Antonio, Texas.

1889.—HILL, ROBERT SOMERVILLE, M.D. Gynecologist to the Laurel Hill Hospital; Senior Councillor of the Medical Association of the State of Alabama; ex-President of the

Montgomery County Medical and Surgical Association; former Surgeon of the Second Regiment, Alabama State Militia. Montgomery, Ala.

1902.—HIRST, BARTON COOKE, M.D. Professor of Obstetrics, University of Pennsylvania; Fellow of College of Physicians, Philadelphia; Gynecologist to the Howard, Orthopedic, and Philadelphia Hospitals; Fellow of American Gynecological Society. 1821 Spruce Street, Philadelphia, Pa.

1900.—HOKE, MICHAEL, M.D., B.E. 268 Peachtree Street, Atlanta, Ga.

1906.—HOLDEN, GERRY R., M.D. Formerly House Surgeon, Roosevelt Hospital, New York City; formerly Resident Gynecologist, Johns Hopkins Hospital, and Assistant in Gynecology, Johns Hopkins Medical School, 223 West Forsyth Street, Jacksonville, Fla.

1891.—HOLMES, J. B. S., M.D. Ex-President of the Tri-State Medical Society of Alabama, Georgia, and Tennessee, ex-President of the Georgia Medical Association; Fellow of the American Association of Obstetricians and Gynecologists. *Vice-President,* 1894. Valdosta, Ga.

1900.—HORSLEY, JOHN SHELTON, M.D. Professor of Principles of Surgery and Clinical Surgery, Medical College of Virginia; Surgeon to Memorial Hospital. *Vice-President,* 1904. 303 West Grace Street, Richmond, Va.

1896.—HUNDLEY, J. MASON, M.D. Associate Professor of Diseases of Women and Children, University of Maryland; President Clinical Society of Baltimore. 1009 Cathedral Street, Baltimore, Md.

1903.—HUNNER, GUY LE ROY, M.D. Associate in Gynecology, Johns Hopkins University; Professor of Genito-Urinary Surgery, Woman's Medical College of Baltimore; Gynecologist-in-Chief, St. Agnes' Hospital; Visiting Gynecologist, Church Home and Hebrew Hospital, Baltimore, Frederick City Hospital, Frederick, Md., and Hagerstown Hospital, Hagerstown, Md.; Consulting Gynecologist, Brattleboro Memorial Hospital, Brattleboro, Vt. 2305 St. Paul Street, Baltimore, Maryland.

1900.—ILL, EDWARD JOSEPH, M.D. Surgeon to the Woman's Hospital; Medical Director, St. Michael's Hospital Gynecologist and Supervising Obstetrician, St. Barnabas' Hospital; Consulting Gynecologist to German Hospital and Beth Israel Hospital of Newark, N. J.; to All Souls' Hospital,

Morristown, N. J., and to Mountain Side Hospital, Montclair N. J.; Vice-President from New Jersey to Pan-American Congress of 1893.   1002 Broad Street, Newark, N. J.

1908.—IRVIN, JAMES S., M.D.   Danville, Va.

1889.—JOHNSON, JOSEPH TABER, M.D.   Professor of Gynecology and Abdominal Surgery, Georgetown University; formerly Gynecologist to Providence Hospital; Chief of Service of Gynecology and Abdominal Surgery, Georgetown University Hospital, and President of the Board of Administration; President of the Woman's Dispensary, and of the Medical Society of the District of Columbia (1887); Member of the British Medical Association; Fellow of the Gynecological Society; President of the Washington Obstetrical and Gynecological Society; Secretary American Gynecological Society, 1886-1890, and President, 1899.   *President*, 1899.   926 Farragut Square, Washington, D. C.

Founder.—JOHNSTON, GEORGE BEN, M.D.   Formerly Consulting Surgeon to the Richmond Eye, Ear, and Throat Infirmary; ex-President of the Richmond Academy of Medicine and Surgery; ex-President of the Medical Society of Virginia; Member of the American Association of Obstetricians and Gynecologists, and First Vice-President, 1896; Member of the Ninth International Medical Congress; Member of the American Surgical Association; Professor of the Practice of Surgery and Clinical Surgery in the Medical College of Virginia and formerly Professor of Anatomy; Surgeon to the Old Dominion Hospital; Consulting Surgeon to the City Free Dispensary.   *Vice-President*, 1892; *President*, 1897.   407 East Grace Street, Richmond, Va.

1908.—JONAS, ERNST, M.D.   Clinical Professor of Surgery, Medical Department, Washington University; Chief of Surgical Clinic, Washington University Hospital; Gynecologist to the Jewish Hospital; Surgeon to the Martha Parsons Hospital for Children; Fellow of the American Association of Obstetricians and Gynecologists.   4495 Westminster Place, St. Louis, Mo.

1902.—JORDAN, WILLIAM MUDD, M.D.   Surgeon to St. Vincent's Hospital; Gynecologist to Hillman Hospital formerly Assistant Surgeon, U. S. Marine Hospital Service. Birmingham, Ala.

1890.—KELLY, HOWARD ATWOOD, M.D.   Founder of Kensington Hospital, Philadelphia; Associate Professor of

Obstetrics, University of Pennsylvania, 1888-89; Professor of Gynecology and Obstetrics, Johns Hopkins University, 1888-99; Professor of Gynecology, Johns Hopkins University; Gynecologist-in-Chief to Johns Hopkins Hospital; Member Associé Etranger de la Société Obstétricale et Gynécologique de Paris; Correspondirendes Mitglied der Gesellschaft f. Geburtshülfe zu Leipzig; Honorary Fellow Edinburgh Obstetrical Society, Royal Academy of Medicine (Ireland), and British Gynecological Society; Member Washington Academy of Sciences; Fellow American Gynecological Society. *President*, 1907. 1418 Eutaw Place, Baltimore, Md.

1907.—KIRCHNER, WALTER C. G., M.D. Superintendent and Surgeon-in-Charge, St. Louis City Hospital. President Medical Society City Hospital Alumni. City Hospital, St. Louis, Mo.

1899.—KOHLMAN, WILLIAM, M.D. 3500 Prytania Street New Orleans, La.

1894.—LEIGH, SOUTHGATE, M.D. Visiting Surgeon to St. Vincent's and Norfolk Protestant Hospitals; First Vice-President Medical Society of Virginia, 1899-1900. 147 Granby Street, Norfolk.

1893.—LEWIS, ERNEST S., M.D. Professor of Gynecology, Medical Department of Tulane University. *Vice-President*, 1895; *President*, 1896; *Member of Council*, 1896-1903. 124 Baronne Street, New Orleans, La.

1900.—LLOYD, SAMUEL, M.D. Professor of Surgery, New York Post-Graduate Medical School; Attending Surgeon to Post-Graduate Hospital and St. Francis' Hospital, and Consulting Surgeon to the Benedictine Sanitarium at Kingston, N. Y. 12 West Fiftieth Street, New York, N. Y.

Founder.—LONG, JOHN W., M.D. Emeritus Professor of Gynecology and Pediatrics in the Medical College of Virginia; formerly Gynecologist to the Old Dominion Hospital and the Richmond City Dispensary; Consulting Surgeon to the Watts Hospital, Durham; Member, ex-Orator, and ex-Vice-President of the North Carolina Medical Society. *Vice-President*, 1902. Greensboro, N. C.

1904.—LUPTON, FRANK A., M.D. 716 North Eighteenth Street, Birmingham, Ala.

1902.—McADORY, WELLINGTON P., M.D. Surgeon to Hillman Hospital. Birmingham, Ala.

1895.—McGANNON, M. C., M.D. Professor of Gynecology, Medical Department, Vanderbilt University; Chief Surgeon, Woman's Hospital. 118 Eighth Avenue, N., Nashville, Tenn.

1893.—McGUIRE, STUART, M.D. Professor of the Principles of Surgery and Clinical Surgery, University College of Medicine; Surgeon-in-Charge, St. Luke's Hospital; Visiting Surgeon, Virginia Hospital; Consulting Surgeon, Virginia Home for Incurables. *President*, 1908. 518 East Grace Street, Richmond Va.

1891.—McGUIRE, W. EDWARD, M.D. Professor of Gynecology, University College of Medicine; Gynecologist to the Virginia Hospital. 411 East Grace Street, Richmond, Va.

1905.—MacLEAN, HENRY STUART, M.D. Professor of Pathology, University College of Medicine. 406 West Grace Street, Richmond, Va.

1888.—McMURTRY, LEWIS S., M.D. Ex-President of the American Medical Association; Professor of Abdominal Surgery and Gynecology in the Medical Department of the University of Louisville; Surgeon to the Louisville City Hospital; Gynecologist to St. Mary and St. Elizabeth Hospital; Gynecologist to Gray Street Infirmary; ex-President of the American Association of Obstetricians and Gynecologists; ex-President of the Kentucky State Medical Society; Corresponding Member of the Gynecological Society of Boston; Fellow of the British Gynecological Society; Ordinary Fellow of the Edinburgh Obstetrical Society; Fellow of the American Surgical Society. *President*, 1891. Suite 610, The Atherton, Fourth and Chestnut Streets, Louisville, Ky.

1888.—McRAE, FLOYD WILLCOX, M.D. Professor of Gastro-intestinal, Rectal, and Clinical Surgery, Atlanta College of Physicians and Surgeons; Surgeon to Grady Hospital; ex-President Medical Association of Georgia; ex-Secretary of Section on Surgery and Anatomy, American Medical Association. *Treasurer*, 1901-1903; *President*, 1904. Peters Building, Atlanta, Ga.

1900.—MacDONALD, WILLIS G., M.D. Professor of Surgery (Adjunct), Albany Medical College; Surgeon to Albany Hospital; Chief Surgeon of South End Dispensary; Fellow of the American Surgical Society. 29 Eagle Street, Albany, N. Y.

1891.—MARCY, HENRY ORLANDO, M.D., LL.D. Ex-President of the American Medical Association; President of the Section of Gynecology, Ninth International Medical Congress; late President of the American Academy of Medicine; Corresponding Member of the Medico-Chirurgical Society of Bologna, Italy; Fellow of the American Association of Obstetricians and Gynecologists. 180 Commonwealth Avenue, Boston, Mass.

1899.—MARTIN, EDMUND DENEGRE, M.D. Professor of Minor and Clinical Surgery, New Orleans Polyclinic; Visiting Surgeon to the Charity Hospital; Consulting Surgeon to the Eye, Ear, Nose, and Throat Hospital; President Orleans Parish Medical Society; ex-Vice-Pesident American Medical Association. 115 Chartres Street, New Orleans, La.

1909.—MARTIN, FRANK, M.D. Clinical Professor of Surgery at the University of Maryland. 1000 Cathedral Street, Baltimore, Md.

1904.—MASON, J. M., M.D. Gynecologist to St. Vincent Hospital. 1915 Sixteenth Avenue, S., Birmingham, Ala.

1899.—MASTIN, WILLIAM M., M.D. Fellow of the American Surgical Association; Member of the American Association of Genito-urinary Surgeons; Surgeon to the Mobile City Hospital. Joachim and Conti Streets, Mobile, Ala.

1893.—MATAS, R., M.D. Professor of Surgery, Medical Department of Tulane University; Fellow of the American Surgical Association. 624 Gravier Street, New Orleans, La.

1896.—MATTHEWS, WILLIAM P., M.D. Professor of Anatomy, Medical College of Virginia; Orthopedic Surgeon to the Old Dominion Hospital. Richmond, Va.

1902.—MAYO, CHARLES H., M.D. Attending Surgeon, St. Mary's Hospital; Member American Surgical Society; ex-President, Western Surgical and Gynecological Association and of Minnesota State Medical Society. Rochester, Minn.

Founder.—MERIWETHER, FRANK T., M.D. Assistant Surgeon, U. S. A. (Retired). Asheville, N. C.

1899.—MICHINARD, P. E., M.D. 624 Gravier Street, New Orleans, La.

1888.—MILLER, C. JEFF., M.D. Professor of Operative Gynecology, New Orleans Polyclinic; Visiting Gynecologist to Charity Hospital. 1719 Jackson Avenue, New Orleans, La.

1907.—MITCHELL, JAMES F., M.D. Surgeon to Providence Hospital. 1344 Nineteenth Street, Washington, D. C.

1901.—MIXTER, SAMUEL JASON, M.D. Surgeon, Massachusetts General Hospital; Consulting Surgeon, Massachusetts Charity Eye and Ear Infirmary; Instructor of Surgery, Harvard Medical School. 180 Marlborough Street, Boston, Mass.

1904.—MORAN, JOHN F., M.D. Professor of Obstetrics, Georgetown University; Obstetrician to Georgetown University Hospital and Columbia Hospital for Women. Washington, D. C.

1903.—MORGAN, JAMES B., M.D. Professor of Anatomy and Clinical Surgery, Medical College of Georgia; Chairman Board of Censors, Georgia Medical Association. 1272 Broad Street, Augusta, Ga.

1902.—MORRIS, LEWIS C., M.D. Professor of Anatomy and Associate Professor of Gynecology, Birmingham Medical College; Councillor of Medical Association, State of Alabama; Vice-President of Tri-State Medical Society of Alabama, Georgia, and Tennessee. *Vice-President.* 716 North Eighteenth Street, Birmingham, Ala.

1900.—MORRIS, ROBERT TUTTLE, M.D. Professor of Surgery, New York Post-Graduate Medical School and Hospital. 616 Madison Avenue, New York, N. Y.

1901.—MULLALLY, LANE, M.D. Professor of Obstetrics and Diseases of Children, Medical College, State of South Carolina; Visiting Physician in Obstetrics and Pediatrics, Roper Hospital. Charleston, S. C.

1905.—MUNRO, JOHN CUMMINGS, M.D. Surgeon-in-Chief, Carney Hospital; Consulting Surgeon, Quincy Hospital and Framingham Hospital; President of the Society of Clinical Surgery; Member American Surgical, American Academy, and of the Association of American Anatomists. 173 Beacon Street, Boston, Mass.

1891.—MURFREE, JAMES BRICKLE, M.D. Formerly Professor of Surgery, University of the South (Sewanee); ex-President of the Tennessee State Medical Society, of the Tri-State Medical Society of Alabama, Georgia, and Tennessee. Murfreesboro, Tenn.

1894.—MURPHY, J. B., M.D. Professor of Surgery, Northwestern University; Professor of Surgery, Post-Graduate School and Hospital; Attending Surgeon, Cook County and Mercy Hospitals. 100 State Street, Chicago, Ill.

Founder.—NASH, HERBERT MILTON, M.D. Consulting Surgeon to the Retreat for the Sick (Hospital), Norfolk, Consultant to the Staff of St. Vincent's Hospital; ex-President of the Norfolk City Medical Society; Member of the State Board of Medical Examiners of Virginia. 296 Freemason Street, Norfolk, Va.

1889.—NICOLSON, WILLIAM PERRIN, M.D. Professor of Anatomy and Clinical Surgery, Atlanta College of Physicians and Surgeons; Visiting Surgeon to Grady Hospital; Senior Surgeon to Wesley Memorial Hospital; Senior Surgeon, St. Joseph Hospital. *Vice-President*, 1900. Prudential Building, Atlanta, Ga.

1896.—NOBLE, CHARLES P., M.D. Surgeon-in-Chief, Kensington Hospital for Women; Consulting Surgeon, Woman's Hospital; Lecturer on Gynecology, Philadelphia Polyclinic. 1500 Locust Street, Philadelphia, Pa.

1890.—NOBLE, GEORGE H., M.D. Dean and Professor of Abdominal Surgery and Clinical Gynecology, Atlanta School of Medicine; Gynecologist of Grady Hospital; Senior Gynecologist, Wesleyan Memorial Hospital, Atlanta; Fellow of the American Gynecological Association and the American Association of Obstetricians and Gynecologists; ex-President of the Medical Association of Georgia; ex-Secretary of the Section of Obstetrics, American Medical Association. *Vice-President*, 1901; *President*, 1905. 131 South Pryor Street, Atlanta, Ga.

1903.—NOLEN, WILLIAM L., M.D. Ex-President, Chattanooga Medical Society. Salem, Va.

1890.—NUNN, R. J., M.D. Savannah, Ga.

1902.—O'BRIEN, MATTHEW WATSON, M.D. Surgeon, Southern and Chesapeake and Ohio Railways; Member of the American Association for the Advancement of Science. 908 Cameron Street, Alexandria, Va.

1901.—OCHSNER, A. J., M.D. Adjunct Professor of Clinical Surgery, College of Physicians and Surgeons; Surgeon-in-Chief, Augustana and St. Mary's Hospital. 710 Sedgwick Street, Chicago, Ill.

1903.—OCHSNER, EDWARD H., M.D. Surgeon to Augustana and St. Mary's Hospital. 710 Sedgwick Street, Chicago, Ill.

1904.—OECHSNER, JOHN F., M.D. Professor of Orthopedic Surgery and the Surgery of Children, Post-Graduate Medical Department, Tulane University of Louisiana; Visiting Surgeon, Charity Hospital. Macheca Building, New Orleans, Louisiana.

1902.—OLIVER, JOHN CHADWICK, M.D. Dean and Professor of Operative Surgery, Miami Medical College; Surgeon to the Cincinnati, Christ, and Presbyterian Hospitals. 628 Elm Street, Cincinnati, Ohio.

Founder.—PAINE, JOHN FANNIN YOUNG, M.D. Professor of Obstetrics and Gynecology in the Medical Department, University of Texas; Gynecologist and Obstetrician, John Sealy Hospital; Fellow of the American Association of Obstetricians and Gynecologists; ex-President of the Texas Medical Association; Fellow of the Texas Academy of Science. 2177 Market Street, Galveston, Texas.

1888.—PARHAM, F. W., M.D. Professor of Surgery in the New Orleans Polyclinic. *Vice-President*, 1899; *President*, 1908. 1429 Seventh Street, New Orleans, La.

1900.—PARK, ROSWELL, M.D. Professor of Surgery, Medical Department, University of Buffalo; Surgeon, Buffalo General Hospital; Member of German Congress of Surgeons, Italian Surgical Society, American Surgical Association, American Orthopedic, and American Genito-urinary Associations. 510 Delaware Avenue, Buffalo, N. Y.

1899.—PERKINS, W. M., M.D. Chief of the Clinic Chair of General Clinical and Operative Surgery, New Orleans Polyclinic; Assistant Demonstrator of Operative Surgery, Medical Department, Tulane University of Louisiana; Visiting Surgeon to the Charity Hospital. Macheca Building, New Orleans, La.

1908.—PETERSON, REUBEN, A.M., M.D. Professor of Obstetrics and Gynecology, University of Michigan; Obstetrician and Gynecologist-in-Chief to the University of Michigan Hospital. Ann Arbor, Mich.

1899.—PLATT, WALTER BREWSTER, M.D. Surgeon to the Robert Garrett Hospital for Children. 802 Cathedral Street, Baltimore, Md.

1889.—POLK, WILLIAM M., M.D. Dean and Professor of Obstetrics and Gynecology, Cornell University Medical College; Gynecologist to Bellevue Hospital; Consulting Surgeon to St. Luke's, St. Vincent's, New York Lying-in, and Trinity Hospitals; ex-President of American Gynecological Society, and New York Obstetrical Society. 7 East Thirty-sixth Street, New York.

1900.—PORTER, MILES F., M.D. Fellow American Surgical Association. 47 West Wayne Street, Fort Wayne, Ind.

1889.—POTTER, WILLIAM WARREN, M.D. Consulting Gynecologist to the Woman's Hospital; Consulting Surgeon to the Buffalo General Hospital; President and Examiner in Obstetrics, New York State Medical Examining and Licensing Board; Chairman of Section of Obstetrics and Diseases of Women, American Medical Association, 1890; President of the Buffalo Obstetrical Society, 1884-1886; President of the Medical Society of the State of New York, 1891; Executive President of the Section of Gynecology and Abdominal Surgery, Pan-American Medical College, 1893. 238 Delaware Avenue, Buffalo, N. Y.

1889.—PRICE, JOSEPH, M.D. Physician-in-Charge of the Obstetrical and Gynecological Department of the Philadelphia Dispensary; Fellow of the American Association of Obstetricians and Gynecologists; ex-Chairman, Section of Diseases of Women and Obstetrics, American Medical Association. *Vice-President*, 1893. 241 North Eighteenth Street, Philadelphia, Pa.

1900.—RANSOHOFF, JOSEPH, M.D., F.R.C.S. Professor of Anatomy and Clinical Surgery, Medical College of Ohio; Surgeon to Cincinnati, Good Samaritan, and Jewish Hospitals; Member American Surgical Association. 19 West Seventh Street, Cincinnati, Ohio.

1890.—REED, CHARLES ALFRED LEE, M.D. Ex-President of the American Medical Association; Professor of Gynecology and Abdominal Surgery in the Cincinnati College of Medicine and Surgery; Surgeon to the Cincinnati Free Hospital for Women; Fellow of the American Association of Obstetricians and Gynecologists; Fellow of the British Gynecological Society; ex-Chairman of the Section on Obstetrics and Diseases of Women of the American Medical Association; Secretary-General of the Pan-American Medical Congress, 1893; Honorary Member of the Medical Society of the State of New York. Corner Seventh and Race Streets, Cincinnati, O.

1900.—REES, CHARLES MAYRANT, M.D. Professor of Abdominal Surgery and Gynecology, Charleston Medical School; Abdominal Surgery and Gynecology, City Hospital; Gynecologist to Shirro's Dispensary. Charleston, S. C.

1899.—RICHARDSON, MAURICE HOWE, M.D. Visiting Surgeon to the Massachusetts General Hospital; Assistant Professor of Clinical Surgery, Harvard Medical School; Mosely

Professorship of Surgery to Harvard University. 224 Beacon Street, Boston, Mass.

1888.—ROBERTS, WILLIAM O., M.D. Professor of Principles of Surgery and Clinical Surgery, Medical Department of the University of Louisville; formerly Secretary of the Surgical Section of the American Medical Association. *President; Vice-President*, 1889. 1520 Third Street, Louisville, Ky.

1901.—ROBINS, CHARLES RUSSELL, M.D. Professor of Gynecology, Medical College of Virginia; Gynecologist to the Memorial Hospital; Surgeon to the Atlantic Coast Railroad. 8 West Grace Street, Richmond, Va.

1889.—ROBINSON, WILLIAM LOVAILLE, M.D. Fellow of the American Association of Obstetricians and Gynecologists; ex-President of the Danville Medical Society; Member of the Medical Examining Board of Virginia; ex-President of Virginia Medical Society. *Vice-President*, 1899. 753 Main Street, Danville, Va.

1906.—ROGERS, CAREY PEGRAM, M.D. Chief of Surgical Staff, St. Luke's Hospital; Consulting Surgeon, Sea Board Air Line Railway. 221 Laura Street, Jacksonville, Fla.

1901.—ROGERS, MACK, M.D. Professor of Anatomy, Birmingham Medical College. 212 Twentieth Street, Birmingham, Ala.

1901.—ROSSER, CHARLES M., M.D. Professor of Surgery, Baylor University, College of Medicine; Consulting Surgeon, Parkland Hospital; Attending Surgeon, Texas Baptist Memorial Sanitarium; ex-Vice-President Texas State Medical Association; Vice-President, Tri-State Society of Texas, Louisiana and Arkansas. *Treasurer*, 1904–07. 432 Gaston Avenue, Dallas, Texas.

1899.—ROYSTER, HUBERT A., A.B., M.D. Professor of Gynecology and Dean of the Faculty, Medical Department University of North Carolina; Gynecologist to Rex Hospital; Surgeon-in-Chief, St. Agnes' Hospital. *Vice-President*, 1907. Tucker Building, Raleigh, N. C.

1909.—RUFFIN, KIRKLAND, M.D. Surgeon-in-Charge of St. Christopher's Hospital. 218 York Street, Norfolk, Va.

1901.—RUNYAN, JOSEPH P., M.D. 203 West Second Street, Little Rock, Ark.

1908.—RUSSELL, WM. WOOD, M.D. Associate Professor of Gynecology, Johns Hopkins University; Associate in

Gynecology, Johns Hopkins Hospital; Gynecologist to Union Protestant Infirmary, Baltimore. Baltimore, Md.

1893.—SAUNDERS, BACON, M.D. Professor of Surgery and Clinical Surgery and Dean of Faculty of Medical Department, Fort Worth University; ex-President, Texas State Medical Association. *Vice-President,* 1903; *Member of Council,* 1908. Ninth and Houston Streets, Fort Worth, Texas.

Founder.—SCHILLING, NICHOLAS, M.D. Cedar Bayou, Tex.

1907.—SCOTT, ARTHUR CARROLL, M.D. Senior Surgeon, Temple Sanatorium. Temple, Texas.

1899.—SHANDS, A. R., M.D. Professor of Orthopedic Surgery in the Medical Department of the George Washington University and in the University of Vermont; Orthopedic Surgeon to the George Washington University Hospital, the Emergency Hospital, and Central Dispensary; Charter Member Washington Academy of Sciences; Member American Orthopedic Association; and Honorary Member of Medical Society of Virginia. 901 Sixteenth Street, N. W., Washington, D. C.

1902.—SHERRILL, J. GARLAND, M.D. Professor of Surgery and Clinical Surgery, University of Louisville; Consulting Surgeon to Louisville Hospital. 633 St. Charles Place, Louisville, Ky.

1893.—SIMONS, MANNING, M.D. Professor of Clinical Surgery, Medical College, State of South Carolina; Surgeon to St. Francis Xavier's Infirmary; Surgeon to City Hospital; ex-President Medical Society of South Carolina; President of the South Carolina Medical Association; Member American Association of Obstetricians and Gynecologists; ex-Vice-President Tri-State Medical Society of Virginia and the Carolinas. *Vice-President,* 1895 and 1900; *President,* 1901. 111 Church Street, Charleston, S. C.

1900.—SIMPSON, FRANK FARROW, M.D. Assistant Gynecologist to Mercy Hospital; Gynecologist to Out-patient Department, Mercy Hospital. 524 Pennsylvania Avenue, Pittsburgh, Pa.

1899.—SMYTHE, FRANK DAVIE, M.D. Surgeon to St. Joseph's Hospital; Assistant Professor of Surgery, Memphis Hospital Medical College; Demonstrator of Operative Surgery; formerly Member of the State Board of Examiners of Mississippi. Porter Building, Memphis, Tenn.

1904.—STOKES, JAMES ERNEST, M.D. Salisbury, N. C.

Founder.—STONE, ISAAC SCOTT, M.D. Clinical Professor Gynecology, Georgetown University; Gynecologist to Columbia Hospital, and Associate Gynecologist to Georgetown University Hospital; Member American and British Gynecological Societies; Honorary Fellow of Medical Society of the State of New York; Fellow of the Medical Society of V rginia; Member Washington Academy of Sciences; Washington Obstetrical and Gynecological Society. 1618 Rhode Island Avenue, N. W., Washington, D. C.

1894.—TALLEY, DYER F., M.D. Associate Professor of Surgery, Birmingham Medical College; Attending Surgeon to Hillman Hospital; Surgeon to the Talley and McAdory Infirmary; Ex-President of the Jefferson County Medical Society; Member of the Southern Medical Association; Member of the Pan-American Medical Association; Member of the Alumni Association of the Charity Hospital of Louisiana; Member of the Board of Censors of the Jefferson County Medical Society; Member of the Alabama State Board of Censors, Committee of Public Health and Examiners; Fellow of the American Association of Obstetricians and Gynecologists. 1801 Seventh Avenue, Birmingham, Ala.

Founder.—TAYLOR, HUGH M., M.D. Professor of Practice of Surgery and Clinical Surgery, University College of Medicine; Surgeon to the Virginia Hospital; ex-President of the Virginia Board of Medical Examiners. 6 North Fifth Street, Richmond, Va.

1898.—TAYLOR, WILLIAM WOOD, A.B., M.D. Gynecologist to St. Joseph's and the Memphis City Hospitals. 246 Randolph Building, Memphis, Tenn.

1892.—THOMPSON, J. E., M.D. Professor of Surgery in the University of Texas. Galveston, Texas.

1890.—TOMPKINS, CHRISTOPHER, M.D. Professor of Obstetrics in the Medical College of Virginia. *Vice-President,* 1903. 116 East Franklin Street, Richmond, Va.

1908.—TORRANCE, GASTON, M.D. Member Surgical Staff, Hillman's Hospital; also the Sisters' Hospital and St. Vincent's; Fellow of the American Association of Obstetricians and Gynecologists. 325 to 328 Woodward Building, Birmingham, Ala.

1909.—TROUT, HUGH HENRY, M.D. Surgeon-in-Chief of Jefferson Surgical Hospital, Roanoke, Va. 1303 Franklin Road, Roanoke, Va.

1888.—TUHOLSKE, HERMAN, M.D. Professor of Surgery, Medical Department, Washington University; Consulting Surgeon, St. Louis City Hospital; Surgeon to St. Louis Polyclinic Hospital, etc. 465 North Taylor Street, St. Louis, Missouri.

1905.—VANCE, AP MORGAN, M.D. Surgeon to St. Mary and Elizabeth Hospital; Consulting Surgeon, Louisville City Hospital. 921 Fourth Street, Louisville, Ky.

1893.—VANDER VEER, ALBERT, M.D. Professor of Clinical, Didactic, and Abdominal Surgery, Albany Medical College; ex-President of the American Surgical Association; ex-President of the American Association of Obstetricians and Gynecologists; ex-President of the Medical Society of the State of New York. 28 Eagle Street, Albany, New York.

1909.—VAUGHAN, GEORGE TULLY, M.D. Professor of Surgery and Head of Department of Surgery in Georgetown University; Chief Surgeon in Georgetown University Hospital; Visiting Surgeon to the Emergency Hospital; Consulting Surgeon to the Government Hospital for the Insane. 1718 I Street, Washington, D.C.

1891.—WALKER, EDWIN, M.D., PH.D. Gynecologist to the Evansville City Hospital; ex-President Mississippi Valley Medical Association; President of the Indiana State Medical Society; Fellow of the American Association of Obstetricians and Gynecologists. 712 Upper Fourth Street, Evansville, Ind.

1905.—WATHEN, JOHN R., A.B., M.D. Professor of Principles and Practice of Surgery and Clinical Surgery, University of Louisville; Surgeon to St. Anthony's, Louisville City, and University of Louisville Hospitals. 628 Fourth Avenue, Louisville, Ky.

1898.—WATKINS, ISAAC LAFAYETTE, M.D. Ex-President of the Montgomery County Medical and Surgical Society. Montgomery, Ala.

1907.—WATTS, STEPHEN H., M.D. Professor of Surgery University of Virginia; Surgeon-in-Chief and Director of the University of Virginia Hospital. University of Virginia, Charlottesville, Va.

1901.—WERDER, X. O., M.D. Gynecologist, Mercy Hospital, Pittsburgh: Professor of Gynecology, West Pennsylvania Medical College; Consulting Surgeon to the South Side

Hospital, Allegheny General Hospital, St. Francis' Hospital, etc. 524 Pennsylvania Avenue, Pittsburgh, Pa.

1888.—WESTMORELAND, WILLIS F., M.D. Professor of Surgery, Atlanta College of Physicians and Surgeons. *Vice President.* 241 Equitable Building, Atlanta, Ga.

1904.—WHALEY, T. P., M.D. Lecturer on Genito-urinary and Renal Surgery, Charleston Medical School; Lecturer on Diseases of Skin, Medical College of the State of South Carolina; Surgeon to Sherra's Dispensary; Visiting Surgeon, Charleston City Hospital. 13 Wentworth Street, Charleston, S. C.

1902.—WHITACRE, HORACE J., M.D. Professor of Pathology and Lecturer on Surgery, Medical Department, University of Cincinnati, also Medical College of Ohio; Surgeon to Christ Hospital; Consulting Surgeon to Speer's Hospital. 22 West Seventh Street, Cincinnati, Ohio.

1900.—WILLIAMS, J. WHITRIDGE, A.B., M.D. Professor of Obstetrics, Johns Hopkins University; Obstetrician-in-Chief, Johns Hopkins Hospital; Gynecologist to the Union Protestant Infirmary. 1128 Cathedral Street, Baltimore, Md.

1907.—WILLIS, A. MURAT, M.D. Instructor in Abdominal Surgery, Medical College of Virginia; Junior Surgeon to Memorial Hospital, Richmond, Va. 405 East Grace Street, Richmond, Va.

Founder.—WILSON, J. T.. M.D. Ex-President of the North Texas Medical Association; President of the Texas Medical Association; Superintendent of the State Hospital for the Insane. *Vice-President,* 1891. Sherman, Texas.

1905.—WINSLOW, RANDOLPH, M.D. Professor of Surgery, University of Maryland; Chief Surgeon, University Hospital; Consulting Surgeon, Hebrew Hospital, and to the Hospital for Crippled Children. 1900 Mt. Royal Terrace, Baltimore, Maryland.

1905.—WITHERSPOON, T. CASEY, M.D. Formerly Professor of Operative and Clinical Surgery, Medical Department, St. Louis University; Member of American Association of Anatomists. 307 West Granite Street, Butte, Mont.

1900.—WYSOR, JOHN C., M.D. Surgeon-in-Charge, Chesapeake and Ohio Hospital. Clifton Forge, Va.

1900.—YOUNG, HUGH H., M.D. Chief of Clinic, Genito-urinary Surgery, Johns Hopkins Hospital. 1005 North Charles Street, Baltimore, Md.

1902.—ZINKE, E. GUSTAV, M.D.   Professor of Obstetrics
and Clinical Gynecology in the Ohio-Miami Medical College,
the Medical Department of the Cincinnati University;
Obstetrician and Gynecologist to German Protestant Hospital; Attending Obstetrician to Ohio Maternity; ex-President
of American Association of Obstetricians and Gynecologists.
4 West Seventh Street, Cincinnati, Ohio.

CONSTITUTION.

ARTICLE I.

The name of this Association shall be THE SOUTHERN SURGICAL AND GYNECOLOGICAL ASSOCIATION.

ARTICLE II.

The object of this Association is to further the study and practice of surgery and gynecology among the profession of the Southern States.

ARTICLE III.

This Association shall adopt and conform to the Code of Ethics of the American Medical Association.

ARTICLE IV.

SECTION 1. Any reputable physician who practises surgery or gynecology, and who is vouched for by two members of the Association and recommended by the Council, shall be eligible to membership in this body.

SEC. 2. The honorary members shall not exceed ten in number, and shall enjoy all the privileges of other members, excepting to vote or hold office, but shall not be required to pay any fee.

ARTICLE V.

SECTION 1. The officers of this Association shall be a President, two Vice-Presidents, a Secretary, a Treasurer, and a Council, elected by ballot.

SEC. 2. The President and Vice-Presidents shall be elected for one year, and the President shall not be eligible for reëlection at any time; the Secretary and Treasurer, each, for five years; and the Council as provided for in the By-laws.

ARTICLE VI.

SECTION 1. It shall be the duty of the President to preside at all meetings of the Association; to give the casting vote; to see that the rules of order and decorum be properly enforced in all deliberations of the Association; to sign the approved proceedings of each meeting, and to approve such orders as may be drawn upon the Treasurer for expenditures ordered by the Association.

SEC. 2. In the absence of the President the first Vice-President shall preside, and in his absence the second Vice-President shall preside.

SEC. 3. In the absence of all three, the Association shall elect one of its members to preside *pro tem.*

SEC. 4. It shall be the duty of the Secretary to keep a true and correct record of the proceedings of the meetings; to preserve all books, papers, and articles belonging to the archives of the Association; to attest all orders drawn on the Treasurer for moneys appropriated by the Association; to keep the account of the Association with its members; to keep a register of the members, with the dates of their admission and places of residence. He shall collect all moneys due from the members and pay to the Treasurer, taking his receipt for the same. He shall report such unfinished business of previous meetings as may appear on his books requiring action, and attend to such other business as the Association may direct. He shall also supervise and conduct all the correspondence of the Association, and edit the TRANSACTIONS under the direction of the Council.

SEC. 5. It shall be the duty of the Treasurer to keep a correct record of all moneys received from the hands of the Secretary, giving his receipt for the same; pay them out by order of the Association as indorsed by the President and attested by the seal in the hands of the Secretary.

SEC. 6. It shall be the duty of the President of the Association to appoint an Auditing Committee, consisting of three members of the Association, whose duty it shall be to examine the books of the Secretary and Treasurer, and report on the same on the last day of the session.

ARTICLE VII.

Vacancies occurring in the offices of the Association shall be filled by appointment of the President until the next meeting. He shall also have the appointment of all committees not otherwise provided for.

ARTICLE VIII.

This Constitution shall take effect immediately from the time of its adoption, and shall not be amended except by a written resolution, which shall lie over one year, and receive a vote of two-thirds of the members present.

ARTICLE IX.

Any member who for three consecutive years fails to attend the meetings or present a paper shall be dropped from the roll of membership.

ARTICLE X.

The membership of the Association shall be limited to two hundred.

ARTICLE XI.

All members who have been in continuous membership for twenty years and have attended fifty per cent. of the meetings shall become life members and be exempt from dues.

BY-LAWS.

ARTICLE I.

The Southern Surgical and Gynecological Association shall meet annually on the Tuesday of the week preceding the week in which Christmas occurs, at 10 A.M., at such place as may be designated at the preceding meeting.

ARTICLE II.

The members present shall constitute a quorum for business.

ARTICLE III.

The annual dues of each member shall be $10, paid in advance.

ARTICLE IV.

The usual parliamentary rules governing deliberative bodies shall govern the business workings of this Association.

ARTICLE V.

All questions before the Association shall be determined by a majority of the votes present.

ARTICLE VI.

The President shall deliver an annual address at each meeting of the Association.

ARTICLE VII.

The Secretary of the Association shall receive at each annual Session a draft from the President, drawn on the Treasurer, for the sum of $500, for services rendered the Association, and to this shall be added the necessary expense incurred in the discharge of his official duties.

ARTICLE VIII.

It shall be the duty of the Secretary, one month prior to the annual meeting, to notify the members of the Association, and urge their attendance.

ARTICLE IX.

The authors of papers shall notify the Secretary, six weeks prior to the meeting, of the titles of their essays, so that they may be incorporated in the preliminary programme.

ARTICLE X.

COUNCIL.

The Council shall consist of five members; and of those elected at the primary meeting, the first shall serve five years, the second four, the third three, the fourth two, and the fifth one year; so that subsequently one member of the Council shall be elected annually to serve five years. No member of the Council shall be eligible for reëlection. The President and Secretary shall be *ex-officio* members of the Council.

This Council shall organize by electing a Chairman and Secretary, and shall keep a record of its proceedings.

The duties of this Council shall be—

1. To investigate applications for membership and report to the Association the names of such persons as are deemed worthy.

2. To take cognizance of all questions of an ethical, judicial, or personal nature, and upon these the decision of the Council shall be final; *provided*, that appeal may be taken from such decision of the Council to the Association, under a written protest, which protest shall be sustained by the Association, and the matter shall then be referred to a special committee, with power to take final action.

3. All motions and resolutions before the Association shall be referred to the Council without debate, and it shall report by recommendation at as early an hour as possible.

ARTICLE XI.

The President shall appoint at each annual meeting a Committee of Arrangements.

ARTICLE XII.

The Council shall have full power to omit from the published TRANSACTIONS, in part or in whole, any paper that may be referred to it by the Association, unless specially instructed to the contrary by the Association, which will be determined by vote.

ARTICLE XIII.

Any member failing to pay his dues for more than one year shall be dropped.

ARTICLE XIV.

No paper shall be read before this Association which does not deal strictly with a subject of surgical or gynecological importance.

ARTICLE XV.

No paper read before this Association shall be published in any medical journal or pamphlet for circulation, as having been read before the Association, without having received the indorsement of the Council.

ARTICLE XVI.

The reading of papers shall be limited to twenty minutes each, except by permission of the Association.

MINUTES OF THE PROCEEDINGS

AT THE

TWENTY-SECOND ANNUAL MEETING

OF

THE SOUTHERN

SURGICAL AND GYNECOLOGICAL

ASSOCIATION,

HELD AT

THE HOMESTEAD,

Hot Springs, Virginia,

DECEMBER 14, 15, AND 16, 1909.

TWENTY-SECOND ANNUAL MEETING.

FIRST DAY.—*Tuesday, December* 14, 1909.

The following-named members were present:

BAKER, JAMES NORMENT

BALLOCH, E. A.

BAUGHMAN, GREER

BLOODGOOD, JOS. E.

BOSHER, LEWIS C.

BOVÉE, J. WESLEY

BROWN, JOHN YOUNG

BRYAN, ROBERT C.

BYFORD, HENRY T.

CALDWELL, C. E.

CANNADY, JOHN E.

CARR, W. P.

CATHCART, R. S.

CLARK, S. M. D.

COFFEY, ROBT. C.

CONNELL, F. GREGORY

CRAWFORD, W. W.

CRILE, G. W.

CULLEN, THOS. S.

DAVIS, JOHN D. S.

DORSETT, WALTER B.

EARNEST, JOHN G.

ELBRECHT, O. H.

FINNEY, J. M. T.

GOLDSMITH, W. S.

GUERRY, LE GRAND

GWATHMEY, LOMAX

HAGGARD, WILLIAM D.

HALL, RUFUS B.

HEFLIN, WYATT

HENDON, GEO. A.

HOLDEN, GERRY R.

HORSLEY, J. SHELTON

IRVIN, JAMES S.

JOHNSTON, GEO. BEN

KELLY, HOWARD A.

KIRCHNER, W. C. G.

LONG, JOHN W.

McGUIRE, STUART

McGUIRE, W. EDWARD

McMURTRY, LEWIS S.

MacLEAN, H. S.

MATTHEWS, WILLIAM P.

MAYO, CHAS. H.

MITCHELL, JAS. F.

MORRIS, LEWIS C.

MORRIS, ROBT. T.

MULLALLY, LANE

MUNRO, JOHN C.

PARK, ROSWELL

PETERSON, REUBEN

PLATT, W. B.

POLK, WILLIAM M.

PRICE, JOSEPH

RANSOHOFF, JOSEPH M.

REED, CHAS. A. L.

ROBERTS, W. O.

ROBINSON, W. L.

ROGERS, MACK
ROYSTER, H. A.
RUSSELL, W. WOOD
SAUNDERS, BACON
SCOTT, A. C.
SHANDS, A. R.
SHERRILL, J. GARLAND
SIMONS, MANNING
STOKES. J. E.
STONE, I. S.

TALLEY, D. F.
TAYLOR, HUGH M.
VANDER VEER, ALBERT
WATTS, STEPHEN H.
WHALEY, T. P.
WHITACRE, H. J.
WINSLOW, RANDOLPH
WITHERSPOON, T. CASEY
WYSOR, JOHN C.

Letters and messages of regret were received from the following Fellows who were not able to attend the meeting: Dr. Herman J. Boldt, Dr. John G. Clark, Dr. W. B. Coley, Dr. G. R. Dean, Dr. John B. Deaver, Dr. H. H. Grant, Dr. Joseph Taber Johnson, Dr. Frank T. Meriwether, Dr. J. B. Murphy, Dr. Miles F. Porter, Dr. Chas. M. Rosser, Dr. F. F. Simpson, and Dr. H. O. Marcy.

Morning Session.—The Association met at 10 A.M., and was called to order by the Chairman of the Committee of Arrangements, Dr. Lewis C. Bosher, of Richmond, Virginia.

After announcing that a Smoker would be held Tuesday evening, and riding or driving parties and golfing on Wednesday afternoon, the President, Dr. Stuart McGuire, took the Chair, and called for the reading of the first paper.

Papers were read as follows:

1. "A Brief Discussion of Some of the Surgical Junk Demanding further Surgical Interference," by Dr. Joseph Price, Philadelphia, Pa., which was discussed by Drs. McMurtry, Vander Veer, Polk, and in closing by Dr. Price.

2. "Adhesion of Sigmoid to Tube and Broad Ligament as a Cause of Pain in Salpingitis," by Dr. Hubert A. Royster, Raleigh, N. C.

This paper was discussed by Drs. Byford, Morris, Cullen, Stone, Carr, and in closing by the essayist.

3. "The Treatment of Advanced Extra-uterine Pregnancy," by Dr. Reuben Peterson, Ann Arbor, Mich.

Discussed by Drs. Byford, Cullen, Morris, Bovée, Kirchner, Royster, Morris (L. C.), Price, Hall, and in closing by the author of the paper.

4. "Advantages of Neglect in Appendicitis Operations," by Dr. Robert T. Morris, New York City.

Discussed by Drs. Carr, Finney, and in closing by the essayist.

On motion, the Association adjourned until 2 P.M.

Afternoon Session.—The Association reassembled at 2 P.M., with the President in the Chair.

5. "An Unusual Type of Bladder Tumor," by Dr. Robert C. Bryan, Richmond, Va. (No discussion.)

6. "Some Observations upon the Surgery of the Knee-joint," by Dr. J. Garland Sherrill, Louisville, Ky.

Discussed by Drs. Shands, Roberts, Whitacre, Wysor, Watts, Winslow, and in closing by Dr. Sherrill.

7. "Ossifying Subperiosteal Hematoma (Myositis Ossificans)," by Dr. John M. T. Finney, Baltimore, Md.

Discussed by Drs. Bloodgood, Ransohoff, Crile, and the discussion closed by the essayist.

8. "A Plea for the More General Use of Cholecystenterostomy in Certain Cases of Pancreatitis," by Dr. Le Grand Guerry, Columbia, S. C.

9. "Hemorrhagic Pancreatitis, with Report of Two Cases," by Dr. Joseph Ransohoff, Cincinnati, Ohio.

10. "Some Recent Observations on Surgery of the Pancreas," by Dr. Joseph C. Bloodgood, Baltimore, Md.

11. "Pancreato-enterostomy," by Dr. R. C. Coffey, Portland, Ore.

These papers were discussed together. The discussion was opened by Dr. Bloodgood, and continued by Drs. Watts, Park, Mayo, Royster, Kirchner, Crile, Munro, Elbrecht, and the discussion closed by Drs. Guerry, Ransohoff, Coffey, and Bloodgood.

12. "Frequency of Cancer," by Dr. Roswell Park, Buffalo, N. Y.

On motion, the Association adjourned until Wednesday, 9 A.M.

SECOND DAY.—*Wednesday, December* 15, 1909.

Morning Session.—The Association met at 9 A.M., and was called to order by the President.

The courtesies of the floor were extended to Drs. White, Hanes, Cooper, Motley, Bishop, and Robinson.

13. "Suture of Recurrent Laryngeal Nerve, with Report of a Case," by Dr. J. Shelton Horsley, Richmond, Va.

Discussed by Drs. Balloch, Carr, Nash, Robinson, Mayo, and in closing by the essayist.

14. "Treatment of Wounds of the Heart, with Report of Two Cases," by Dr. Walter C. G. Kirchner, St. Louis, Mo.

Discussed by Drs. Kelly, Stone, Davis, Brown, Vander Veer, Lloyd, White, Watts, Ransohoff, and in closing by the essayist.

The President appointed on the Auditing Committee Drs. J. Garland Sherrill, Louisville; Dr. D. F. Talley, Birmingham, and G. D. Baughman, Richmond.

15. "Skin Grafting," by Dr. A. C. Scott, Temple, Texas.

Discussed by Drs. Price, Vander Veer, Winslow, Connell, Finney, Ransohoff, Horsley, Crile, Cullen, and in closing by the essayist.

16. "Circumscribed Serous Spinal Meningitis,'' by Dr. John C. Munro, Boston, Mass.

Discussed by Drs. Robinson, Kirchner, Mayo, and in closing by the essayist.

17. "Abdominal Section for Puerperal Eclampsia," by Dr. Lane Mullally, Charleston, S. C.

Discussed by Drs. Robinson, Peterson, Stone, Price, and in closing by the author of the paper.

NOTE.—No afternoon session was held, the time allotted for it being spent in riding or driving parties or golfing.

Evening Session.—The Association reassembled at 8 P.M., with the President in the Chair.

18. "Anatomical, Pathological, and Clinical Studies of Lesions Involving the Appendix and Right Ureter, with Special Reference to Diagnosis and Operative Treatment," by Drs. John Young Brown and William Engelbach, of St. Louis, Mo.

The paper was discussed by Drs. Kelly, Mayo, Polk, Coffey, Matthews, Reed, and the discussion closed by Dr. Brown.

19. "Latent and Active Neurasthenia in its Relation to Surgery," by Dr. Stuart McGuire, Richmond, Va. This was the title of the President's Address.

20. "Diagnosis of Hyperthyroidism, or Exophthalmic Goitre," by Dr. Charles H. Mayo, Rochester, Minn.

Discussed by Drs. Crile, Bloodgood, and in closing by Dr. Mayo.

21. "Hypernephromata (Illustrated with Lantern Slides),"
by Dr. Louis B. Wilson (by invitation), Rochester, Minn.

Discussed by Drs. Cullen, Munro, and in closing by Dr.
Wilson.

22. "Incision to Expose the Kidney," by Dr. Howard
A. Kelly, Baltimore, Md.

Discussed by Drs. Coffey, Cullen, Vander Veer, Bovée,
Matthews, and in closing by the essayist.

On motion, the Association adjourned until 8.45 A.M.
Thursday.

THIRD DAY.—*Thursday, December* 16, 1909.

Morning Session.—The Association met at 8.45 A.M.,
with the President in the Chair.

23. "Clinical and Experimental Research into Nitrous
Oxide and Ether Anesthesia," by Dr. Geo. W. Crile, Cleveland, Ohio.

Discussed by Drs. Reed, Horsley, Kelly, Coffey, Haggard,
Mayo, and in closing by the author of the paper.

24. "Some Observations on Gallstones, with Reference
to Cancer of the Gall-bladder," by Dr. Albert Vander Veer,
Albany, N. Y.

Discussed by Drs. Lloyd, Mayo, Sherrill, Elbrecht, Crile,
and in closing by the essayist.

25. "Acute Diffuse Peritonitis from Spontaneous Rupture
of Pyosalpinx," by Dr. J. Wesley Bovée, Washington, D. C.

Discussed by Drs. Elbrecht, McMurtry, Stone, Byford,
Sherrill, Clark, Morris, and in closing by the essayist.

26. "Some Therapeutic Adaptations of Cecostomy and
Appendicostomy," by Dr. Chas. A. L. Reed, Cincinnati, Ohio.

Discussed by Drs. Mc Murtry, Coffey, Sherrill, Polk,
Hanes (by invitation), and in closing by the essayist.

27. "Successful Enucleation of a Tumor from the Motor
Cortex," by Dr. Stephen A. Watts, Charlottesville, Va.

Discussed by Drs. Kirchner and Munro.

28. "Further Report on the Surgical Treatment of Epilepsy; Some Interesting Facts in Brain Surgery," by Dr.
W. P. Carr, Washington, D. C.

Discussed by Drs. Horsley, Gavin, Mayo, Kirchner, and
the discussion closed by the author of the paper.

29. "Some Cases of Surgical Shock, with Remarks,"
by Dr. J. G. Earnest, Atlanta, Ga.

S Surg   D

On motion, the Association then adjourned until 2.15 P.M.

Afternoon Session.—The Association reassembled at 2.30, with the President in the Chair.

30. "Symptoms and Ultimate Treatment of Hydatidiform Degeneration of the Chorion, with Report of a Case," by Dr. J. Ernest Stokes, Salisbury, N. C.

Discussed by Drs. Cullen, Haggard, Kelly, Hendon, and Peterson.

At this juncture Dr. Hubert A. Royster presented the report of the Auditing Committee, stating that the committee had examined the books of the Treasurer and Secretary and had found them correct, leaving a balance in the Treasury of $1843.79.

On motion of Dr. I. S. Stone, seconded by Dr. J. Wesley Bovée, the report of the Auditing Committee was adopted.

The Secretary read the report of the council, as follows:

REPORT OF THE COUNCIL.

To the members of the Southern Surgical and Gynecological Association the Council hereby makes the following recommendations:

1. That Article IX of the Constitution, providing that a member shall forfeit his membership if he fails to attend three consecutive meetings, be amended by substituting the word "five" consecutive years for three consecutive years.

2. That the deaths of Dr. Thaddeus A. Reamy, of Cincinnati, an honorary member, and of Dr. O. L. Shivers, of Marion, Ala., be appropriately recorded.

3. That the resignations of Dr. E. C. Dudley, of Chicago, Dr. John A. Wyeth, of New York, and Dr. J. Riddle Goffe, of New York, be accepted.

4. That the six vacancies in the constitutional limitation of membership be filled by the following applicants:

Dr. George Tulley Vaughan, Washington, D. C.

Dr. H. E. Trout, Roanoke, Va.

Dr. Joseph Graham, Durham, S. C.

Dr. Frank Martin, Baltimore, Md.

Dr. Herbert P. Cole, Mobile, Ala.

Dr. Kirkland Ruffin, Norfolk, Va.

5. That Nashville, Tenn., be nominated as the next place of meeting, and Dr. Rufus E. Fort be made Chairman of the Committee of Arrangements.

6. The following members are nominated for the respective offices:

President, Dr. W. O. Roberts, Louisville, Ky.

First Vice-President, Dr. Joseph C. Bloodgood, Baltimore, Md.

Second Vice-President, Dr. Lewis C. Morris, Birmingham, Ala.

Treasurer, Dr. William S. Goldsmith, Atlanta, Ga.

The office of Secretary holds over.

For the vacancy in the Council caused by the expiration of service of Dr. L. S. McMurtry, Dr. Stuart McGuire was nominated.

All of which is respectfully submitted,

H. A. KELLY,
BACON SAUNDERS,
STUART McGUIRE,
GEORGE BEN JOHNSTON,
L. S. McMURTRY,
W. D. HAGGARD.

It was moved and seconded that the report be adopted.

Dr. J. Wesley Bovée, of Washington, in speaking of Article IX of the Constitution, said he thought if any member was interested in the welfare of the Association he ought to be willing to attend its meetings oftener than once in five years in order to continue his membership, and for any member to absent himself for four consecutive years was more than a progressive association should expect, because there were too many good men on the outside waiting to become members. If it was seen fit to prolong the three-year limit, he thought the Association should compromise on four.

Dr. Lewis S. McMurtry, of Louisville said that the correspondence of the Secretary, which was submitted to Council, shows that if the three-year limit was enforced at this meeting it would work a hardship on a great many of the Fellows who had been veritable wheel-horses in the building up of the Association to its present proud position. Some of the older members might not be able to attend on account of being sick themselves or on account of having serious illness in members of their families; hence the enforcement of the three-year limit would be a hardship to many. Another year the Council could adopt a plan similar to that which the American Surgical Association established, namely, an honorary or seniority list for men who had served a long time and could not attend the meetings regularly. This Association could make such a provision another year if it saw fit to do so. That is, transferring the oldest members to this list and relieving them from the payment of dues, thus leaving vacancies in the active list to be filled by new members. He thought some arrangement of this kind should be carefully considered by the members, because they did not want to take men who had served and honored the Association for twenty or more years and drop them from the list of membership.

Dr. Bovée said it was in the power of the Association to excuse any member or to suspend any action of its regulations by unanimous consent. He was willing to have the matter lay over for further consideration, but was absolutely opposed to increase in the length of time.

Dr. Hubert A. Royster, of Raleigh, N. C., agreed with Dr. Bovée that the three-year limit was long enough, and he did not think the members would improve matters by making it five years.

Dr. I. S. Stone, of Washington, moved that the clause in the Constitution be amended so as to read "temporary suspension for one year," where a member had gone for three years without reading a paper.

Dr. William D. Haggard said the report should be disposed of in a constitutional and parliamentary manner. It could not be temporarily waived aside. If the members would reflect a little, it would be seen that if the three-year limit went into effect this year it would eliminate thirty-three members, and he felt sure the members did not want to do this, and that on further consideration of the matter they would take the view that had actuated the best judgment of the Council. He did not see any possible objection to letting the matter go for two years. In that time some of the present members might not want to retain their membership, while others might pass into the beyond. A good waiting list was a healthy thing to have. It showed that those who were not members appreciated the great importance of the Association and its work. After mature reflection his deliberate conclusion was that if the term could be limited to five years it would be more satisfactory, for the reason that if a man did not attend the meeting once in five years he ought to be dropped. The Association had been in existence for twenty-two years, and was considered one of the most successful and strongest organizations of its kind in this or any other country. He hoped the recommendations of the Council would be adopted.

Dr. Henry T. Byford, of Chicago, said there was either a misinterpretation of the report of the Council or else the report was unconstitutional, because the Constitution distinctly stated that "any member who for three consecutive years fails to attend the meetings or present a paper shall be dropped from the roll of membership."

According to the construction of that article of the Constitution we must expel them and not let them hang over another year. The amendment cannot be retroactive. Therefore, the motion made by Dr. Stone was just as constitutional as the motion that was made to adopt the report of the Council. We could lay aside any article of the Constitution by unanimous vote, when the voting was done by ballot. Action could be taken now, or that part of the Constitution by vote could be suspended for one year if the vote of the Association was unanimous. Accordingly, Dr. Byford moved that action in reference to this part of the Constitution be suspended until next year.

Seconded.

Dr. Stone accepted this, and said he did not want the Association to commit itself to the idea of extending the period to five years. He wanted the members to express themselves after mature thought, and by letting the matter go over for one year and the members in the meantime having time to think about it, next year they would be able to vote more intelligently.

Dr. McMurtry thought the wishes of Dr. Stone would be conserved by adopting the recommendations of the Council.

Dr. Samuel Lloyd, of New York, said that if the Association was going to provide for the retention of those gentlemen in the membership who were affected by the constitutional provision presented, it would be necessary to sustain their membership pending the approval of the Association of the constitutional amendment. In his judgment any other way of getting at the matter would be absolutely unconstitutional and unparliamentary, and it would require the approval of the amendment contained in the report of the Council to retain these men.

Dr. Lloyd then moved as an amendment, which was seconded and accepted, that pending the vote of the Association on the report of the Council, Article IX of the Constitution be suspended.

Carried.

The President then put the original motion to adopt the report of the Council as amended, which was carried.

The President appointed Drs. Howard A. Kelly and Randolph Winslow to escort the President-elect to the platform.

Dr. McGuire, in introducing his successor, said: "It is unnecessary to introduce Dr. Roberts to you. He has been a member of the Association for twenty years or more. I congratulate him on his election to the Presidency of this Association. I want to congratulate the Association on the fact that it has chosen a man who can carry out its work efficiently and faithfully." (Applause.)

Dr. Roberts, in accepting the Presidency, said: "Any gentleman would feel highly honored at being elected President of this Association, but I assure you that no one appreciates this honor more than I do. I attended the first meeting of this Association twenty-two years ago. It was held at Birmingham, Ala. The father of our Secretary, Dr. Haggard, was the presiding officer on that occasion, and the celebrated surgeon, Dr. Hunter McGuire, the father of the out-going President, was elected President for the ensuing year. Many of the men who were present at that meeting and who did excellent work in this Association, like these two great men, have passed to the beyond. I have been a regular attendant upon the meetings of this Association ever since then, and I have always gone home from the meetings delighted at having been present and at having heard the papers and the discussions.

"In thanking you, gentlemen, for the honor you have conferred upon me, I assure you that I will try to attend to the duties of the office to the best of my ability." (Applause.)

31. "Acute Abdominal Conditions in Infants," by Dr. Randolph Winslow, Baltimore, Md.

Discussed by Drs. Crile, Hall, Connell, McGuire, Munro, Stone, Johnston, Vander Veer, and Wysor.

32. "Acute Gastromesenteric Ileus following Operation for Ulcer of the Stomach," by Dr. T. Casey Witherspoon, Butte, Mont.

Discussed by Drs. Connell, Kirchner, and in closing by the author of the paper.

33. "Extraperitoneal Drainage after Ureteral Anastomosis," by Dr. J. E. Cannady, of Charleston, W. Va.

Discussed by Drs. Kelly, Bovée, and in closing by the author of the paper.

34. "Iodine Sterilization of the Skin,". by Dr. I. S. Stone, Washington, D. C.

Discussed by Drs. Kelly, Bovée, Witherspoon, and in closing by the essayist.

35. "A Tumor Developing from the Iliopsoas Bursa Opening into the Hip-joint and Containing Large, Free, Cartilaginous Masses,". by Dr. Thos. S. Cullen, of Baltimore, Md.

Discussed by Drs. Munro, and the discussion closed by the author of the paper.

36. "A Simple Method of Excising Varicose Veins,". by Dr. W. S. Goldsmith, Atlanta, Ga., was read by title.

As there were no more papers to be read, Dr. I. S. Stone said that he had never been more highly entertained at any meeting of any association of physicians or surgeons in his life than during the last three days. He was not saying this for himself, but in conversation with all of the members with whom he had conversed during this time he had learned from them that this was one of the best, probably the best, meetings in the history of the Association both from a social and scientific standpoint. Accordingly, he moved that a vote of thanks be extended to those who had prepared the program, as well as those who had conducted the affairs of the Association for the last year. Further, he moved that thanks be extended not only to the retiring President, but to the other officers who had so ably and efficiently performed their duties, as well as to those who had provided so well for the entertainment of the members and their guests.

This motion was duly seconded and unanimously adopted by a rising vote.

There being no further business, either scientific or otherwise, to come before the meeting, on motion the Association then adjourned to meet at Nashville, Tenn., in December, 1910.

W. D. HAGGARD,
Secretary.

ADDRESS OF THE PRESIDENT.

LATENT AND ACTIVE NEURASTHENIA IN ITS RELATION TO SURGERY.

By Stuart McGuire, M.D.,
Richmond, Virginia.

WE have met at this the twenty-second annual session of the Southern Surgical and Gynecological Association, some to learn, some to teach, and all to secure a well-earned vacation, and for a time, at least, be free from the complaints of nervous and exacting patients. This being the case, some of you may think that in choosing as the subject for a presidential address, "Latent and Active Neurasthenia in its Relation to Surgery," I have shown a lack of tact by introducing a topic which brings to mind unpleasant experiences, which for the occasion you wish to forget. I trust this will not be the case, and hope there will be found, if not in what I write, at least in what you read between the lines, something which will be of practical value.

Specialists usually divide functional neurotic disorders into hysteria, neurasthenia, and hypochondria.

Hysteria is a special psychical state often produced in certain individuals by suggestion, and capable of being relieved by persuasion. It is a condition of nervous instability, stigmatized by emotional storms, crises, contractures, and

S Surg   1

paralyses, by a craving for sympathy, a desire for an audience, and a tendency to pose.

Neurasthenia is a fatigue neurosis due in part to malnutrition, and in part to functional overexertion, occurring in persons with an hereditary or acquired predisposition. It is characterized by exhaustibility of the nervous system, slight exertion causing prostration and bringing on the various distressing symptoms from which the patient suffers.

Hypochondria is a mental disease marked by obsessions, depressions, and morbid fears concerning the health of the individual. It is not very common, is easily diagnosticated, and is usually incurable.

Hysterical patients give a great deal of trouble before an operation, but do very well after the ordeal is over. A nervous woman who describes her symptoms with hesitating vivacity, who desires to discuss every detail of her operation and subsequent treatment, and who is possessed of exaggerated fears of complications which may develop, or of the ultimate result which may follow, usually, after the operation is over, becomes a model patient. Her imagination enters upon fresh fields; she becomes hopeful and courageous, and begins at once to plan a new life of activity.

Neurasthenic patients usually discuss their cases calmly and logically: they describe their symptoms systematically, and employ technical terms correctly. They complain of nearly every organ in the body. The essential feature of their clinical picture is fatigue, exhaustion, and incapacity for prolonged physical or mental exertion. They suffer from general weakness, headache, backache, and insomnia. Their mental condition is one of hesitation, doubt, and indecision. They do not reach conclusions, and are unable to fix their attention for any period of time. They usually have digestive and sexual disorders, and often grossly exaggerate the importance of their symptoms. They frequently have psychic depressions, shown by irritability, introspection and selfishness. They are firmly convinced as to the nature of their disease, and come to the surgeon for what they believe to be a necessary operation.

Hypochondriac patients are the victims of what is often a hopeless psychosis. The individual is possessed of the idea that she has some strange and horrible malady. She soon wears out the patience of her family and friends, and in order to secure a sympathetic listener, and to demonstrate to the community the serious nature of her disease, she goes from surgeon to surgeon, and from hospital to hospital, offering herself as a bloody sacrifice to her curious obsession, and glorying in her martyrdom.

As simple hysteria is easily recognized and controlled, and as pure hypochondria is usually unmistakable and incurable, I will dismiss these two subjects and devote the time at my disposal to neurasthenia. I shall not limit the term to the definition given by the scientific neurologist, but shall employ it in the broad sense in which it is used by the practical surgeon. This is necessary because, while in theory it is easy to distinguish between hysteria, neurasthenia, and hypochondria, in practice it will be found that the symptoms of two or more of them are often present in the same patient at the same time. Thus, one writer says all hysterical patients are neurasthenic, but all neurasthenics are not hysterical. Name and classify neuroses as you please, the trail of the serpent is over them all.

None of us want neurasthenics as patients, but all of us have them constantly in our practice. Some of them are referred to us by the general practitioner; some come to us from other specialists; and some develop their pernicious symptoms under our personal observation and treatment. In deploring the frequency of neurasthenia, and in criticising practitioners in other departments of medicine for the occurrence of the disease, it should be remembered that we, as surgeons, are responsible for the development of a large number of these cases. A surgical operation injudiciously performed, or carried out without proper precautions on a susceptible patient, will frequently be the beginning of a neurosis, and terminate in the condition known as traumatic or surgical neurasthenia.

It is the object of this address, first, to emphasize the importance of refusing to operate on a neurasthenic patient unless the symptoms can be clearly shown to be due to organic disease; and second, to impress the necessity, if an operation is undertaken on a patient with either latent or developed neurasthenia, to protect the nervous system from psychical and physical shock, not only by a proper preliminary preparation, but by careful and often prolonged post-operative and post-hospital treatment.

A surgeon cannot be expected to be an expert neurologist, but for his own happiness, if not for his patient's welfare, he must study functional neurotic disorders, as well as organic diseases. He must learn to know his limitations, as well as recognize his abilities; and to estimate the possible injurious effects as well as the probable beneficial results to be expected from surgical intervention. He must remember that the patient does not come to him primarily to be cut, but to be cured; and that an operation is not a success unless the individual is restored to health, not only physically, but also psychically; not only anatomically, but also symptomatically. In surgery the main question is no longer one of mortality, but one of morbidity. In endeavoring to forecast the end results of an operation, the mental and nervous condition of the patient must be carefully considered. If neuroses exist, without anatomical disease, an operation will do no good, and may result in harm. If neuroses are found coincident with pathological lesions, an operation may prove of great benefit; but in relieving the physical disease, care must be taken to avoid increasing the nervous disorder. If neuroses are present, reflex in character and due to remediable causes, an operation may be undertaken with assurance of complete success. In other words, the surgeon should divide these cases into three classes: the first to be avoided; the second to be undertaken with caution; and the third to be cheerfully given the relief to which they are entitled.

Of the class to be avoided, because the neurasthenia has no organic basis, Goodell says: "The sufferer may be a jilted maiden, a bereaved mother, a grieving widow, or a neglected wife, and all her uterine symptoms—yes, every one of them—may be the outcome of her sorrow, and not of her local lesions. She is suffering from a sore brain and not from a sore womb." Here an operation will not relieve, but will aggravate, the symptoms.

Of the class to be undertaken with caution, because the neurasthenia is merely coincident with anatomical disease, it is often a question whether the patient had better endure the evils he has, or fly to those he knows not of. An illustration of where one of our greatest surgical philosophers elected the first course is quoted from Mumford's recent article: "Said John Hunter to a patient with a chronic running sore who was brought to him for consultation: 'And so, sir, you have a chronic running sore?'

"'Yes, Mr. Hunter.'

"'Well, sir, if I had your chronic running sore, I should say, "Mr. Sore, you may run and be damned."'"

In other cases it may be deemed best to operate—not to cure the neurasthenia, but to relieve the pathological condition. Great care must be exercised to avoid increasing the nervous weakness by the very means used to cure the physical discomfort. This is especially true in patients who have been previously the subject of other operations.

Of the class where the neurasthenia is directly due to anatomical disease, it may be said that if the diagnosis can be made and the cause removed, the patient will be cured. Often the symptoms are obscure and misleading, and much patient investigation will be necessary to reach the proper conclusion. A distinguished modern surgeon relates the following experience occurring in his early professional life. One of his friends developed digestive disturbances and came to see him with periodical regularity. He first treated him along accepted lines; then gave him all the samples of proprietary medicine left at his office, and as he did not improve, he decided that the man was a neurasthenic. One day he was hurriedly called to see him, and found he had acute appendicitis. He operated on him, and hoped that by taking out the appendix he had not only relieved the immediate danger, but had also removed the cause of his previous symptoms. Much to his disappointment, the patient, after leaving the hospital, complained as before, and he was therefore confirmed in his opinion that he was a neurasthenic. Later, the patient developed jaundice and symptoms of cholecystitis. He was operated on a second time and a number of gallstones removed, and it was again hoped that the cause of his trouble had been diagnosticated and relieved. Before he left the hospital, however, he began to have his old pains, and then the surgeon said he knew he was a neurasthenic. Despite his failure to secure relief, the patient persisted in coming to the office, and one day called just after the installation of an x-ray apparatus. More to test the new instrument than with any expectation of benefiting the patient, a skiagraph was made of his abdomen, and it was found that he had a stone in his right kidney. A third operation was performed, the stone removed, and from that time to this the patient has been absolutely well. This is not a unique case. All of us have had similar, if not quite such aggravated, experiences. The story is told to impress the fact that even an apparently hopeless neurasthenic should not be condemned without a trial, as some of them may be cured provided a correct diagnosis is made.

The means employed by surgeons to distinguish between hopeless and curable neurasthenia cover the entire field of diagnostic medicine, and cannot be discussed. The precautions to be observed in operating on a patient who is likely to develop neurasthenia will now be considered.

Two separate and independent preliminary examinations

should be made of every surgical patient: the first for the purpose of diagnosis, or the determination of the condition to be corrected; the second for the purpose of prognosis, or the determination of the safety of the operation, and the probability of a complete cure resulting from it. To do this satisfactorily it will usually be found necessary to secure the aid and coöperation of several specialists. Few busy surgeons have the time or skill to make the necessary physical examination of the heart and lungs, or the laboratory investigation of the urine, blood, and stomach contents, to say nothing of the special work which is sometimes required of the bacteriologist, ophthalmologist, neurologist, Röntgenologist, and other experts. Patients will not object to frequent and prolonged examinations, but will be inspired with confidence in the surgeon by the realization that nothing is taken for granted, and that every effort is being employed to ascertain the nature of their trouble and the best method to effect a cure. In fact, the laity are now so educated in medical matters that failure to give a case a thorough preliminary examination is a cause for criticism and distrust.

An important exception to this, however, is in the case of a young, unmarried woman who complains of pelvic symptoms. She may be of neurotic temperment, and, owing to backache and painful menstruation, become convinced she has uterine or ovarian disease, when, in fact, she has no local trouble. On the other hand, she may have cervical stenosis, uterine displacement, or ovarian cystoma. In such a case a physical examination should be made to ascertain whether the trouble is neurological or gynecological. In order to minimize the psychical shock and to avoid physical pain, the examination should be made under a general anesthetic. If her symptoms are found to be due to some defect of her nervous system, she should be positively assured she has no local lesion, and be referred to a suitable attendant for general treatment. If, on the other hand, her symptoms are found to be due to actual disease of the pelvis, she should be given the surgical relief her case demands. Noble has emphasized the fact that virgins rarely suffer from traumatism and infection of the genital organs, and when pathological disease exists they almost invariably demand operative treatment. Repeated examinations, local applications, and other manipulations do them little good, and often convert them into chronic nervous invalids. The "pelvic woman" of the old author is the "sexual neurasthenic" of the modern writer.

The preparation of a patient for operation should be both physical and psychical. In the past much attention has been paid to the first, and but little to the second. We now recognize that we have overdone starvation, purgation, and sterilization, and have neglected to study the patient's mental attitude to the operation, in order to lessen apprehension, if it is unduly present; to inspire confidence, if it is lacking; and to lay the foundation for a philosophy which will be needed during convalescence.

The surgeon's first efforts should be directed to relieving the patient's dread of going to the hospital. The laity are being rapidly educated to a just appreciation of the advantages afforded by such institutions, but some people still regard them as a cross between a prison and a pest house. The easiest and most effective way to overcome this belief is to induce the patient to enter the hospital several days before the date fixed for the operation. In the environment of a well regulated sanatorium excitement and fear will soon be replaced by calmness and hope.

The surgeon should see the patient daily. His bearing should be kindly but not oversympathetic. The patient should not be the object of commiseration because of the anticipated operation, but the subject of congratulation because her case is one that can be cured by surgery. She should be made to realize that operations are but an incident in the day's work, and that, while her case will receive al needful attention, she is not the most important individual in the hospital. Care should be taken, in talking to her, not to magnify the importance of her lesions or the difficulty and danger incident to their correction. The relatives and friends should, of course, be informed of the facts in the case, but the patient should not be burdened with doubts and fears. It is also well to avoid giving unnecessary information about the etiology and pathology of her disease, or to describe the different methods by which her abnormality might be corrected. While she will listen eagerly to any statement with reference to her case, and will enter into a discussion of what is best to do for her, she realizes that she does not fully comprehend what has been said to her by the surgeon, and is worried by the responsibility she has assumed in the opinion she has expressed to him.

It is, however, important at this time that the surgeon warn the patient against certain symptoms, complications, and sequelæ which may develop after the operation, telling her that while they entail no danger and will not affect the final result, it is well that she should realize their possibility, in order that, if they develop, she may know they were foreseen. For instance, a patient to be operated on for hemorrhoids should be told that possibly she will require catheterization for a day or two; a patient with a goitre, that her throat will feel sore, and it will hurt her to swallow; a patient with gallstones, that a drain will be used for a week or ten days; and a patient with fibromyoma of the uterus, that artificial menopause will follow, with symptoms such as usually occur at the "change of life." A word of warning before the operation will be found to be worth more than an hour's explanation afterward to prevent discouragement from ordinary sequelæ, whose significance and importance are not understood.

Finally, the patient's fear of the anesthetic should be relieved by reassurance, reason, or ridicule. A badly frightened patient should never be sent to the operating room.

Psychical shock is a greater factor than traumatic shock in the production of surgical neurasthenia.

Some patients are in good nervous and physical condition and require practically nothing but the mechanical correction of a local trouble. Others are as bad off nervously as they are physically, and often will be more benefited by a modified form of rest cure than by the operation itself. Most surgeons recognize this fact, but are often unable to carry out the principles of seclusion, rest, full feeding, bathing, massage, and electricity, as taught by Mitchell, because of the present attitude of the public to surgery. Not many years ago an operation was considered, in the words of the marriage ceremony, as something not to be entered into unadvisedly or lightly, but discreetly, soberly, and in the fear of God. Today it has come to be regarded as a comparatively trivial event, and the principal dread is the surgeon's fee. In the old days it was understood that a patient requiring a serious operation would have to remain two or three months in a hospital. At present, patients enter the hospital one day, are operated upon the next, begin to ask when they can go home before they stop vomiting, and usually are permitted to leave before it is wise for them to do so.

Nearly all surgeons admit the injurious results which frequently follow the premature discharge of a case from the hospital, but most of them try to evade responsibility by attributing the evil to the unreasonable insistence of the patient to be permitted to return home. The fault, however, is not with the laity, but with the profession. Patients would consent to longer detention in the hospital just as submissively today as they did some years ago, if they believed it to be necessary. The fault is with a few surgeons who, for various reasons, have entered into a competition to see who can get their cases out quickest, and have thereby set a precedent which others have followed. Some have been actuated by a desire to save the patient time and money; others by a desire to advertise themselves. The public is prone to estimate the ability of a surgeon by the apparent rapidity of the recovery of his patients, and to make comparisons between different operators on the basis of the length of time they keep their patients in the hospital. This is not surprising, as even some of the profession do not seem to fully realize that, all things being equal, a wound will not heal quicker for one man than it will for another, and the number of days a surgeon keeps a patient in bed is not a measure of his surgical dexterity, but of his surgical judgment.

In order to appreciate the dangers to a patient of premature discharge, it is necessary to contrast the conditions of hospital and home life. The change is as decided and the influence as great to either sex, the man on returning home being confronted by financial obligations and business complications, and the woman by family cares and domestic duties.

By way of illustration, we will take the case of a woman. While in the hospital she is free from responsibility, and has comforts and conveniences which are often as new as they are delightful. Her room is clean and well heated; dainty meals are served with clock-like regularity; and an electric bell commands the services of an attractive and efficient nurse. Other patients recovering from more serious operations inspire her with courage, and she emulates their example and tries to surpass them in rapidity of progress. It is like playing a game to see who can get well first. Above all, she is conscious of being under the watchful eye of the surgeon, and appreciates the fact that complications, if they occur, will be promptly corrected.

Now compare the condition of this woman when she returns home. At the very outset she has to meet either injudicious sympathy or unreasonable expectations. Sometimes her friends and relatives, by a combination of commiseration and indulgence, induce her to believe that she has been the most unfortunate woman on earth, and is therefore entitled to lead a life of invalidism for the remainder of her existence. Or, again, her husband and family may show in their manner, if they do not express it in words, the conviction that she ought to be in good working order after so much money has been spent in repairing her, and, as a result, she feels impelled to exert herself to discharge duties for which she is not physically competent. During the woman's absence from home the domestic economy often gets sadly out of gear. Undesirable relatives have come to make visits; servants have grown slack and impudent; children have been spoiled and pampered; and the husband's sexual appetite has not been gratified. As a consequence, in the first few days after her return, she has to snub her mother-in-law, discharge her servants, clean her house, cook her dinner, spank her babies, and resist or yield to her husband's advances.

If she lives in the country, as is often the case, the contrast between hospital and home life is even greater. The house is often inadequately heated; servants are generally unreliable and incompetent; food is usually indigestible in character and monotonous in variety; outdoor exercise is difficult to practise; a bath can only be obtained by bringing in a wash-tub and heating water in a kettle; and an evacuation of the bowels can only be effected by an excursion to the garden, along a grass-grown path overhung with box-wood bushes, and by the exposure of a vulnerable portion of the anatomy to the chilling wintry blasts. Is it a wonder that the woman becomes neurasthenic and fails to get well?

What has been said with reference to the short stay of patients in the hospital, and the conditions which frequently exist at home which work adversely to their recovery, makes it plain that those interested in their welfare should thoughtfully consider the situation and endeavor to remove the evil. The remedy obviously consists in the patient's remaining longer under the care of the surgeon, and on returning home being placed under the close supervision of the family physician.

A patient should not be detained an unnecessary time in the hospital, as it is not only a waste of the individual's time and money, but also tends to the creation of invalidism. A patient should not be dismissed too soon, as failure to secure the expected benefit from the operation may lead to discouragement, which finally results in well-established neurasthenia. Convalescence is a question of temperament, and must be psychical as well as physical. People are coming to regard surgeons as mechanics, and patients as machines which are to be repaired. They must be taught that the operation is not everything, and that the after-treatment is often of equal importance. They must be made to understand that the operation merely corrects an abnormal condition and puts Nature in a position to effect a cure; that often the first effect of an operation is injurious, and that the beneficial results are only experienced after the system recovers from the shock and readjusts itself to new conditions; that sometimes it takes weeks, months, or even years for this to be accomplished. They must be impressed with the fact that surgical patients are not well because their wounds have healed, but should remain in the hospital until they have regained to a certain extent their physical strength and nervous equilibrium, and that, after returning home, for a time they should lead a life of prudence and restraint.

The surgeon usually attempts to direct the treatment of patients after they return home by giving them verbal instruction when they leave the hospital, and by subsequently corresponding with them, but the end desired can be more effectually and properly secured by referring the patient back to the family physician. The reason verbal instructions are not satisfactory is because they cannot cover all eventualities, and are frequently not understood. When a surgeon takes charge of a new case he is on his mettle both to make a good impression and to solve the diagnostic problems presented. Consultations are usually held with other members of the staff, and for a day, at least, the case receives more attention than any other patient in the hospital. The diagnosis made, the operation performed, the danger period passed, and convalescence established, it is only natural that the surgeon's time and thoughts are occupied with more recent cases, so when the time comes to say good-bye and give parting instructions, he simply utters a few perfunctory injunctions, tells her to be patient and prudent, and to write him if she has any untoward symptoms. The patient's expectation and disappointment are often apparent, but she hesitates to ask the many questions which are uppermost in her mind for fear of wearying or irritating the busy man, the value of whose time she has been taught to respect.

The reason subsequent treatment by mail is not satisfactory is because patients usually fail to give important facts, and either exaggerate or underestimate their symptoms. Also because the surgeon cannot remember their idiosyncrasies and peculiarities, and even if he prescribes correctly, his advice lacks the personal element of suggestion which is so essential to make it efficient.

How much better it would be if the patient were examined before she left the hospital, and told that the operation which had been performed had satisfactorily corrected the condition which had given rise to her symptoms, but that she was not well and that it would require some months of proper living to restore her to full health and activity. She should be directed, on returning home, to place her case in the hands of her family doctor. This would safeguard the patient's future welfare, and would overcome to a large extent the growing feeling on the part of the general practitioner that he is not always fairly treated by the surgeon. Few surgeons are willing to turn patients over to a physician immediately after a serious operation. Complications are often so sudden and dangerous, symptoms so slight and misleading, diagnosis so difficult, and correct treatment so essential, that no one except a man who has had long and constant experience in the management of this special class of cases is competent to have charge of them. When, however, the danger of the operation is over, and the subsequent treatment consists in regulating the various functions of the body, restoring lost flesh and strength, and reëstablishing nervous and mental equilibrium, the family physician becomes the safer adviser.

With the rapidly increasing· amount of surgery and the consequent number of convalescent patients under treatment, an educational move ought to be instituted for the study of the many peculiar factors involved. Papers ought to be written and discussions ought to be participated in by both surgeon and family doctor, taking up the various details and discussing them from their different standpoints, until finally there is evolved a consensus of opinion with reference to the very many important points in the treatment of these patients. These should include the question of a proper dietary; of the best method of regulating the bowels; of treating bladder irritation; of the number of hours of sleep, and of the necessary periods of rest during the day; of the amount of exercise that is permissible, whether steps are injurious, how soon the sewing machine may be employed, or house work taken up; the question of driving, riding horseback, dancing, swimming, and athletic contests; the sort of clothing to be worn, whether corsets are injurious or an abdominal binder necessary; the question of prudence at menstrual periods and the relief of pain often experienced at that time; the treatment of headache, the administration of tonics, nervines, and hypnotics; the use of baths, massage, and electricity; the protection of wounds; the employment of douches; the use of tampons; the period at which sexual relations may be resumed—these and a hundred other questions all require consideration in order that they may be settled.

When surgeons appreciate the influence of neurasthenia

on the result of an operation, and the influence of an operation on the production of neurasthenia; when the family physician is educated in the details of posthospital treatment and given legitimate work with proper compensation, then and not until then will there be harmony in the profession and the greatest good accomplished to the greatest number of patients.

A BRIEF DISCUSSION OF SOME OF THE SURGICAL JUNK DEMANDING FURTHER SURGICAL INTERFERENCE.

By Joseph Price, M.D.,
Philadelphia.

You do me a great honor by placing me first on your splendid program.

I greatly disapprove of fault-finding and complaining. I am in the fullest sympathy and interest with that great progressive, educational wave now going over this country and the entire world—our present progress drives us to specialties. We cannot keep up with the present startling progress and advance of the world.

My colleague, Dr. McMurtry, wrote me on December 9— he never permits a gynecological sparrow to fall unnoticed— "Dear Joe, One hundred years ago (December 9, 1809) today Ephraim McDowell did the first abdominal section, and I celebrated quietly the centennial by doing a McDowell operation (large ovarian cystoma complicated by uterine fibroma subserous) at the same hour of the day (10 A.M.). I know you were celebrating appropriately the Centennial in Philadelphia." Our mutual friend, McMurtry, was quite correct—I unfortunately had on the operating table surgical junk. The patient entered my office on the 7th and asked me to reopen her abdomen and to correct, if possible, a distressing condition that she could bear no longer—her abdomen had been opened three times, a pelvic operation followed by two gall-bladder operations. She complained

S Surg 2

bitterly of that griping sensation in her epigastric region, followed by nausea and starvation. In the short period of six days I have reopened four abdomens for post-operative, pathological, and operative sequelæ many of us are quite familiar with.

Large numbers of these patients are objects of pity and mercy, all are objects of charity—one of the number had had her abdomen opened eight times. Fortunately, late operations were complete procedures, the reproductive organs and appendix were gone, leaving only a ventral hernia, omental and bowel adhesions to be freed. One of the late operators drained her gall-bladder, leaving a fistula and distressing adhesions. I freed the stomach, bowel, and other adhesions, exposing the gall-bladder, disorganized and charged with pus; its clean removal will probably result in cure. It was my distinguished friend, Dr. Lewis S. McMurtry, who first urged the importance of all doctors and specialists of serving a practical apprenticeship in a good hospital or dispensary under an industrious master.

Dealing with surgical junk requires more than the ordinary hospital apprenticeship. A distinguished operator remarked, while finishing an operation, Gentlemen, you have to do a hundred of these operations before you learn how—meaning primary procedures.

It would have been interesting to have heard what he had to say about 100 repeated operations for adhesions or partial and incomplete surgery.

McDowell's first patient recovered rapidly, lived a healthy, physiological life, conceived and bore children—a son went to Congress.

The operations done by the pioneers in abdominal surgery were free of operative sequelæ. The percentage of recoveries was good in the country.

The first operation done by ——— Baynum, Ephraim McDowell, Nathan Smith, John Light Atlee, and others recovered speedily and lived to a good old age.

I have had the opportunity of seeing a large number of patients operated upon by the first school of abdominal surgeons, an interesting group of patients. None of them complaining of those common symptoms of modern operations.

The high death rate in the hands of some few operators explains surgically the distressing condition of the few that do recover, but demand more surgery.

A distinguished specialist in gall-bladder disease lost four patients in a series of five. I re-opened the abdomen twice in the fifth patient. I thought I could relieve him by freeing adhesions in the first attempt.

In the second I removed his diseased gall-bladder and placed his viscera in normal relation. He is now useful, healthy, and comfortable.

Junk surgery will shorten the lives of the old surgeons if they have the courage to do it; it will also poison their reputation; it gives a mortality that few operators can stand.

The young, unschooled surgeon cannot do it—cannot begin it or complete it. It results disastrously both to his reputation and to his patient; again he is counselled not to attempt it.

On the 6th I received a letter from a young surgeon, asking me to take a patient or tell him how to deal with it. She had had two or three gall-bladder operations followed by fistulæ, and is now septic and asks for relief. I wrote him, "I don't want her; hands off." He saw me the following day for instructions. Go ahead, remove the gall-bladder, if you can find it, and drain. He is a painstaking young surgeon, but I am satisfied he will not find that gall-bladder.

Some years ago a valued friend gave me a picture of McDowell's first ovariotomy, and quoted on the back of it from McDowell: "I sincerely trust that the merely mechanical surgeon will never attempt the operation."

Some few years ago I walked into the clinic of a genius and an artist in surgery, in Richmond, Va. He is now presiding. He had before him a patient—surgical junk—fistula and chronic obstructions. What he had to say was characteristic of the inheritance and of the masterful teacher; it was brief and surgically correct: "You must look and go beyond the fistula," correct the snarls, the obstructions, the adhesions, give the bowel its normal lumen; the obstruction will vanish and the fistula close. He condemned all efforts at relief by simply dealing with the fistulæ from the skin end. The procedure was simple and rapid. He demonstrated the vital importance of the first subject to be taught in the new university, recently endowed with a gift of $1,000,000. Thirty-two subjects to be taught, thirty-two specialties; the first on the list mentioned is cleanliness. He aided in the simple detail of protecting the field of operation with gloved hands; he then cast away the gloves, gathered up the cluster of adherent bowel, freed the obstructions, and closed the fistula. Every step of this procedure was a lesson in surgery.

Mr. President, it is needless to detail the variety of pathological complications from the pelvic basin to the pyloric orifice of the stomach in the great variety of surgical afflictions found between those two points, but if dealt with scientifically, according to our surgical lights, junk will not be the result. Again, in the suppurative forms of disease of the the pelvic viscera, about the head of the cecum, and on up to the suppurations about the liver, the advanced thinkers and workers have given us perfected procedures, and if practised completely and scientifically, but few uncomfortable sequelæ will follow.

It is exceedingly rare to get junk from the operating tables of the experts. I rejoice that there is prolonged and painstaking effort on the part of the well-schooled to correct the common errors and calamities.

Our precise knowledge of pathological calamities and the early efforts at relief now give us about a nil mortality.

Many years ago we rejoiced in our wonderful progress

in pathology and diagnosis and the splendid results in early procedures. We had every reason to rejoice that the young surgeon with his apprenticeship on the opposite side of the table, his refined knowledge of pathology and diagnosis would give him the patients early for simple completed procedures, and that hereafter extensive complications, pathological invasions, and disorganizations would not be permitted.

Dr. Deaver righteously rebuked the internist, the new specialist in pathology, diagnosis, and therapeutics, for his prejudice to surgery. Probably no one living or dead has more precise knowledge of living pathology and what can be accomplished by early surgery than that past master in practical surgery, John B. Deaver.

The perfect results in stab and gunshot wounds are uniformly successful throughout the country. A good number of the patients fortunately fell into the hands of the young surgeons with extensive mutilations. It is rare to have patients ask for more surgery after gunshot and stab wounds. The entire character of the female dispensary services has changed—the patients entering daily would alarm an old operator.

Some years ago I wrote a brief paper with the title, "Major Gynecological Operations Due to Tinkering."

Incomplete procedures, a remaining diseased tube or ovary, is a common error in the primary procedure. Large numbers apply after the first, second, or third, or multiple operations. The patient then starts along the hospital highways for a fresh but not complete procedure.

String bag snarls of small bowel with general adhesions of the sigmoid to everything in the pelvis and an interesting fixation of the cecum. Some with a history of removal of the appendix once, twice, or thrice. We often find it after it has been many times removed—well up behind the cecum and buried.

The repair of lesions about the sigmoid, primary and

repeated, are difficult and important procedures. All intestinal surgery demands experimental schooling; freeing bowel adhesions following the septic operation, imperfect surgery, bad drainage, leave and give sequelæ demanding further relief.

Fistulæ are not so common. Operators are abandoning the incomplete operations that favor them. They practise the incision and puncture and drainage methods or palliative methods; the results are about always incomplete. The teacher, artist, or musician who has that needless suspension or fixation done largely for remunerative purposes goes perfectly wild about the bladder and fixation discomfort. You cannot halter up an important organ in the peritoneal cavity as you would a horse or cow; it is dangerous to halter the cow or horse, but it is torture to try to halter a vital organ. Last week two little Quaker teachers entered my office, told me they would have to give up their jobs if they were not relieved; both had vesical and pelvic discomfort and occasionally severe paroxysms of pain; they had been the rounds of a number of specialists; about all their special organs had been tinkered with, without relief. I told them that the uterus would have to be freed. They wailed, "Is it possible I have to go through with all that again?" We must have more prolonged hospital apprenticeship in our young men at the hands of skilful operators. All of our graduates should go through a hospital. The *public hospitals, like the private hospitals,* should be made clinical schools, and from this clinical schooling on top of a thorough scientific education we will get a new class of practitioners, better pathologists and better diagnosticians.

The resulting thoroughness, scientific and clinical, will give us a stronger profession with better judgment and a confidence in his community that he does not possess. Doctors with better educations will give us the patients early, while the troubles are simple—free of invasion and infection—simple operations demanded, extensive and complicated procedures rare.

In about all of our early operations we are pleased with the simplicity and the absence of complications and happy over the results.

All junk surgery is uncertain; it may be simple or it may be too complicated for completion. Good numbers of masterful operators have been prompted by their good judgment to give up their prolonged and painstaking efforts.

DISCUSSION.

DR. LEWIS S. MCMURTRY, of Louisville.—This paper should not be allowed to pass without discussion. I am sure Dr. Price in his inimitable style has called the attention of the Association to one of the very greatest evils prevalent at this time, and I take it what he alludes to especially is the incomplete operations that are being done, and the large number of men who are operating in the abdomen, without proper training. When this association was organized, it was far more difficult for men who were not qualified to operate in abdominal surgery than at the present time. Let me illustrate this point: You take any well-appointed hospital in any of the cities of this country, and even in smaller towns and they have a well-appointed operating-room. They have an operating-room nurse who is thoroughly qualified to pre-pare patients for all operations, and who understands the technique of modern aseptic surgery. An operator who has no operative skill can put on a pair of sterilized rubber gloves, and if the preparation has been done by a well-qualified nurse, he can open the abdomen, stir around in there a good deal, and the patient may not die. Twenty years ago if an operator undertook to do this kind of work, the patient would die of sepsis. He could not clean his hands; he did not have the facilities of the modern hospital, and sepsis followed. At the present time there are more men doing tyro-surgery in the abdomen than ever before. There are men without any apprenticeship undertaking major surgical operations, and I think it is this class of surgery Dr. Price has characterized as "junk;" surgery done by men who are not qualified is usually incomplete and unsatisfactory; if the patients survive they come to other surgeons with complicated conditions. The men who are doing abdominal surgery constantly seem to

have tired of inveighing against this abuse of surgery, but I believe it is the duty of an association composed of men who have served a long time at this work, and who know the bad results that come from such work as Dr. Price has described— it is the duty of these men publicly and privately to protest against men entering upon this work without being properly qualified to do it.

DR. ALBERT VANDER VEER, of Albany, New York.—It is gratifying to have one who has had such a long and large experience as Dr. McMurtry to open the discussion on this valuable paper. It has been my good fortune to see a great deal of Dr. Price's work almost from the beginning, and I have seen him operate at various times since, and I have seen a number of other operators' work. But I have said to my students and said to the internes in my hospital that there are few men who have maintained the same simplicity in operating that Dr. Price has from the beginning of his surgical work. That is one strong reason why he has succeeded so well.

Dr. McMurtry referred to one point that I do not hesitate to speak of and to emphasize somewhat, namely, the importance of establishing small hospitals in small villages. In these places there are some prominent citizens who want to show their kindness toward the community, and they undertake to build a hospital, and immediately out of six or seven physicians living in that small town, four or five of them become operators at once. They become surgeons. They undertake abdominal surgery, and I feel, as I said in our State Society on one or two occasions, that here enters an element of risk. What is more distressing than to get a telephone message like this: "Doctor, I am going to operate tomorrow on a case of fibroid tumor of the uterus; I have not got instruments enough, I will come down this afternoon and want you to loan me enough instruments to carry this operation through." Out of that class comes a certain amount of surgical junk, or incomplete operating to which Dr. Price has alluded. The chances are that an accurate diagnosis has not been made, and the operator is doing his first operation, or probably does one in about eighteen months, and undertakes to do operations with which he is not entirely familiar. These are the cases that pass along eventually to the larger hospitals for further operations to be done along the lines indicated by Dr. Price, in order that they may be completely cured. I always feel we have a certain amount of risk in encouraging abdominal work in hospitals of this kind, but in every other respect encourage them. Now, Dr. Price must remember that in cleaning up the abdomen and going on with the work with which he is familiar, some of us older men have endeavored to do the same thing along the lines of getting at a correct diagnosis, and then doing as complete an operation as possible and which has resulted in that kind of surgery, which has reflected great credit upon American abdominal surgeons. But recently, say within ten or fifteen years, there has been a sort of feeling in the minds of some younger surgeons to do as many operations as they could upon a particular patient and completing the diagnosis. In that respect they sometimes err. The result has been that the work along toward the end has been incomplete, and I have seen a number of such cases that Dr. Price refers to, many of them having terminated in what he has called surgical junk. Such a paper as Dr. Price has presented here is one to which we ought to pay more attention at the present time. It is the kind of paper which should be read by the younger operators of today, and I am sure if they were to do so it would result in great good to them. It does us all good to have this question brought up, and I hope it will be discussed more freely. I felt a little reluctant in saying anything at the beginning of the session, yet I feel we should discuss this paper very freely, and Dr. Price is entitled to a great deal of credit and to a great deal of consideration for having presented the subject in such a sensible and clear light as he has done.

DR. WM. M. POLK, of New York City.—I am one of the chief sinners, and I rise in a contrite mood. I have been brought to task many a time by Dr. Price and it seems to me that he is administering one of those same lessons, which I have benefited by in times gone by. The trouble with some of us is we have been endeavoring to work out pathological problems on live subjects, and in so doing we have left conditions within the abdomen in our endeavor to preserve structures, that really had no business there, and in so far as I have been a sinner in that direction, I am free to confess that probably I deserve all that the distinguished gentleman has said. Beyond this, I am particularly obliged to him, because it opens up this whole field of surgical work. One great difficulty I encounter is the insistence of people on being operated upon.

I find that the average person has been so well educated that their minds are made up as to what they wish their physicians to do long before they interview him, and if he fails in any way to fall in with their preconceived notions they at once turn elsewhere. Now, it is no excuse that you should be debarred from executing your conception of what is proper, because the individual happens to have a different notion; but we all know perfectly well that there are a great many of the younger members of the profession who have not got stiffness of spine that comes with age, that kind of ankylosis of the vertebral column, which is so beneficent in its influence and which does come with age and with experience and which acts as a barrier to too much operating. I feel that this question is, as Dr. Price has very aptly said, something we cannot trifle with.

Dr. Price has alluded to what I may term the spread of the craze for medical education. Perhaps I am wrong in using the word craze, because it may suggest to you that I am not in sympathy with it. It is not simply education in the lecture hall, but education in our common everyday life and to be imparted by the leaders of our profession. This, it appears to me, is one of the favorable demands of the situation. But this is not an opportunity for moralizing, and yet I think I am correct when I say that we are absolutely responsible for the dissection of this state of affairs. We are responsible for the state of affairs I have endeavored to picture, and self-righteousness will not help the situation one bit. We have simply got to get down to first principles, to what our knowledge of the given situation teaches us is, the truthful thing to tell our people, whether they be our patients or medical students, and when we have reached that frame of mind we will get somewhere, but we will not move one inch in the direction Dr. Price's paper leads us, until we make up our minds to rid our own minds of the junk that is within them.

Dr. Price (closing).—We have here this morning an exceptional gathering of scientific men—a beautiful, practical, class of men who have contributed so much to the saving of human life and the relief of suffering along these peculiar lines, so beautifully alluded to by Dr. Polk. The most of us know very well that Doctor Polk is incapable of sinning in surgery, and more than a quarter of a century or perhaps half a century he has labored and toiled earnestly to put others to work along righteous lines in the relief of suffering and in the saving of human lives. Dr. Polk is perfectly unconscious of the fact, I think, that he has during his long professional career saved many lives and made good workers out of bad ones.

Let us take the work of Bernutz and Goupil, or of Mr. Tait, or of the advanced thinkers and workers of Europe, and we will find in the transactions of the American Gynecological Society the presentation of the suppurative forms of pelvic disease, conditions described, which antedate the researches of Bernutz and Goupil, or a revision of the treatment of pelvic disease. You will find in one page a criticism of what they did or what they tested at Bellevue, and the patients went away and came back, and what these surgeons found, was a beautiful scientific allusion to the methods of dealing with advanced lesions. You have in that one page instruction of a precise, accurate character. You have instructions for the advanced operators in pelvic disease on that one page. I allude to this to call your attention to a class of men who hesitate, and you know what the Bible says about men who hesitate. Dr. Polk has labored long and earnestly in hospital work, and along clinical lines of instruction. He has been instructing large numbers of men how to make diagnoses and how to correct accidents in connection with parturition and how to deal with the suppurative forms of disease. This belongs to the advanced surgeons and workers.

Then we have another class of workers here this morning— men who have a scientific bend of mind; men who are lovers of pathology and lovers of good surgery—men who practice the best surgery that people can possibly have in their respective communities. I can remember very well that more than a quarter of a century ago Dr. McMurtry was laboring along the lines of apprenticeship in dealing with infections of a puerperal nature. He was laboring along the lines of new hospitals, because the hospitals in those days were little better than pest houses and alms houses. That was a part of the work of the new man, it was part of the work of Sims and others whose names might be mentioned. These men saw the necessity of creating private hospitals. But what happens to men who are advanced thinkers and workers like Dr. Vander Veer? He works in the old hospital, and creates a new one. These new hospitals really rob us of the best type of practitioners. In all of the new hospitals in this country nowadays you will see the brightest pathologists, the men who have been taken from our colleges and hospitals. For instance, in Albany they build a magnificent hospital, supplying it with every modern convenience and equipment to suit every specialty of medicine, and they take pathologists and laboratory men from Philadelphia and elsewhere to enable them to carry on their work more efficiently on the most modern or up-to-date lines. Their principal aim is to do good scientific work and in so doing it simply means they are robbing us of good clinicians. The specialties and the rich women are robbing us of some of our brightest minds. We need specialists. We need surgeons. Take this body of surgeons and we know all of them are capable of doing the best possible work and of achieving the best possible results. There is nothing in my paper which suggests adverse criticism of the work of any member of this Association, as all of you are doing the best surgical work. Moreover, you have surgical consciences. No one is more cognizant of what you have done and what you are capable of doing than I am; but there are certain sections of this country which have not been educated up to the refinement of early surgical work.

ON ADHESION OF SIGMOID TO TUBE AND BROAD LIGAMENT AS A CAUSE OF PAIN IN SALPINGITIS.

By Hubert A. Royster, M.D.,
Raleigh, North Carolina.

PAIN in pelvic disease bears no relation to the size of the lesion. Conditions accompanied with most intense suffering often present no changes that are palpable, while the largest masses may give rise to little or no annoyance. For this reason, in seeking for a cause of pelvic pain, it is important to keep in mind complicating conditions, entirely apart from the reproductive organs, and to study these either as separate affections or as allied to pathology in the pelvis. We have got bravely over the "ovarian neuralgia" obsession, and we are rapidly learning that the ovary is not the only origin of pain in the inferior somatic segment of the female. Few affections of the ovaries can be differentiated from their associated diseases.

The Fallopian tube is the most frequent seat of imflammatory disease in the pelvis. It is the narrowest portion of the channel from the vulva to the ovary and is the least resistant to infection. Pain, then, is more concerned with salpingitis than with ovaritis, whether attended by a gross lesion or not.

Too many times the ovary has been regarded as the offending organ and needlessly removed. In some instances a diseased tube has been blamed as the sole cause of pain, while other factors produced by the salpingitis, or arising independently of it, may be overlooked.

Somewhat less than three years ago I made a clinical observation that bears upon this question. Mrs. S., aged thirty years, married seven years, had given birth to one child about a year before. Previous to that she had had an abortion performed on account of pernicious vomiting. Several weeks before I first saw her the same procedure had been again gone through with for the same reason. For two or three years she had suffered from typical tubal dysmenorrhea (pain beginning a week before the flow and continuing throughout the period); intermenstrual pain was constant and referred chiefly to the left iliac region; there had been several slight attacks of "pelvic peritonitis;" defecation was particularly distressful. Almost every day the patient was taking morphine or heroin. Examination revealed extreme tenderness in either side of the pelvis, especially in the left. A diagnosis of chronic salpingitis was made. At operation (March 28, 1907) both tubes, tortuous and thickened, were removed. This removal was considered justified in view of the history. The ovaries were what are called "cystic." I removed the left and excised two thirds of the right one. In bringing up the left tube for inspection I found that the sigmoid flexure was adherent to its fimbriated end and also to the upper surface of the broad ligament. These adhesions were carefully divided, and the raw areas were closed by fine catgut sutures. The result was all that could have been expected. The patient immediately improved, but not until six months had passed was she really relieved. She is now entirely well, menstruating regularly without pain.

I have records of eight similar cases, in which the sigmoid adhesion was apparently the sole source of left-sided pelvic pain. I am convinced that the condition is one to be reckoned with. Its association with salpingitis or other disease in the pelvis cannot, as a rule, be determined beforehand, but it may be suspected in the absence of other lesions to account for the suffering and more especially in the presence of painful defecation. This has been a constant symptom in the instances which I have observed.

When discovered the adhesion must be dealt with as seems proper in the given case. After snipping the bands which fix the sigmoid to the broad ligament, there are left two triangular raw surfaces, one on the bowel and the other on the ligament, with their bases together; these form a diamond-shaped area. The peritoneal edges are then closed over this space by continuous catgut, applied from below upward. The sigmoid is thus allowed to drop lower down into the pelvis away from the tube and ligament—a maneuver which, in my opinion, must be executed to secure permanent relief. Covering all denuded places is not less important. In one patient, who had also a chronic cystitis (cured by a vaginal cystotomy), I failed to close the raw area as well as I should have done, and she is still now and then having pain on defecation, undoubtedly because of the reforming of adhesions. This is the only case of the nine that, so far as I know, has not been relieved.

A very interesting case in the series was that of a young lady who had been first curetted, and who then had a large cystic left ovary removed through the vagina for dysmenorrhea with only fitful mitigation of her suffering. Six months after the last operation I opened her abdomen and found an old dense adhesion of sigmoid to left broad ligament and a more recent fixation of the tube. Removal of this structure and releasing the sigmoid has cured the patient of pain. We are thus afforded another striking bit of evidence, if any were needed, of the superiority of the abdominal over the vaginal method of operating.

Now I feel very sure that the condition, which I have endeavored to describe here is independent of the observations of Mr. Arbuthnot Lane and also of the work of Dr. Clark. The former has referred in his paper on "Chronic Intestinal Stasis" (*Annals of Surgery*, July, 1909) to "pain in the sigmoid segment" due to "irregular anchoring by adhesions" and also to "pain in the fixed left ovary."

In his view any pelvic lesions present may be secondary to the intestinal stasis; he recommends excision of the large bowel. Clark has studied left-sided pain in women, and attributes much of it to the "redundant sigmoid" (*Penna. Med. Jour.* April, 1909), which is analogous to Hirschsprung's disease, but which Clark thinks is due to an unequal growth of the large intestine after birth. He advises resection of the sigmoid or suturing it to the parietal peritoneum (sigmoid-opexy).

With neither of these views does my observation either coincide or conflict. The three conditions are clearly distinct. The point I wish to emphasize in the clinical picture, as I have seen it, is this: the sigmoid adhesion referred to may or may not be a result of pelvic disease, but the pain is produced by the adhesion and is not directly due to the pelvic pathology. It is worthy of further comment that this condition is best managed by dropping the sigmoid and not by hanging it up.

DISCUSSION.

DR. HENRY T. BYFORD, of Chicago.—These cases are not so very rare. In a patient who has pelvic disease I always ask her whether she has pain on defecation. Then I ask her if she has any mucus in the stools. I think we often find mucus in the stools, but not the abundant mucus which comes from a general colitis, nor the stringy mucus with a tendency to tenesmus that comes from an inflammation low down in the rectum. When they are constipated these patients usually have pain when the bowels move. If the pain is in the left iliac region there will usually be found adhesions of the sigmoid flexure. But if the pain is in the sacral region we will upon making a vaginal examination find one of the appendages adherent lower down behind the uterus, or perhaps it can be felt hanging over the utero-sacral ligaments. In the class of patients referred to by the author of the paper, with pain in the iliac region and the appendages adherent in that region we would seldom operate through the vagina unless the uterus were to be removed at the same time. We would not even have to consider it. We operate through the vagina only in cases in which the ovaries can easily be felt from below, and are more evidently accessible from below.

In regard to the size of the sigmoid flexure, I think these cases are apt to occur in women who are constipated a great deal, and who have a distended colon or distended sigmoid flexure, and the giving of laxatives in small quantities and perhaps strychnin, and other remedies that tone up the alimentary canal, with proper diet, would be sufficient. Of course my remarks have reference to simple cases.

DR. ROBERT T. MORRIS, of New York City.—There is one place where the surgeon should allow adhesions to remain. He should allow them to remain in his subliminal mind— always have the idea of them ready to bring forward for action. There is no one thing so frequently overlooked in my experience as peritoneal adhesions, and their insidious influence.

From what Dr. Royster has said, he likes to close raw surfaces with continuous suture. I believe we can certainly save time by one of two methods. The commonest one which I have used is that of sprinkling aristol over the raw surfaces, and waiting a moment until lymph coagulates and engages the aristol in a mesh, and that presents a mechanical obstacle to adhesion formation, and it is satisfactory in my experiments with animals.

The other is the use of the sterilized animal membrane. That takes a little longer, but in such a case as Dr. Royster has described this morning, aristol powder would be engaged in the lymph coagulum, presenting an excellent mechanical obstacle to re-adhesion.

DR. THOMAS S. CULLEN, of Baltimore.—I have at the present time a patient who has complained for five or six years of a severe and constant pain in the left lower abdomen. On opening the abdomen we found the uterus perfectly normal. The tubes and ovaries showed no alteration whatever. There was no thickening of the ureter, and we were at a loss to explain the cause of the discomfort. Finally, in making a closer examination of the sigmoid we found it to be adherent to the entire left broad ligament, the adhesions extending as far forward as the round ligament. We adopted the same procedure as Dr. Royster has described, that is, we freed the adhesion as thoroughly as possible, and closed the raw surface of the broad ligament by continuous catgut, and the raw surfaces of the rectum by interrupted sutures.

Dr. I. S. Stone, of Washington, D. C.—I suppose I have left as much surgical junk in my experience as many others, and I would not like to know how much I have left, because I have not only seen some of my own patients on whom incomplete operations were originally done, but the patients of other surgeons who have left similar conditions. There is a great deal of difference in the point of view. It is a question whether or not the patient of Dr. Price, on whom eight operations were performed before he operated on her, would not eventually have gone to some one else, even after Dr. Price had performed the operation he mentioned.

I think there is something in Dr. Polk's remark that patients are apt to get into the habit of being operated on. For instance, patients frequently come to my office and tell me that they have been operated on two or three times, and not only that, but have seen two or three physicians in regard to the propriety of another operation. We are going to a great deal too much trouble in separating adhesions, for we must remember that when we open the abdomen of a patient two or three times and find organized adhesions each time, we will probably not relieve that patient of her trouble. In opening the abdomen of patients who have been cured of tubercular peritonitis, and allied conditions, we can never hope to separate all adhesions in such cases. It would be folly to try it; and I must take issue with Dr. Royster, because in many of these cases the most extensive adhesions may exist in any part of the intestinal tract, one organ being thoroughly adherent to its fellow without causing any pain on defecation, or any pain at any time. Where are we to stop in separating adhesions when we have such cases as these?

Not long ago a patient came to see me in Washington, who had been operated on abroad. She gave a history of pain in the scar of a former operation, which was done by an eminent surgeon in Paris. Three physicians held a consultation in regard to this case. There was pain in the cicatrix, and that was about all the woman could tell. Two out of the three physicians voted in favor of opening the abdomen to liberate adhesions. When the abdomen was opened there was a slender adhesion of the omentum. The family was told that adhesions were found and separated. What else could they be told? The patient suffered after this operation the same as she did before. The operation did her no good.

I find I am getting most excellent results in operating on patients and placing the viscera in the very best possible condition I can, for the continuous passage of flatus and feces. I separate adhesions of the sigmoid and in some cases have been astonished to find not only the greatest improvement as regards pain and local distress, but in the general improvement of the patient when the sigmoid has been sutured up out of the pelvis, where there should be continuous passage of flatus and gas, instead of more or less obstruction being caused by circular fold or duplication of the sigmoid in the pelvis. Such a practice has given me more satisfaction than the mere separation of adhesions.

DR. W. P. CARR, of Washington, D. C.—We have all seen cases in which there were many adhesions and no pain. On the other hand, we have seen cases in which there were slight adhesions and great pain. I have come to the conclusion that it is the character and the situation of the adhesions and not the amount of them that cause trouble. I think we have more pain in cases where there is a small but strong adhesion attached to a small area of some movable organ so that the traction is concentrated on one point. Whereas, in the extensive adhesion of a large surface the weight is sustained without pain. It is my experience that the most painful adhesions were where a small band was pulling on one point of a movable organ. I have relieved the pain by separating adhesions not larger than a slate pencil. On the other hand, large adhesions, especially around the liver and stomach, often produce no pain at all.

DR. ROYSTER (closing).—I am very glad that Dr. Byford has mentioned the occurrence of a discharge of mucus, as I think that is very important. The question then arises in such a case: Is not the intestinal condition the cause of the adhesion, rather than the pelvic disease? I think in these cases where the adhesion is due to intestinal stasis, mucus is a prominent symptom, but where it is secondary to pelvic disease mucus is not a prominent symptom.

I probably took advantage of Dr. Byford in giving a shot at vaginal work. The point I tried to impress was that there are some operators who would remove an ovary through the vagina if they took it to be the cause of pain, but who would leave behind a tube adherent to the sigmoid.

I agree with Dr. Cullen that in many cases the interrupted

suture would be better than the continuous suture, both for the closing and lengthening of the space between the sigmoid and the ligament.   The endeavor should be to get pronounced dropping of the sigmoid.

With reference to the remarks made by Dr. Stone as to general adhesions in the abdomen and separating them, I wish to say that I presented a condition which is specific and that had definite symptoms, rather than general adhesions, and I think Dr. Carr explained the point at issue.   Where we have a small painful adhesion which causes a certain condition, by releasing it we relieve the patient.

THE TREATMENT OF ADVANCED EXTRA-UTERINE PREGNANCY.

By Reuben Peterson, M.D.,
Ann Arbor, Michigan.

In extra-uterine pregnancy rupture occurs in the great majority of cases during the first, second, or third months of gestation. Furthermore, rupture of the ectopic sac almost always means death of the fetus from separation of the ovum or placenta from the wall of the tube. Occasionally enough of the placenta remains attached to the tube wall to nourish the fetus and permit of its further development. Still more rarely the pregnancy may go on to term without rupture. That these two last terminations are exceptional is demonstrated by the experience of most operators of even large experience who rarely meet with more than one case of advanced extra-uterine pregnancy in their operative lifetimes. Again, the frequency of extra-uterine pregnancy beyond the sixth month is shown by the work of Sittner.[1] This author, after a most exhaustive search through the literature, has been able to collect only 165 cases, occurring between the years 1813 and 1906, where the fetus was alive and viable when the patients were operated upon. Hence every case of this comparatively rare condition should be reported, since the operator cannot depend upon his own experience. When called upon to treat such cases his treatment must necessarily depend

---

[1] Sittner, A. Ergebnisse der in den letzten 20 Jahren durch Koeliotomie bei lebendem Kinde operierten Fälle von vorgeschrittener Extrauterinschwangerschaft. Arch. f. Gynaek., 1907–8, lxxxiv, 1.

upon the accumulative experience of others. The work of Sittner referred to above is a storehouse of information, practically containing everything in the literature of advanced extra-uterine pregnancy with viable fetus. Every one interested in this subject is under great obligations to this author, since the thoroughness with which he has performed his task makes repetition unnecessary.

The following case was briefly reported before the Chicago Gynecological Society at the meeting of December 18, 1908, and may be found in the transactions of that Society in the *American Journal of Obstetrics*, April, 1909, p. 651.

Mrs. M., aged thirty-three years, primipara, married nine years, menstruated normally the early part of June, 1908. She flowed in July, but not naturally, as there were irregular discharges of blood during the remainder of that month and August. At times she flowed enough to just soil a napkin; at other times it came with a gush, two or three teaspoonfuls at a time, and bright red in color. Life was felt first about the middle of October, and has been quite noticeable ever since, but always in the left side. The patient has had a great deal of abdominal pain for the last two or three months, and has not felt well. About the middle of November she began to suffer from headache, dizziness, disturbance of vision, and edema of the lower extremities. Examination of the urine at this time showed a considerable quantity of albumin and numerous casts. The headache and eye symptoms have grown progressively worse in spite of treatment. She has had colicky pains in the abdomen ever since August, although these pains have been much worse since October. She thought they were due to the contractions of the uterus. During the early part of August the abdominal pains were exceptionally severe, and were ascribed to peritonitis.

I saw the patient December 12, 1908, in consultation with Dr. T. E. Sands, of Battle Creek, Michigan, at the Nichol's Hospital in the same city. Examination showed the patient to be well nourished, but quite anemic. There was a marked puffiness of the eyelids and edema of the extremities as high up as the knees. The breasts showed the ordinary signs of pregnancy. The shape of the abdomen was peculiar. Instead of the ordinary dome-shaped swelling of pregnancy, the suprapubic region was quite flat, the abdominal swelling increasing toward the umbilicus, where it ended in a kind of peak. The abdomen was exquisitely tender, interfering greatly with palpation. What appeared to be a fetal head could be made out in the left flank. The fetal back and extremities were also to the left of the median line. Fetal movements and heart sounds were also distinct on the same side. Extra-uterine pregnancy was suspected, but a positive diagnosis could not be made. The sensitive abdomen made a more thorough examination impossible. Examination under anesthesia showed the cervix soft, low down in the pelvis, and patulous, easily admitting the tip of the finger. It was continuous with a soft, elastic, immovable mass reaching across the posterior part of the pelvis. No definitely enlarged uterus could be made out above the pubes. The fetal head located in the left flank could be easily palpated through the vagina, and the fetal parts could be readily mapped out. An incarcerated, retroverted uterus with stretching of the anterior wall due to pregnancy was considered a possibility. A sound was passed backward and to the left, a distance of five and one-half inches. It could not be passed to the right until it was withdrawn and then it passed in that direction for the same distance. The anterior and posterior cervical walls were incised enough to allow of the introduction of the finger, when it was seen that we had to deal with an empty, enlarged bicornate uterus. The diagnosis of extra-uterine gestation being established, the abdomen was opened in the median line by a five-inch incision. The sac lay immediately beneath the incision and the placenta led down to the right tube, the greater portion of it being in the posterior cul-de-sac, but not attached to it. The sac was ruptured, and there was a small amount of free blood in the peritoneal cavity above the fetus, which lay almost entirely to the left of the median line. The membranes were slightly attached to two loops of small intestines. The cord was clamped and the child removed. It only breathed a few times after removal. The adhesions to the intestines were carefully loosened, the infundibulopelvic ligament and uterine end of the tube clamped, and the placenta removed. It was easily freed from its few adhesions. The sac was also removed entire except for a few shreds attached to the intestines. The uterus together with the other tube and ovary were buried in adhesions, and it was thought best to remove them. A complete hysterectomy was accordingly performed, drainage being secured by gauze leading out through the vagina. The abdominal incision was closed in the usual manner without drainage. The patient had a good pulse at the completion of the operation, and at no time suffered from shock. The abdominal incision healed by primary union, and the patient made a good recovery.

Pathological Report. This report was not complete because the specimen was preserved in kaiserlin for museum purposes.

A fetus 32.5 cm. long; greatest diameter of head, 22 cm.; bisacromial diameter, 14.5 cm.; bitrochanteric diameter, 7 cm.; length of cord, 22 cm.; length of nails, 3 mm.; occipito-bregmatic, 9 cm.; parietomental, 11 cm.; bitemporal, 6.5.

It is a male fetus without malformation, with the exception of a marked pes valgus on either side—right side greater than left. There is a fine hair on head averaging 1 cm. in length. Sutures all open. Boundaries of fontanelles not well defined. Orifices of body are normal. No lesions nor other abnormalities.

A bicornate uterus 11 cm. long in the median line, 12 cm. long from extremity of either horn to external os. A partition 5 cm. long partially separates the two horns. The uterus is 10.5 cm. broad in greatest diameter, 5 cm. thick in greatest diameter.

In the above case we had to deal with the most common form of secondary abdominal pregnancy, where the rupture of the tube had been followed by the escape of the fetus into the abdominal cavity, enough of the placenta escaping destruction to allow of the further development of the fetus. Of the 43 cases of advanced extra-uterine pregnancy collected by Sittner in his last article, published in 1908, there were 6 intact tubal pregnancies, while in 3 the ovaries were intact, 3 being classified as primary abdominal pregnancies. The gestation sac was ruptured in 29 tubal and one ovarian pregnancy. In one instance the fetus had been set free **by tubal abortion.**

In the case reported, the placenta and sac were only slightly adherent, and were so movable as to allow of a preliminary clamping of the blood supply of the side on which the placenta was situated, in this way rendering the operation almost bloodless.

The pain which was a marked symptom of this case may be explained in part by the contractions which usually are **an** accompaniment of ectopic pregnancies, and in part to the adhesions, although they were not extensive enough to account for the discomfort the patient experienced. Albuminuria with casts in connection with an ectopic pregnancy is not particularly common so far as my reading and experience go. Nicholson[1] mentions the presence of albumin and casts in a patient upon whom he operated at term for an extra-uterine pregnancy. But in his case the fetus was macerated, and the patient had a temperature with an increased pulse rate. It is more than probable that the urinary condition in this case was due to the sepsis.

[1] Nicholson, W. R. Extra-uterine *Pregnancy* at Term. Amer. Jour. Obst., 1908, lvii, 801.

The bicornate uterus was a coincidence, and had nothing to do with the ectopic gestation; still it complicated the diagnosis, especially since the broad fundus was retroverted and adherent. Of course, the true condition was at once revealed when the cervix was bisected and the finger passed to the fundus.

In this case there was only one thing to do as far as treatment was concerned. The patient was pregnant either within the uterus or outside of it. Her condition was serious, in that her urine was becoming progressively worse in spite of treatment, while her headaches, eye symptoms, and general edema showed that she was not far removed from an eclamptic attack. The only course to pursue under these conditions was to terminate the pregnancy wherever situated, and this we were prepared to do when the patient was anesthetized for examination.

The mode of procedure is not so apparent when symptoms of intoxication are absent in a case of advanced extra-uterine pregnancy. During the first few months the indications for operation are positive in extra-uterine gestation. There may be some discussion as to the advisability of operating immediately after rupture has occurred, on account of the additional shock entailed by the operation. But the indication is clear to remove the extra-uterine gestation sac, if this can be done safely. The chances of rupture, primary or secondary, and death from hemorrhage are so great that, as far as the mother is concerned, the indications are to remove the products of conception at once by operation. And in the first half of pregnancy the fetus may be considered a negligible factor, since its chances of escaping death through rupture or malnutrition in an extra-uterine pregnancy are slight.

In a case of advanced extra-uterine pregnancy, where probably rupture has already occurred without causing the death of the fetus, the question is a little different. The placenta in a case of secondary abdominal pregnancy is more firmly attached, hemorrhage is less liable to occur, and the chances that the fetus will reach the age of viability infinitely greater.

Shall the extra-uterine child, approaching the age of viability, be given a chance for an independent existence by postponing the operation until just before full term? Before the operator answers this question affirmatively he will want to know the risk to the mother postponement of the operation entails. How often does rupture, primary or secondary, occur in cases of advanced extra-uterine gestation? If it be of frequent occurrence, the question is settled once and for all. If hemorrhage occurs even as frequently or is as menacing as in placenta prævia, there will always be found those who, even with the patient under the best surroundings, will consider it unjustifiable to allow the pregnancy to continue. On the other hand, the tendency of modern obstetrics is to be more and more conservative about terminating pregnancy, unless the mother's life be in great danger. If Sittner's figures are approximately correct, hemorrhage from rupture in cases of advanced extra-uterine pregnancy is not particularly common, since operation was performed for this reason alone only 8 times in 165 cases, or in 4.8 per cent. Thus, it would seem as if Sittner were correct when he claims that the danger of hemorrhage after the fifth month is not so great that the life of the child need not be considered.

But is the extra-uterine child of much value after it has been saved? No operator would want to advocate additional risks to the mother if the chances were largely in favor of such children being so weak and puny that they die shortly after being delivered. The same would hold true if the majority of such children are malformed and crippled so that even if they survive the critical period of infancy they are doomed to lead more or less pitiable existencies. Here again we must turn to Sittner for facts. He is able to report upon 122 children delivered through operation in cases of extra-uterine gestation. Of these, 63, or over half, lived beyond the first year, six lived to be over six years of age, one reaching the age of nineteen.

Sittner's statistics on deformities and lack of development in children are also interesting. Of 93 children, only 10 were seriously deformed, in 5 the deformities being so extensive as to cause death. Most of the deformities mentioned are of the head and extremities. Compression of the skull has been noted a number of times, probably due to the absorption of the liquor amnii and pressure. Hence it may be concluded that while deformities are not uncommon with extra-uterine children, they are not so frequent as to preclude attempts at saving their lives by operative measures, performed at times most favorable to the children.

Still, even with these two questions disposed of, the surgeon will hesitate to postpone operation if by so doing he is increasing the technical difficulties of the operation to such an extent as to greatly add to the danger of the mother. In other words, how are the two bugbears in the operative treatment of this class of cases, hemorrhage and sepsis, affected by the postponement of the operation. Although in the case reported above the control of the hemorrhage was a very simple matter, for the placenta was so situated as to allow the ovarian and uterine arteries to be easily clamped, such is not always the case. Taylor has called such a placenta "ball-like" in contradistinction to the "discoid" variety, which has only one surface free from vascular attachments. It is from this latter kind of placenta that the terrific hemorrhages arise when attempts are made to detach it. Leaving the placenta behind after removal of the child Sittner considers a good criterion of the difficulties of the operation. He finds that the operator was forced to leave the placenta in the latter part of pregnancy in about the same percentage of cases as in the earlier months of the viability of the child. Thus, the danger of waiting, so far as hemorrhage is concerned, need not decide us against such a procedure.

Again, the postponement has been overdone for fear of

hemorrhage, some advocating operation weeks after the death of the fetus, thus giving time for the placenta to become loosened. To the modern abdominal surgeon there is something repugnant in this mode of procedure. While he plans to avoid hemorrhage in every possible way, he is not in the habit of dodging an operation for fear of it. Instead, he devises means for the control of the hemorrhage. If one method fails, he employs another. Especially true is this where another, although more frail, life is at stake. I am not belittling the hemorrhages one may get during the attempt to remove a placenta without first controlling its blood supply. I have had too many cases of placenta prævia not to have a good respect for hemorrhage from uncontrolled sinuses. Still the problem before the abdominal surgeon is to devise means whereby the placenta can be removed in every case, and before the death of the child. He must do this because the patients do so much better when this has been accomplished. To quote Sittner again, in 95 cases, from 1813 to 1906, the placenta was removed, with a maternal mortality of 21.05 per cent., in comparison with a mortality of 57.1 per cent. in 70 cases where the operator, for one reason or the other, was obliged to leave the placenta behind.

Preliminary securing of the bloodvessels supplying the placenta is almost essential in the discoid variety of placenta. This can be easily accomplished unless the placenta and sac are in such a position that the ovarian and uterine arteries are covered up. Ordinarily one can dissect off the super-imposed mass, but not so with the placenta. If it lie in such a position, it is better to let it alone and attack the uterus from the other side. Tie off the opposite ovarian and uter-ine arteries, cut across the cervix, secure the opposite uterine artery, then the remaining ovarian artery can probably be clamped. Removal of the placenta after the securing of hemostasis is not especially difficult, even in the presence of adhesions to pelvic organs and intestines. In case the above plan of controlling the blood supply of the placenta seems impracticable for any reason, it may be possible to tie the internal iliacs, then compression of the aorta above the origin of the ovarian arteries will be sufficient to secure hemostasis. Werder suggests the use of Halstead's apparatus for compression of the aorta or compression of this artery by means of rubber protected forceps similar to those used in intestinal work. The reason, in my opinion, why the question of hemostasis in extra-uterine cases has not been better worked out, is that each operator has had too few cases whereby the technique could be improved. This is one of the instances where, in a way, the technique must be improved from a priori reasoning, so far as each individual operator in concerned. Moreover, it is' obligatory on the surgeon who may be called upon to operate upon such patients to have his plan of action already outlined, else it may mean the losing of his patient.

Where for any reason it becomes impossible to remove the placenta, the best results have followed the stitching of the sac to the abdominal wall and protecting it, together with the placenta, from the peritoneal cavity by gauze packing. Here is an instance where dependent drainage through the vagina should be secured if possible. Many cases have been reported where abdominal drainage proved inefficient, yet the patient was saved through vaginal drainage.

Taylor's suggestion, where the placenta cannot be removed, to depend upon the asepticity of the operation and leave behind the placenta after closing the abdomen without drainage, may be all right theoretically, but practically it does not appeal to one, nor has it been particularly successful in those cases where it has been tried.

CONCLUSIONS. 1. Wherever conditions permit, operation for the removal of the gestation sac is indicated in the first half of an extra-uterine pregnancy, since,

2. At this period the mother is in great danger from rupture and sepsis, and

3. The chances for the survival of the fetus are very poor.

4. During the latter part of an extra-uterine gestation the chances of rupture and a fatal hemorrhage are very much less (4.8 per cent), and

5. The chances of the survival of the fetus are very much greater.

6. While malnutrition and malformation of the extra-uterine child are more common than with the fetus under normal conditions, they are not frequent enough to contra-indicate attempts at saving its life.

7. Hence, under favorable surroundings, when the patient can be watched, she should be allowed to go to within two or three weeks of term before operation.

8. Since the maternal mortality is more than twice as great after operation in advanced extra-uterine pregnancy where the placenta is left behind,

9. Its removal should be one of the cardinal principles of each operation.

10. In the "discoid" variety of placenta, where only a small surface of this organ is not attached, the blood supply must be controlled, either by tying the vessels, or by com-pression of the aorta before an attempt be made to remove the placenta.

11. When for any reason removal of the placenta is impossible, the sac should be stitched to the abdominal wall and the placenta shut off from the peritoneal cavity by gauze.

12. Dependent drainage through the vagina should be secured whenever possible.

DISCUSSION.

DR. HENRY T. BYFORD, of Chicago.—The fact that a placenta that can be separated at the end of five months can probably be separated at term is no reason why it should be allowed to go to term. The separation of that placenta at eight or nine months would present more danger than its separation at five months.

With regard to the risk to the mother, if we can save a few more mothers this way by operating early, some of those mothers would probably conceive again and provide enough children to offset the few that can be saved by allowing the pregnancy to go on. If it were the case of my wife, I should not be so anxious to have a full-term child born, as I do *not* care for any cripples in my family, who would become a burden to me and probably a detriment to the race. I do not believe that the statistics given by the essayist are sufficiently comprehensive. I am sure that there are more healthy, well-formed adults that have been born of mothers who have survived previous ectopic gestation of four or five months duration, than there are who have been developed outside of the uterine cavity. Therefore I would determine the pregnancy in these cases as soon as possible for the benefit of the mother and have absolutely no regard for the life of the child. If the child were already viable a short delay for its benefit might be justifiable.

DR. THOMAS S. CULLEN, of Baltimore.—I have been very much interested in Dr. Peterson's paper and can agree with what he has said. It is certainly rather rare to find the fetus in the early months of pregnancy, but I have in the hospital at present a woman from whom we got the fetus at about the third month. In this case, as we opened the abdomen, the fetus popped out, and lived for fully fifteen minutes. The development of the hands and feet was perfect.

With regard to a bicornuate uterus, in one case, prior to operation we had felt a small uterus and a large tender mass to one side. We had also had the characteristic hemorrhage seen in extrauterine pregnancy—due to pregnancy in the opposite horn.

There is some diversity of opinion as to the question of delaying operation in these cases, hoping that a viable child may later be obtained. Within the last month I have had a patient in whom an extra-uterine pregnancy had advanced to the third month and at operation we found two fistulous openings between the small bowel and the sac. It was necessary to resect two and one-half inches of bowel. I have not had the opportunity of running the sections through; but there was no bleeding from the fistulous opening and there was very little organization of tissue. Each opening was nearly 1 cm. in diameter.

The only live child at term that I have observed was in Chrobak's clinic in Vienna in 1893. In that case the child had clubbed hand and clubbed feet. It lived but a few minutes after removal from the abdomen.

In 1907 I reported a case[1] of abdominal pregnancy; I did not know at the time of the operation what I was dealing with. There was a large mass that filled two-thirds of the abdomen; over the surface was the transverse colon, and the omentum everywhere was adherent. The uterus was normal in size. There was a pus tube on the right side. In removing the large tumor from the left side we thought we were dealing with a dermoid. When the specimen was opened, however, we found a full term extrauterine pregnancy, which had lain in the abdomen for four years. It was adherent to the mesentery of the transverse colon. In this case we turned the colon in on itself, made a sort of funnel, and established vaginal drainage. The final outcome was perfectly satisfactory.

DR. WALTER C. G. KIRCHNER, of St. Louis.—A little more than a year ago I had a case which illustrated many of the points that have been brought out by Dr. Peterson in his paper. It was a case in which pregnancy went on to term. It was an extrauterine pregnancy, and it was interesting to note that the conditions simulated very much those of normal pregnancy. When first observed it was found that the patient had a tumor-like mass on the right side in the ovarian region, which grew, became central, and the surgeon, who saw her at the time, advised operation. She feared this condition and fell into the hands of a number of physicians who treated her for miscarriage and for pregnancy. The tumor was of such a nature as to incapacitate her and she was obliged to remain almost constantly in her room. This forced her to take special care and to allow the intra-abdominal condition to develop in the

---

[1] Abdominal *Pregnancy* of *Four* Years' *Duration.* Jour. Amer. Med. Assoc., May 4, 1907.

S Surg

best possible way. When pregnancy was at full term, the usual labor pains came on, as she thought. She had previously had eight children, and stated that her condition and symptoms were similar to those she had previously experienced, and the physician thinking she was in false labor decided to wait. She came to the hospital three days later with a prolapsed uterus and greatly edematous cervix. An emergency existed, and section was made. A cystic-like sac filled the abdomen; the placenta was adherent anteriorly to the inner side of the sac, and a healthy and living child was delivered. This child weighed six and three-quarter pounds, and was well developed. With the exception of a slight asymmetry of the head, there were no deformities. The child is now over a year old, and is in good health. The sac was quite easily enucleated except for a few adhesions, omental and intestinal. The appendix was adherent to the sac.

The conclusions at which we arrived were, that, inasmuch as both tubes were normal, we were dealing with an ovarian pregnancy. The case was interesting from the fact that the pregnancy went on to term; that the conditions simulated normal pregnancy, and that the child is not deformed. The left ovary was left, but in the hurry of the operation the left tube was removed. Had this not been done, the mother would be in a condition where future pregnancy would be probable. The argument that in all these cases pregnancy should be terminated does not always hold good. because in this instance we had a healthy child, with no deformity.

DR. ROBERT T. MORRIS, of New York City.—I would like to ask if Dr. Peterson has any statistics showing the cause or causes of death in cases in which the placenta was left?

I have felt with regard to the internal secretion of the placenta that there was a tendency to the formation of coagulates as soon as the cord was tied, and the peritoneum will absorb aseptic beef-steak.

DR. J. WESLEY BOVÉE, of Washington, D. C.—I was not prepared for the statement of Dr. Peterson in regard to the safety of waiting until nearly full term pregnancy has occurred, that is, with regard to the deformity of the child. My impression relative to the amount of deformity was that it is much greater than his statistics show. I have never operated on a living full term or nearly full term ectopic pregnancy. I have, however, operated on two advanced cases. In one of them there were several points of interest.

About seventeen years ago, on the old plantation of Wakefield, Westmoreland County, Virginia, a woman was taken in labor (full term labor), as it was supposed, and a midwife was with her. A doctor was called to see her; but the labor stopped after a day's labor pains. No child was born. Six years later, however, she had a full term child, the delivery being normal. Three years after that Dr. Willie, Washington, brought her to me for operation and it was found that the fetus lay behind the peritoneum. It was removed by bringing the posterior peritoneum forward and depressing the abdominal wall, stitching the posterior peritoneum to the anterior layer of the peritoneum, around the incision, then incising and removing it. This seemed advisable, because she had passed some days before one of the parietal bones of the fetus by rectum, and it proved advisable in this case because for the next two weeks after operation all the bowel movements came through the abdominal wound and none through the anus. The fistula gradually closed, leaving a hernia.

In the other case I was confident it was one of retroperitoneal pregnancy. That was a case in which pregnancy had gone on for eleven months with a dead fetus. There was suppuration in the sac. That woman died thirteen days after operation from pulmonary tuberculosis. My impression is from this work that the sooner we operate on cases of ectopic pregnancy the better it is, except in very late cases. In every advanced case I would operate as soon as I could after seeing them. I would not wait, if possible, for the development of the fetus at term, because I am not prepared to believe that the statistics Dr. Peterson has given us are really exact. My impression is that the proportion of malformations is much greater than the author has given in his paper.

DR. H. A. ROYSTER, of Raleigh, North Carolina.—I have had three full term extrauterine pregnancies, and they have been recorded elsewhere. Briefly, I wish to mention them. In neither one of the three was the diagnosis made during the life of the fetus, and the women all got well. The first one was complicated with intra-uterine pregnancy at term, and in this case I had to marsupialate the sac on account of the intestinal adhesions. The second one was mistaken for a normal pregnancy, and the woman allowed to go two months beyond term. She was in a dreadful condition, from which she was saved by desperate means. In a third case the fetus had been in the abdomen for four years. The case was regarded as one of fibroid tumor, movable, and somewhat shrunken.

I am not prepared to say that the point made by the essayist is correct, simply because I do not know; but his statistics seem to furnish us a sound basis.

DR. LEWIS C. MORRIS, of Birmingham, Alabama.—Just a few months ago I had a case which has not been reported, and which presents some points of interest. The woman had gone to full term, but no diagnosis had been made. Labor pains had started, and it was thought she was in normal labor until it was found by examination that nothing presented at cervix, when an obstetrician made a diagnosis of abdominal pregnancy. She was sent to the hospital five days after false labor with this diagnosis. The physician in charge stated that the fetus was living during the time of the false labor pains. The woman lived seven miles from Birmingham; was sent across the country to the hospital in a wagon, and left home in a good condition. When she entered the hospital she was found to have a rapid pulse and some evidences of hemorrhage. I was telephoned for and as I walked into the operating room I found that the resident physician had just done a postmortem Cesarean section with the idea of saving the child. The child died soon after the onset of the false labor; its body was peeling; there was separation of the placenta, probably the result of the transit across the mountains from her home to Birmingham.

This case illustrates in a very striking way that waiting in these cases after the onset of labor is attended with great danger, particularly waiting for the placenta to shrink before operating. The delayed operation in these cases is attended with considerable risk.

DR. JOSEPH PRICE, of Philadelphia.—We are so familiar with the calamities attending cases of extrauterine pregnancy that it has prompted all active surgeons to operate on these cases early, whether they are seen early or late; the condition is one which demands early operative interference. If recognized early, counsel is recommended, and we have become so expert in the diagnosis of abdominal calamities and conditions, that from the cardinal symptoms in extrauterine pregnancy we can make a correct diagnosis in 99 cases out of 100, and if we work early we avoid a high mortality. Most of us are familiar with the fact that the mortality still remains high. There are many physicians who wait in these cases and make earnest efforts to bring about reaction, but they find that these patients do not react and die. The results from these persistent efforts to bring about reaction are not as good as those obtained from early surgery.

In regard to infection, when the placenta is very much like a beef-steak, and becomes virulently septic, the removal of it will give us a ghastly hemorrhage; the patient disappears under such a hemorrhage at term, and the men who attempt to remove the placenta at term in a case of ectopic gestation will have a hemorrhage that will give them such alarm as they have never had before; but the moment they loosen up the placenta with gauze and make efforts at establishing drainage then infection or sepsis begins, and the patient escapes narrowly with her life. I recall two cases in which the children were saved by early operation; one by my brother, and the other by Dr. Bonifield. These were two fine, healthy looking children. But such children are very scarce after such operations have been undertaken. The man who works early and completely is the one who saves the largest percentage of cases.

This paper is valuable, and particularly so from a statistical point of view. We have had a number of valuable articles bearing on this subject from time to time, one by Dr. Hayd, of Buffalo. Let us take, for instance, the classical case of Dr. Mann, of Buffalo, on whom an operation was done twenty-five years ago. In this case, the operator operated in the midst of extensive complications; the intestine was resected, and an old sac was removed, and a lot of debris from this neglected ectopic gestation. The woman made a recovery, conceived, and bore a child afterward.

Mr. Hutchinson collected fifty cases showing the progress of these cases of degenerating ectopic pregnancies, going through every viscus. In some ten or fifteen of them bones came through the bladder or rectum or at other points.

DR. RUFUS B. HALL, of Cincinnati.—The remarks made by the last speaker induce me to emphasize one or two points. I agree with Dr. Price that if we wait to try to save the life of the child, we wait for complications that are dangerous to the mother. It is self-evident that the earlier operation is done after the diagnosis has been made, the better it is for the mother. Of course, whether the operator shall wait for the viability of the child and try to save its life, must depend in the future, as in the past, on the judgment of the operator.

These discussions all add something to the sum total of our knowledge of the subject. Few men have enough cases of their own from which to draw definite conclusions in regard to adopting any set rule in dealing with this class of cases.

I rise particularly to emphasize one remark made by the essayist, namely, after all, for the good of the mother in these far advanced cases, it would add more to her safety than anything else he suggests in the paper if the hemorrhage can be controlled. If we expect to save these mothers in the far advanced cases, then we must remove the placenta. In those cases in which it is impossible to remove it we must have a high mortality, say 60 per cent. or more, from sepsis, because the placenta must slough, and we cannot provide for drainage, and that is where the danger comes. I am convinced that a larger number of these patients can be saved than are saved if the plan were adopted to sacrifice the uterus, as suggested in the paper, where the placenta is located in the pelvis, where it does not get its blood supply high up from the mesentery. Where it gets its blood supply from the pelvis, if the posterior uterine artery is tied, and the uterine artery on the side on which the placenta is placed, or the ovarian artery alone is ligated on the side of the placenta, hemorrhage is controlled before we commence to remove the placenta. Then there is hardly any hemorrhage which takes place from separating the placenta, and you get the blood supply from the vessels that are situated higher up which is easily controlled. If this one point is looked after we will save these patients. That method was suggested to me many years ago in removing broad ligament cysts and subperitoneal cysts of the ovary. Hemorrhage can be controlled in that way, and you can make a bloody operation on old broad ligament cysts a bloodless operation in this way, and it does well and to the great advantage in far advanced cases of this kind.

DR. PETERSON (closing).—I was not prepared to have the members of the Society agree that the proper procedure is to delay operation in cases of advanced extrauterine pregnancy until the eighth and a half month in order to give the fetus a better chance for life. In fact before I began a statistical study of this subject, from my own experience in cases of early ectopic pregnancy I was opposed to the idea of waiting. But it is difficult to set aside certain statistics which show the advantage of postponing operation.

Doctor Bovée's doubts as to the accuracy of Sittner's statistics can easily be settled, since this indefatigable worker has abstracted each of the one hundred and sixty-five cases upon which his conclusions are based. For my own part a study of his articles has led me to the conclusion that the statistics are accurate. They show that only a small percentage of the extrauterine children are crippled, for out of 93 only 10 were deformed. Out of 122 children, 63 lived beyond the first month, and nearly 20 per cent. lived beyond the first year. With these facts before us, as abdominal surgeons we are unable to ignore the life of the child. If we do, then it is more or less of a confession that for the fear of hemorrhage, which after all is not apt to be much greater at eight and a half than at five months, we give up all hope of saving the child. These elective operations are performed two or three weeks before term when that time can be definitely determined.

The placenta does not always suppurate when left behind, as Dr. Price has stated. In some of these cases the abdomen has been closed after removal of the child. If the operation has been aseptic and no sepsis develops later from the hollow viscera, the placenta may be absorbed without suppuration. But the chances of asepticity are slight, so that the placenta should always be removed if possible.

The more we study this subject the better able will we be to control hemorrhage, which at times, it must be confessed, may be very severe. Whether this control shall be by compression of the aorta or preliminary ligation of the vessels or both combined will depend upon circumstances. At any rate a study of the cases shows that in the discoid variety of placenta, preliminary hemostasis is an absolute necessity.

ADVANTAGES OF NEGLECT IN APPENDICITIS OPERATIONS.

BY ROBERT T. MORRIS, M.D.,
New York City.

MOST of us who are at this meeting have been reared under the principles of the third or pathological era in surgery. The keystone of our work has consisted in preventing the development of bacteria in wounds, and of removing bacteria and their products ar far as possible from wounds. Our conscientious devotion to the latter led us into methods of work which often damaged our patient seriously and unnecessarily. We did not know this until Metchnikoff and Wright showed us the way in which the patient protected himself against infections by means of his phagocytes and opsonins. At the present time we know that the patient in order to manufacture phagocytes and opsonins must be in the best possible physical condition which can be maintained under the circumstances of his infection. Many of the details of our method of work under the principles of the third or pathological era resulted in lowering the patient's vitality to such a point that he could not manufacture his own resistance materials well. We are now entering into the light of the fourth or physiological era, in which we are to conserve in in every possible way the normal resistance of the patient in order that he may be enabled to call out his own normal resistance factors for meeting infections.

There is no one field in surgery perhaps in which contrast between the third and fourth eras of surgery is so distinctly outlined as in our appendicitis work in cases with acute infection.

If we neglect to wash or wipe away all of the pus when the abdomen is opened, we give the patient an advantage in avoidance of the shock and loss of time incidental to this part of the work. As a matter of fact, much of the pus is actually sterile, because no matter how badly it may smell, the bacteria have committed suicide with their own toxins, some of which, mercaptans and sulpher ethers, cause the most nauseous odor. The active colonies of bacteria are chiefly in the living tissues in the vicinity, and these we cannot possibly remove, therefore the idea of getting rid of the nearly harmless pus is based upon our gross idea of cleanliness, rather than upon the knowledge which we actually possess today.

If we neglect to make long incisions and multiple incisions, which in the third era of surgery were thought to be necessary for removing the products of infection, we again give the patient an advantage in avoidance of shock.

If we neglect to wall off the normal peritoneal area with pads of gauze, and if we neglect to put extensive drainage apparatus in the area of infection, the patient has the advantage of missing the shock and the ileus, and superabundant adhesions, which were often the result of the application of these resources.

If we neglect to do injurious work formerly thought necessary for exposing an adherent cecum, in order to apply some fanciful treatment to the stump, the patient again has a good advantage.

Simple ligation of the stump we know today is all that is necessary, and where it would cost the patient too much to expose the base of the appendix, we can simply snap on a pair of forceps at that point, pull away the appendix, or what remains of it, and take off the forceps the next day. I make it a rule to remove the appendix in all cases, but if the patient is nearly moribund, he will have an advantage if we neglect to do the work requisite for removing the appendix. This will apply to only a very small percentage of our cases, but in this small percentage the patient will have the advantage given by our neglect.

Fecal fistula does not occur nearly so often as one would anticipate, probably because of the closure of small lumens through atmospheric pressure, but when fecal fistula does occur the patient will have a great advantage if we neglect to keep the fistula clean. Our methods for cleansing a fistula interfere with nature's method for carrying on repair with new cells, because these are destroyed very frequently by the resources which we employ, directed by our desire for gross cleanliness. The use of peroxide of hydrogen is very harmful when used for cleaning fecal fistulæ, because it destroys new repair tissue about as rapidly as it destroys pus. Under normal conditions connective tissue is formed in the walls of the fistula. This always has a natural tendency to contract, and such a natural contraction will obliterate the fistula better if we do not meddle conscientiously.

As soon as patients are out of bed and able to get about, I allow them to play golf, ride horseback, or engage in any physical exercise while the fistula is still open, asking them simply to wear external pads of gauze for ordinary neatness' sake.

If we neglect to separate all of the adhesions in the vicinity of the area of infection, the patient has an advantage, for adhesions when separated immediately re-form under the conditions of acute infection, and they may re-form in such a way as to angulate loops of bowel which were not angulated in the course of protective adhesion formation as conducted by the peritoneum.

If we neglect to have the patient wear an abdominal supporter after he is out of bed, we allow the tissues to carry on a complete repair, which they may fail to do if they find that our apparatus is relieving them of that necessity. There is no objection in some cases to wearing a supporter for a very short time, if we get our patient up early, because at that time the strain upon the tissue undergoing repair may result in an undue amount of reactionary inflammation. The point which I wish to make is, that the patient will have an advantage if we neglect to advise him to wear an abdominal supporter for weeks, or, as I have sometimes known, for months after operation. In my experimental work with animals with reference to the necessity for wearing abdominal supporters after operation, it was found that we not only caused unnecessary annoyance in many cases, but that supporting apparatus was actually harmful.

DISCUSSION.

DR. JOSEPH PRICE, of Philadelphia.—I am satisfied that there will be a spirited discussion on this subject. Probably Dr. Morris has forgotten what he said in his reply to Dr. Murphy at Atlantic City, when this subject was under discussion, and the question of starvation came up. At that time Dr. Morris remarked, if I remember rightly. "Oh! God, these patients have enough trouble without starvation."

Keith, of Edinburgh, that great and past master who did all he could toward perfecting hysterectomy, had a series of forty-five hysterectomies, with three deaths, and lamented the fact that his death rate was so great. He had labored long in this field, and had made every endeavor to establish as perfect a technique as possible, from which he deviated very little. I lament that Dr. Morris has deviated very much from his former methods of practice. Nevertheless, he has given us a beautiful opportunity to discuss every phase of this subject at this time. Some four years ago, after Dr. Morris had done so much in surgery in the East in rendering a life saving service to those patients who were afflicted with appendicitis, he got into the habit of calling the appendix the little assassin, and urged surgeons to remove it when it was the cause of so much trouble, and in operating on cases of appendicitis he found not only an infected appendix, but one or two gangrenous windows in it, and one or more concretions in a puddle of filth. Today he is not so radical in his methods of practice as he was in years gone by. In other words, he does not favor the removal of the appendix in as many cases as he did formerly.

Again, I want to condemn unqualifiedly any stump operation of whatever character, as I think we are too far advanced to leave one-sixth or one-eighth of the appendix, and allow the patient to suffer subsequently from trouble with the stump. It has taken one patient to my knowledge ten years to recover from physical and mental distress incident to stump disease from a chronic infection of a buried ulcer. We have a surgeon in this room who suffers from pericarditis, the result of stump disease.

We have with us Dr. Munro, of Boston, who came to Philadelphia not long ago and read a classical paper on "Retroperitoneal Infections Due to Appendicitis." I fear we have overlooked the importance of that paper, and the valuable lessons it teaches. I mention these things with a view of emphasizing the importance of doing as thorough and complete work as possible in removing the appendix.

After Dr. Morris had done so much in reference to the surgical treatment of appendicitis years ago in urging early operation and the complete removal of the appendix, whenever it was possible to do so, and had written a good deal on the subject, a homeopath replied to him by saying that the appendix had a function; that it had a pump-handle function; that it played up and down and pumped the contents of the cecum, so that the fecal matter traveled on; and that the olive oil lubricated the handle of the pump, etc. As a result, a wave of sweet oil passed all over America and killed lots of lovely children.

Dr. Keen critized his own work at the Denver meeting, but alluded to the therapeutics of Nothnagel, the prince of clinical lecturers, to cold storage and the ice pack, and quoted Nothnagel as having said that 95 per cent. of these patients recovered by cold storage. How absurb! Nothnagel would not go to see an operation performed by any one of the distinguished surgeons present for the removal of a gangrenous appendix, with two concretions in it, and receive an object lesson upon that living pathology. And that is true of the so-called internists all over the country.

My brother was called at the eleventh hour to operate on a lovely little child, who had been in the hands of a prominent clinician and teacher at the University of Pennsylvania, and who had resorted to the sweet oil treatment. My brother removed the appendix and saved the life of the child. The sweet oil treatment was pretty generally adopted at that time by internists; and then came cold storage, and the reading of a paper by one of the best surgeons of the world in which he advocated starvation and rest in cases of appendicitis. This was unfortunate. After all, there is not a single therapeutic method which will compare with the rapid and clean extirpation of a gangrenous appendix, and the removal of the pathological products. This good work was begun in this state (Virginia) by the father of our distinguished President—Dr. Hunter McGuire. He regarded appendicitis as a virulent disease, and fulminating appendicitis was an expression used long before this led to the infectious forms of the disease. A clean removal of the appendix is a simple operation. I tried my best to teach that this operation is one that can be done by the dummiest doctor behind the cotton-gin, or behind the saw-mill, with two little needles or forceps, and I think I have succeeded. You can make a simple toilet with normal salt solution. You can cleanse the infected zones with normal salt solution, and establish drainage. So much for that.

A few years ago at the Johns Hopkins Hospital drainage was condemned. It was considered an admission of bad surgery. There was some truth in that; but right on top of that a patient came in dying, with his abdominal cavity laden with pus. They opened his abdomen and found the viscera bathed with pus. They opened both loins, established drainage, and the man got well, and then they ceased to say that drainage was an admission of bad surgery.

DR. W. P. CARR, of Washington, D. C.—Dr. Morris is certainly right in one respect, and that is, in bad cases we must fit the operation to suit the condition of the patient. In a great many cases that are operated on the patients will not stand more than fifteen or twenty minutes' work. I have seen many patients recover very well after a simple opening has been made, letting out the pus, without anything further being done, except to put a catgut ligature around the appendix, and remove it, if it is possible to do so, and these patients would not have stood any prolonged operation, probably not more than ten minutes. I think we ought to bear in mind the condition of the patient and fit the operation to it.

In removing the appendix it is not always possible to do so in an ideal way. There are many cases of appendicitis where the appendix and the cecum around the base of the appendix are both thick and cheesy, and it is impossible to do anything like turning in the appendix or putting in stitches which would hold. In a case of that kind I have put a catgut ligature around the appendix and removed it, and the patient did just as well, although some of them have had a fecal fistula which usually only lasted for a few days before it closed. Where drainage is used, there is danger of hernia following, and if the patient's condition will bear it, I think it is better to drain through the flank and close the abdominal wound. It is easy to do, and it means simply a few minutes additional work. It is a question to be decided by the condition of the patient at the time of the operation. There is too much tendency to map out an operation and go ahead with it irrespective of how the patient is doing, and what condition he is in.

Dr. J. M. T. FINNEY, of Baltimore.—I hesitate very much to take part in this discussion, following as I do those who have preceded me with their wide experience in such matters; but I really cannot sit quiet without raising, at least, a word of protest against some of the statements I have heard made this morning, and some of the interpretations which have been given to certain phenomena which have been observed.

In the first place, I should take exception to the title of the paper just read, and particularly to the word "neglect." If by that word the reader of the paper means to describe certain practices which he has related to us, I should take vigorous exception to it, and should venture to substitute for "neglect" the word "observance," meaning the observance of certain fundamental principles of surgery. It seems to me, if anything has been settled or can be accepted as settled today, it is that unnecessary handling of tissues, unnecessary trauma inflicted upon abdominal organs is a surgical sin; the unnecessary application of certain irritating antiseptic solutions to the peritoneal surface is also a surgical sin. As I understand it, these gentlemen are blaming a system for the faulty application of it by certain men who from ignorance or some other reason have sinned, not only against surgery, but against that particular system.

Mr. Lawson Tait has been referred to as a striking illustration of the men who have habitually violated surgical principles. I should raise strong objection to that. Mr. Tait was simply a pioneer along certain lines. He saw light before others did, and simply put into practice certain methods without really knowing just what he was doing, because he was far in advance of some other members of the profession.

I want to take exception to the slur, if I may characterize it as such, which has been cast upon antiseptic surgery. If there is any one thing this profession of ours should be proud of, it is the great results which have been accomplished by antiseptic or aseptic surgery. If you will observe carefully the work of various operators who practice aseptic surgery, according to their idea of it, you will find that they are constantly violating certain cardinal principles in that system. You watch their results and you will see that 90 odd per cent. of their cases do well. A small per cent. of their patients do not do well. What is the explanation of it? It simply shows what the resistance of the tissue is to infection. Ninety odd per cent. of the cases will take care of themselves in spite of what the surgeon does. It is the hundredth case we are playing for, and if we are perfectly honest with ourselves we will have to admit it, and there is where the value of the aseptic system, properly carried out shows itself. The ninety-nine will take care of themselves, often in spite of what you do, rather than because of what you do.

There is one or two other points which I would like to refer to. One is with reference to the closure of intestinal fistulæ. Everybody knows that a fistula of the large intestine will usually heal of itself if let alone; but a fistula of the small intestine will practically never close without operation. That is a point I should like to emphasize.

A great deal can be said with regard to the management of the stump in cases of appendicitis. Personally I want to be considered as one or those who always ligates the stump; I have always done so, and from an experience of over two thousand cases in which this method has been used, I cannot, after careful study, find a single instance in which the slightest degree of trouble can be referred to the stump. Again, it seems to me we are blaming a system for the faulty application of it. If ligation of the stump is properly carried out, it is followed by the most satisfactory results, and we do not have that percentage of cases of serious, perhaps fatal post-operative hemorrhage which we will find in studying the statistics from those clinics in which ligation of the stump has not been practised.

DR. MORRIS (closing).—With reference to the matter of stump treatment, I did not suppose anyone would have much trouble from that source. My principle has been to remove the appendix completely and regularly, as a rule.

In regard to drainage, and this has reference to the remarks made by Dr. Price, I use a small drain so as to shock the patient as little as possible, by using the smallest drain which will suffice for the purpose.

In regard to fecal fistula, it does not occur so frequently as I had anticipated in cases in which we simply snap on a pair of forceps close to the cecum, and do not stop to ligate the stump. Once in a while one will see it, but not often.

Dr. Finney takes exception to the word "neglect" in the title of my paper. The context will care for that; but the word "neglect" related to the idea of the pathological era; that we must remove all bacteria and all products of infection, no matter what happens to the patient. I am as firm a believer in aseptic surgery and antiseptic surgery now as in the past when I brought about a storm of disapproval by fighting for it. Today in opening the knee-joint or in opening the cranial cavity I wear my cap, mouth guard, and rubber gloves religiously, but in opening the abdomen in a case in which there is infection of the appendix, gangrene and pus, I may as well wash my hands after operation as before, and do not wear gloves. They are a handicaps in that sort of case. We are all after the hundredth case to which Dr. Finney referred.

In regard to fistulæ, my remarks had reference to cecal fistulæ. I referred particularly to the common history of fistulæ from the large bowel, and that in fistulæ from the small bowel we have a different problem to deal with. The fistulæ with which we commonly have to deal are the cecal, and these have done much better under the treatment of neglect than where they have been carefully treated for weeks and months. I find in conversation with my nurses they have said to me, "we have used the utmost care in treating these fistulæ; we have injected peroxide of hydrogen; we have washed them out with salt solution; we have done this and that two or three times a day sometimes, and yet these fistulæ have continued for weeks and occasionally for months." It has been my experience that when I have simply used an external dressing of gauze in these cases and have done nothing to the fistulæ, cell repair has been carried on naturally; the new cells have not been disturbed by the cleansing methods, and these fistulæ have closed spontaneously and quickly by that simple method of dealing with them. Instead of keeping the patient quiet I have him play golf, ride horseback, or climb mountains if he wishes, before the fistulæ is closed.

SOME OBSERVATIONS UPON SURGERY OF THE KNEE-JOINT.

By J. Garland Sherrill, *M.D.*,
Louisville, Kentucky.

For some years I have been greatly interested in affections of the knee-joint, especially of the non-tuberculous type, and have noticed a marked tendency upon the part of many members of the profession to follow in their management of these cases the treatment recommended twenty years ago. It has seemed to us that while the minority of the profession has given careful and extended study to the pathology and treatment of these troubles, a large percentage has not considered the subject as worthy of more than passing notice. This condition of affairs should not be allowed to continue, for the knee-joint comes into constant use, and any disturbance to its mechanism at once proves crippling to the individual.

In presenting this paper before this body we do so with an apology for making no original contribution to the knowledge of the subject. My hope is to excite a discussion among the members which will place what is known in this connection into crystalline and concise form, so that we may have a proper foundation for a correct line of treatment. Even excluding the very frequent tuberculosis of this joint, we find a very large array of traumatism and diseases which, together with the deformities following in course of an inflammation of the joint, give us much food for contemplation and investigation. When one considers the complicated arrange-ment of the knee, its numerous and strong ligaments, the many synovial folds, the articulating surfaces, their manner of contact, the shallow deepening cartilages, the function of the joint, and its easy exposure to traumatism and insult, it is not surprising that it is frequently the source of annoyance and distress, but the surprise lies in the fact that such affec-tions are not much more frequent.

Our remarks will be limited to those minor and so called trifling affections which, while not endangering the life of the patient, very seriously cripple him and impair his useful-ness. Many of these conditions have as their chief causative factor traumatism in a greater or less degree. The limits of this paper will prevent more than brief consideration of the various conditions which result in interference with or aboli-tion of the function of the joint. Of the major traumatisms, fracture of the patella is of chief importance. This may be a very simple injury, if, for instance, the fracture is incom-plete and the fragments are not separated. This rare type has come under my observation only once. On the other hand, a compound fracture of this bone becomes a most serious accident. The result, after the so-called expectant treatment of fracture of this bone, may be sufficiently good to insure fair functional use of the limb. The results of the open operative treatment, however, are so much better that in healthy young patients and under proper surroundings the open method is strongly to be advised. We do not advise operative treatment in patients who are for any reason poor surgical risks, as sufferers from cardiac, pulmonary, or renal disease; nor would we advise it in the aged, or where there is little or no separation of the fragments.

The ill effects of infection of the joint are so serious that no one who has not so perfected his technique as to be able to avoid inflammatory reaction in clean wounds should attempt any surgery about the knee-joint. With such a perfection of technique one can fearlessly attack this structure.

Our plan of treatment in fracture of the patella consists in a semilunar incision across the front of the joint at or just below the site of the fracture. Any clots of blood present are removed and all bleeding vessels controlled. The lacerated tendon of the quadriceps muscle is then sutured on each side and over the patella with chromic catgut. The fascia and skin are then closed with catgut without drainage. After the wound is dressed the limb is placed in plaster of Paris. The results of this plan are uniformly good. The patient makes a speedy recovery and retains the usefulness of the limb. Passive motion is advisable in the third week, and the patient can walk upon the limb before the end of the fourth week. The fractures of the femur and tibia are always the accompaniment of very severe violence, and ought to be treated according to the general principles for use in such injuries. Passive motion should be instituted early.

Another disabling affection is what may be termed habitual dislocation of the patella. This tendency to repeated luxation of the patella to the outer side of the joint results in part from the anatomical form of the external condyle and in part from the direction of the femur toward the joint; in part from the relaxation of the ligamentum patellæ and quadriceps, and finally from trauma as an exciting cause. Patients suffering from this condition never feel secure in the erect posture, but are always in dread of the knee giving way. The patella tends to slip out upon extension and to return to its normal situation on flexion of the leg. In some instances this movement of the patella is accompanied by rather sharp pain. We record a case herewith in which first one and then the other patella was dislocated as result of trauma, with the persistence of dislocation in each case. The patient was a young lady of twenty six years, referred to me by Dr. Currey, of West Virginia. She gave a history of an injury to the right knee about four or five years ago, since which time she has suffered considerable pain and has noted a slipping of the patella away from the joint upon motion. This prevents her walking well. She later injured the left knee and developed a similar trouble there.

DIAGNOSIS. Double habitual luxation of the patella outward. Operation, September 13, 1909: A five-inch curved incision was made, convexity posteriorly along the inner side of the knee, through the skin, subcutaneous tissue, and the tendon of the quadriceps muscle. The cut edges of this tendon were overlapped by drawing the inferior margin under the superior by mattress sutures, while the patella was drawn forcibly inward. A second row of sutures coapted the free edge of the wound in the tendon with the inferior flap. Approximation of the skin and fascia was made without drainage. Sterile dressings were applied and the limb incased in plaster, extending from the malleolus to the upper third of the thigh. Passive motion following this procedure showed no displacement of the bone. Both knees were treated the same way, and the patient left the infirmary at the end of the second week. She is still wearing a support for the knee.

It is somewhat difficult to determine the reason of the persistence of this dislocation. The patient's limb is normal in direction and has no tendency to genu valgum, and beyond the slight relaxation of the parts around the joint and the fact that she had an injury there is nothing we can consider as a causative factor. It is probable that the loose condition of the quadriceps tendon is congenital and it only needed the traumatism to produce the dislocation. Several plans of treatment have been proposed to correct this tendency, one of which consists in the dissection of a narrow strip from the quadriceps tendon parallel with the patella on its inner side and the transplantation of this flap into an incision made on the outer side of the patella to receive it; the incision on the inner side of the patella is then approximated by sutures. The method used in our case was the one described by F. E. Bunts in *Surgery, Gynecology, and Obstetrics*, August, 1909.

The so-called internal derangements of the knee were

described more than a hundred years ago by Hey. Several
conditions are now mentioned under this head as (1) dislocation of the semilunar cartilages; (2) loose bodies in the joint;
(3) fat tabs in the joint. All of these conditions result in
interference with the function of the joint, and all present
some symptoms in common—pain upon motion with occa-
sioual fixation of the joint, tenderness, and usually hydrops.

Bennett reports 750 cases in which effusion in the joint
following injury was recurrent, either spontaneously or after
another injury, generally so slight that its effect on the normal
joint probably would not have been noticed. The larger
number of these cases were the result of displacement of
part of the semilunar cartilage. In the total number of 428
cases the symptoms pointed to the inner side being concerned
in 304, the outer side in 113, and both sides in 11. It was
also noticed that when the outer semilunar cartilage seemed
at fault the symptoms of pain and locking were referred to
the popliteal space in at least half the cases.

Dislocation of the semilunar cartilage proves very troublesome to the patient and frequently causes great pain as well as
fixation of the joint. The internal cartilage is affected more
frequently than the external, and the dislocation may be partial
as a folding of the cartilage upon itself, or the entire cartilage
may be separated. The causative factor is in most cases a
sudden torsion of the tibia, although a blow driving the tibia
backward in moderate flexion might produce it. The diagnosis is to be made by the sudden fixation of a previously
healthy joint accompanied by a sharp pain with subsequent
restoration of function, and later a recurrence of the symptoms. Effusion into the joint may follow the injury, and in
some cases the cartilage may be felt in front of the joint near
the margin of the tibia. Pressure over its former attachment
will elicit pain and soreness. The latter is a valuable point
in the diagnosis of this condition from loose (extraneous)
bodies in the joints. Treatment for this condition is either
palliative or operative. Pressure of the thumb over the

dislocated cartilage while the joint is slightly flexed and extended, followed by support with an adhesive plaster bandage, will allow comparative comfort. For those cases with a recurrent interference with the function, removal is indicated, and very superior results can be obtained by the use of a method employed by Sir Alfred Fripp, of Guy's Hospital. He places the limb in flexion and makes an inch long incision about one-half inch internal to and parallel with the inner margin of the patella. The edges of this small opening are strongly retracted by two small hooks and the joint cavity is inspected, giving a surprisingly good view of its structures. The cartilage is then removed, its remaining attachments to the tibia being severed with a small sharp knife. Nothing is allowed to come into contact with the joint except the knife and forceps, the cavity being neither washed nor sponged. He quickly closes the opening with three silkworm-gut sutures passed preferably from within out, thus approximating all the layers. A gauze dressing is applied and over this is a very voluminous layer of absorbent cotton. The latter acts as a support to the knee. Mr. Fripp insists upon these patients being out of bed on the second day, and by the end of the second week they are well. This method is much preferable to the transverse incision or the long lateral incision formerly in use, and it does away with protracted convalescence.

Loose bodies in the joint occur with some degree of frequency, varying in number from 1 to 40 or even 100; they may exist with but little disturbance of function, or may excite great disability. The mode of formation and causative factors are not well understood. Hunter thought them due to the deposit of ossific material upon coagula left in the joint after injury. Others thought them to result from pieces of cartilage torn off by violence from the semilunars; still others have believed them to result from congestion of the fatty tabs on the synovial membrane which have entered the joint and have allowed the lime salts from the joint fluid to collect or be deposited in them. The latter method seems to have been the method of formation in the case recorded herewith. A very small vascular band connected the larger of the two bodies with the synovial membrane. About the point of attachment of this band to the body there was a dark red congested area through which it evidently received some nourishment. The small body was not attached. Another method by which these loose bodies might form is by a process described by Mr. Paget, who says that after an injury an exfoliation takes place "without acute inflammation, just as a tooth after a blow may be slowly detached from its alveolus and cast out." Subsequently a similar process has been described by König, and later by Barth, and more recently by Ludloff as "osteochondritis dissecans," in which exfoliation of bone and cartilage occurs.[1] This exfoliation, according to Ludloff, always occurs on the convexity of the inner condyle near the site of the attachment of the posterior crucial ligament. König assumed that because he had proved that one of these bodies could not be forced off the bone by direct thrust a circulatory disturbance must account for its origin. Barth, on the other hand, believed that traumatism was the most important factor. Ludloff went fully into the study of three cases clinically and made a number of dead-house experiments, and concludes that, from studies on the bodies of children and adults, sufficient traumatism could not be applied to tear the posterior crucial ligament if the other joint structures remained intact. After section of the lateral ligaments he was able to tear off the posterior crucial ligaments by overextension and internal rotation of the tibia. With these facts in mind and in the absence of a history of such severe trauma, the lateral ligaments uninjured and showing no evidence of having been injured, the conclusion was reached that trauma in this form was not the cause. He described a small vessel springing from the internal articular

[1] Dr. *K.* Ludloff, Archiv f. Chir., Berlin, 1908, Band lxxxvii, Heft 3, S. 552.

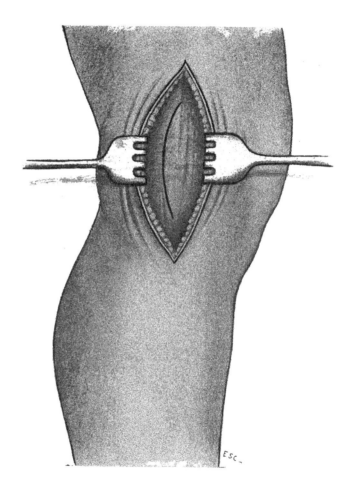

FIG. 1.—After F. E. Bunts.

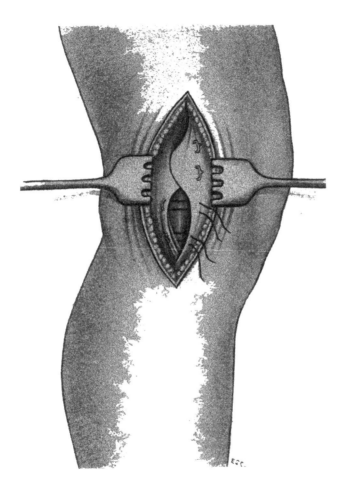

Fig. 2

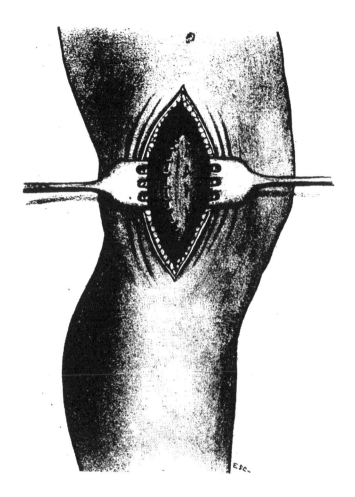

FIG. 3.—After F. E. Bunts.

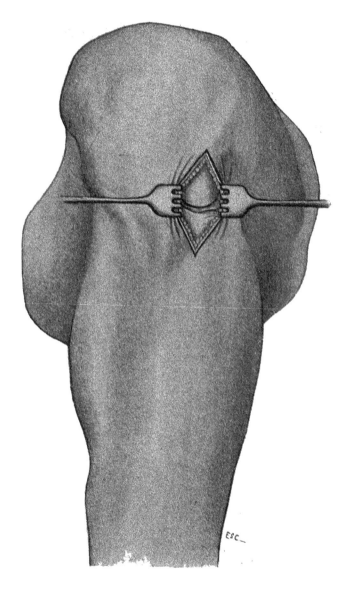

FIG. 4.—Incision for dislocated cartilage. Method used
by Sir Alfred Fripp.

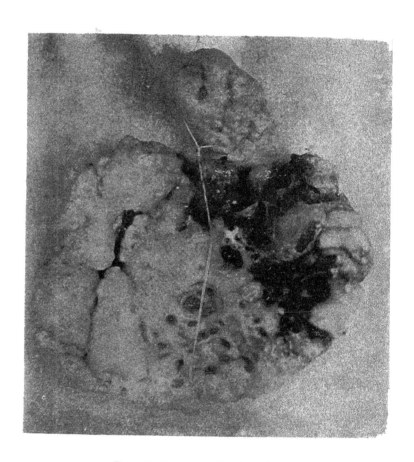

FIG. 5.—Loose bodies from knee.

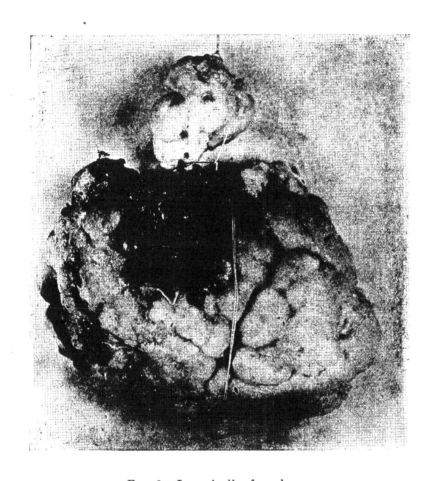

Fɪɢ. 6.—Loose bodies from knee.

artery and passing between the crossed bands on the posterior crucial ligament to supply the inner condyle and finally ending in the joint without anastomosis. When this vessel is damaged part of the inner condyle at the site of the attachments of the posterior crucial ligament must be deprived of circulation. He found that this vessel could not be injured as it passed along the posterior crucial ligament, but when the weight of the body was momentarily placed upon the hyper-extended limb, as for instance in stepping off the last step of a dark stairway, the posterior ligament was made tense, the artery clamped in the narrowed opening, and at the same time the internal condyloid eminence of the tibia strongly pressed against the inner and upper limits of the fossa inter-condyloidea. By such repeated and trifling traumatisms as are scarcely recollected by a hard-working individual, the circulation to this part can be disturbed. He declares the free bodies in the joint to result not from a severe trauma, contusion, or distortion, nor upon the basis of arthritis deformans, nor from a destructive process involving the whole joint, but by insignificant, oft-repeated tearing of the knee-joint through overstretching and inward rotation, damaging the internal articular artery. A disturbance of the circulation of the external part of the internal condyle in the region of the insertion of the posterior crucial ligament causes a disturbance of nutrition and death of a limited area of bone. After the death of the piece of bone the overlying cartilage is poorly nourished and is separated; the fragment lies in its place until all the attachments are loosened, or until some other traumatism separates it. He believes that in one of his cases the process continued for seven years before the body was finally extruded into the joint. He thinks his findings reconcile the claims of König for vascular disturbance, and those of Barth of trauma as a causative factor.

The following, taken from my case book, is a fairly illustrative case of this condition:

E. C., white, aged forty-seven years, male; referred to us

on November 13, 1907, by Dr. Graham, of Jeffersonville, Indiana. History of a blow upon the right knee thirty-three years ago from the kick of a horse, which the patient thinks caused a separation of a fragment from the head of the tibia. Three years ago the joint began to trouble him considerably. He has felt a large floating body for a long time, and recently can feel another. The joint is swollen and locomotion impaired.

EXAMINATION. Marked synovial swelling and extension of the sac, with two movable bodies readily felt above the patella. On November 16, 1907, an incision two inches long was made over the outer part of the synovial pouch through the quadriceps parallel to its fibers and two bodies were removed. The first was large, concave on its under surface, convex on the upper, about two inches in its widest part. It was unevenly rounded and presented marked irregularity of surface, with pits underneath and rounded prominences on its upper surface and edges. These prominences were smooth and covered with glistening white firm material like cartilage. The color of the whole piece was white except near the point of attachment by a single pedicle to the synovial fringe. For a space the size of a quarter it was reddish purple in color.

The smaller body was the size of a hazelnut and presented the same rounded irregularities; it was white in color and quite firm. A quantity of thick synovial fluid escaped when the sac was opened. The wound was sutured in three layers, several layers of gauze applied to the knee, and bandaged. Over this a voluminous layer of cotton was applied and a very snug roller. Healing took place in five days with the joint normal size. No evidence of tuberculosis. A portion of the tissue from the joint and some of the synovial fluid was examined by Dr. John E. Hays, who reported that the tissue was granulation tissue, non-tuberculous. The fluid taken from the cavity was sterile. No growth on media after forty-eight hours.

Hoffa, Benjamin Tenny, and others have described the disturbances produced by hypertrophied tabs of fat within the joint. These conditions usually occur in fat patients, the excessive amount of fat being pinched in the movements of the joint causing an increased circulation and an increased deposit of fat. The patient does not walk, owing to the pain experienced, and from this very fact the amount of fat increases; thus efforts at locomotion become more painful.

Among the late results of inflammatory lesions at the knee ankylosis is the most important, since it leaves the patient permanently crippled. We will not enter upon the discussion of the various causes of ankylosis; formerly this conclusion to an inflammatory case was considered quite satisfactory provided the limb became ankylosed in extension. It has long been taught, and with some reason, that a leg which was straight and fixed at the knee and painless was more useful functionally than one which was movable in part but painful. Within more recent years there has been an effort upon the part of some to obtain a painless and yet movable knee-joint in cases of ankylosis. Schuh, in 1853, attempted by dividing a synechia to free the patella, but nothing being interposed the ankylosis recurred. In 1893 Helferich excised the condyle of the inferior maxilla and interposed a flap from the temporal muscle. In 1899 he proposed to free the patella and to interpose part of the vastus internus between it and the femur, but did not perform the operation. Verneuil had, in 1860, made the same suggestion. Cramer, in 1901, operated upon seven cases of fixation of the patella alone, with six successes. Chlumsky found that in not a single case (fourteen in ten years) treated in Breslau Surgical Clinic was there improvement in mobility of the joint after the usual methods of treatment. Finding no better results in the literature of the joints, he undertook to clear up the question. He found that after forcible extension and flexion repeatedly done under anesthesia there was each time an increase of the deposits of bony and fibrous tissue and the cases were uniformly worse than before operation. With a knowledge of the good results of Mickulicz, Helferich, and others along this line by the interposition of a flap of muscle or fascia, he concluded that the procedure was not possible in the large joints either through failure of preservation of the interposed tissue, or because of technical difficulties. He therefore experimented with a number of foreign bodies, using silver, zinc, rubber, celluloid, cambric, and layers of collodion. He obtained mobility in some of these cases, but in none for more than four and one-half months. Ankylosis with extrusion of the foreign body occurred. He then used absorbable material, decalcified bone, ivory, magnesia, but with very unsatisfactory results.

Murphy, in 1905, reports his experiments along this line, and relates a number of cases in which he interposed muscle and fascia between the separated joint surfaces. Murphy says the points to be considered in treatment are the type of ankylosis, the tissues involved, and pathological lesion producing the ankylosis. He advises plastic elongation of the tendons in the extracapsular variety of fixation, and says that tenotomy with forcible extension fails to give free motion in the joint. He also advises the exsection of the sheath of the tendon where tenovaginitis has existed. After this is done the tendon is to be surrounded or covered by a layer of connective tissue. Cicatrices either from phlegmons or burns should be extensively dissected and their places supplemented by large cutaneous flaps with considerable fat attached. He lays great stress upon the complete dissection of the capsule when the latter is closely adherent to the bone. Liberation to easy and free motion without tension on tendon capsule or ligaments is essential. In the knee when the capsule and periarticular tissues have been involved in the pathological processes, the posterior ham-string tendons and the quadriceps and patellar tendons, with the crucial ligaments, are the only attachments which should be allowed to remain. He considers that his failures were due to the fact that he did not remove a sufficient portion of the ligaments and capsule of the joint.

William S. Baer, in *Johns Hopkins Hospital Bulletin*, September, 1909, discusses the use of animal membrane placed between the articulating surfaces of ankylosed joints, and reaches the following conclusions, which he considers as suggestive rather than definite: That a certain amount of mobility may be obtained if the material interposed will remain intact thirty or forty days. He says chromicized pig's bladder will do this. Cargile membrane is absorbed in ten to fifteen days, and therefore fails. Four cases of ankylosis of the knee recorded by him show two recoveries without mobility, one with 75 degrees and one with 3⁓ degrees of motion.

Hoffa (*Zeitschrift f. Orth. Chir.*, Band xviii) says that, while other joints could be successfully treated by the interposition of muscle and fascia, the amount of motion, 15 degrees, which he obtained, did not justify the additional risk.

Huguier, in 1905, says that, notwithstanding the exceptional cases, we must conclude that at the present time, at least, we are not justified in attempting to establish mobility of an ankylosed knee by an orthopedic operation.

Weglowsky (*Zentralbl. f. Chir.*, April 27, 1907) transplanted cartilage at the elbow, and through a subsequent pneumonia was able to examine the result. The perichondrial surface was smooth, even, and shining; the cartilage was enlarging and passed without definite margin into the surface of the humerus, and was well preserved throughout its extent. We believe that while there is room for development along this line, more especially in other joints than the knee, in the latter at least, unless the operation promises more and requires less interference than in the cases reported, we should advise resection and fixation of the knee.

DISCUSSION.

DR. A. R. SHANDS, of Washington, D. C.—I do not know that I can add anything of particular interest to this subject but there was one point in the beginning of the paper with which I do not agree exactly, and that is hesitation on the part of Dr. Sherrill in entering the knee-joint. While it is a brave procedure, I do not hesitate to open the knee-joint any more than I would to open the abdominal cavity. I have been opening knee-joints right along, especially in cases of obstinate synovitis, and I do not hesitate to do it freely. In many cases of recurrent synovitis, the joint has never been emptied of synovial fluid. The accumulated synovial fluid forms a mass similar to that found in the bottom of an old vinegar barrel, and that is what causes recurrence.

Speaking of floating bodies in the knee-joint, I had a case with a similar history to the one mentioned, but not extending over so many years. The patient was a young man who wrenched his knee in a foot-ball game. The following day a traumatic synovitis developed from which he recovered in the course of time under palliative treatment, but he had a recurrence of this trouble. He had been treated for rheumatism with many remedies, and finally after eight years, the knee becoming much enlarged and containing a great deal of fluid, from the history given I concluded it was one of two things, namely, a lipoma which was pinched from time to time, causing the traumatic synovitis, or a floating body in the joint was the cause of the trouble. At the site of the incision made over semilunar cartilage, as soon as I got my finger in the joint I felt a foreign body which was a floating cartilage the shape of a large lima bean.

In regard to the treatment of fracture of the patella, for the same reason the joint should be opened in case of trouble. I recently operated on a man and fastened the fragments together, a perfect recovery resulted. It is unnecessary to do it with wire. A purse-string suture of kangaroo tendon will do, suturing around, the suture being brought out at the same point.

DR. W. O. ROBERTS, of Louisville.—I agree with what Dr. Sherrill has said in reference to the treatment of fractures of the patellar. I have had a good deal of experience in treating these fractures, and have long since given up the use of metal appliances for holding the fragments together. Like him, I use the open method in the treatment of these cases where we have the advantages of a suitable infirmary.

As to dislocation of the patella, the case he has shown is interesting. Strange to say, I have seen but two cases of dislocation of the patella. In one of these there was a lateral displacement, and reduction was accomplished without any difficulty. It never recurred. The other was a vertical displacement of the patella. The man had also a fracture of the femur. I expected to have had a good deal of difficulty in reducing the dislocated patella, but did not. He got well, but it was a long time before he got motion in the knee-joint on account of a fracture of the thigh. We could not resort to passive motion, which otherwise would have been done, but eventually the man secured good motion at the joint.

As to loose bodies in the knee-joint, sometimes they give a good deal of trouble in their removal, because of the fact they slip away from us and it is hard to find them again. I shall never forget an experience I had in my early professional career, where I attempted to remove one of these foreign bodies in a young man at his residence. I cut down on it and just as I grasped it with forceps, it slipped away. I worked over this case for half an hour, when the loose body popped out on the other side of the knee. I stuck a needle through it, then cut down on it, and removed it.

DR. HORACE J. WHITACRE, of Cincinnati.—I did not get here in time to hear all of Dr. Sherrill's paper, but should like to mention two cases of loose semilunar cartilage, one in a boy, aged ten years, in which the cartilage was disorganized and entirely removed. The second case was one in which the cartilage appeared to be in fairly good shape, and was sutured in place. The boy has remained in good condition except that he has some pain in this knee from time to time on vigorous exertion, but he has not had any further displacement. I thought I would merely give you the results in the only two cases which I have operated on for displaced cartilage.

I judge from the paper the author does not believe much in osteoplastic work, and I wish to report some cases in which this has been done. I believe fully in our ability to create some sort of new joint, and get motion which will be painless and useful; I likewise believe that this operation can be done in the knee. The operation finds its best application in the socket joints, particularly in the maxillary articulation, in the hip, shoulder, and elbow. In the three cases done by myself the operation was performed after the method recommended by Dr. Murphy, and all are walking without crutch or cane, and they have movable knees.

The first case, a young lady, has a flexion of 90 degrees. Once in a while, after prolonged exertion or a long walk, she has some pain in the knee. Her occupation is that of builder in a millinery store, and she gets along without much limp.

In the second case I removed too much bone. In attempting to get a freely movable line between the two bones, I took off more bone than I should have done, and left the patient with a slightly relaxed joint. This girl has a flexion of more than 90 degrees. She was a trained nurse before operation, and has since done some nursing, but is now married. By shortening the ligaments a much better result might be secured, but she does not feel she wants to undergo that operation. At any rate, she has a movable knee, which will work without any support, although it is not a strong knee.

The third case was one in a school teacher [who has a satisfactory joint, the operation having been done about eighteen months ago, and she is most enthusiastic about the condition of her joint. I have recently received a letter from her, and judging from her description think that she has about forty-five degrees flexion. She brings the foot back far enough to get it out of the way when she sits. This woman likewise walks well, and performs the ordinary duties of teaching.

My only case of arthroplasty in the shoulder is as yet too recent to report upon, but this young man had an ankylosed shoulder, and a fairly satisfactory operation was done. The flap of fat-bearing fascia was made to completely surrounded the head of the humerus, as was done in the other cases, and I hope for a result. I mention these cases as further evidence in the claim that it is possible to create a movable, painless joint.

DR. JOHN C. WYSOR, of Clifton Forge, Virginia.—I want to report a rather unusual case of floating bodies in the knee-joint. I have had several such cases in railroad men. In the case I wish to speak of the man was from Kentucky, and had his knee injured in a railroad wreck some twelve or fifteen years before I saw him. When he came to me he walked fairly well, except that on occasion he would fall or be unable to proceed farther owing to locking of joint. I discovered floating bodies in the knee-joint, and operated on him. The interesting point is the number of cartilages which were found, some of them being partially ossified. I found fifteen of these floating bodies in his knee-joint, which varied in size from the end of my little finger to more than an inch in diameter. I had a handful which looked like a quail's nest if laid in the leaves. They were all white. The largest one was under the quadriceps tendon, was almost square, being a little over an inch square, half an inch in thickness, and was bony, and the bony projections came out through the cartilage in various places. We got a very good result in this case, so far as the function of the knee was concerned, and he rejoiced that the knee-joint did not become locked.

DR. STEPHEN H. WATTS, of Charlottesville, Virginia.— Dr. Sherrill has said very little about the transplantation of joints in cases of ankylosis. I have been very much interested in this subject of late, although I have not had an opportunity to make use of the method.

I recently had a case of fracture-dislocation of the elbow-joint in which I had hoped to transplant the big toe joint from some amputated extremity. Unfortunately there was no case requiring amputation in the hospital at the time, and, after waiting some time, I finally had to resort to resection. As luck would have it, a case of senile gangrene of the foot which required amputation entered the hospital the day after the resection was done. I had looked up the subject extensively in connection with this case and was impressed with the work of Lexer and others in Germany. These results are interesting and quite striking in some instances, but we all feel as though we should like to see these cases and note the amount of pain they have when the joint is used. It is rather astonishing when we find that we can transplant long pieces of the pipe bones and that they live and perform their function.

The animal experiments of Axhausen are very interesting. He has shown that we can make use of periosteum-covered bone from the same individual, from an individual of the same species or of a different species. He found, however, that the living periosteum-covered bone from the same individual rather than from another individual of the same species, is the best material, for in the former case the cells are nourished by the same tissue fluids to which they have been accustomed. He finds another very interesting thing, namely, that the production of new bone is more active at the ends of the transplanted pipe bones, for here the specific cells of the periosteum are directly exposed to the tissue fluids, which nourish them; therefore he suggests that in transplanting large pieces of the long pipe bones we make longitudinal incisions in the periosteum in order that the fluids may gain access to the specific cells. He also finds that the marrow cells are capable of new bone formation and suggests that the transplanted bones be split in order that the marrow be apposed to the surrounding tissues and thus acquire their nourishment.

Another interesting thing in modern surgery is the transplantation of pieces of bone to splint an old ununited fracture.

DR. RANDOLPH WINSLOW, of Baltimore.—Our attention was called this morning to the dangers connected with abdominal surgery when this work is undertaken by so many unprepared and unqualified persons. Now, the knee joint, of all joints particularly, is infinitely a more dangerous location than is the abdomen. Infection is much more readily conveyed and much more difficult to get rid of, so that while this work is perfectly proper in the hands of men who are fully prepared and amply qualified to do it, the notion should not go out to the young men all over the country, to the country physician, or the city physician, that they are perfectly competent to open knee-joints, to suture fractured patellas, or to do the various operative procedures recommended for pathological conditions about the knee-joint. Personally, I teach my students that nine-tenths of those who go into the practice of medicine are utterly unqualified to undertake to treat fractures of the patella by means of the open method, and that they should confine themselves to the use of apparatus, or they should take their patients to some one who is properly equipped and qualified for this work.

The remarks of Dr. Shands were interesting to me. In a fracture of the patella it is by no means necessary to wire the patella, or to drill holes in the bone in the vast majority of cases of fracture of the patella. The aponeurotic tissues covering the patella, after having been trimmed off, can be used for suturing the fragments together. Dr. Shands spoke of using chromicized catgut or kangaroo tendon for suturing the fragments; or silver wire, or silk-worm gut sutures, or silk may be passed around the patella, or may be used for bringing the fragments of the patella together. For a good many years in infective conditions about the knee-joint and even in conditions in which there is no infection, or where the infection is slight, I have been accustomed to open the joint, especially in cases of hydrops articuli, and in conditions of gonorrheal arthritis, etc., irrigating it with salt solution and then with 5 per cent. solution of carbolic acid, and then again with salt solution, and the results have been extremely good. In these relaxed joints, where the person is scarcely able to walk, where the joint is distended with liquid, this method of treatment in my hands has caused a prompt disappearance of the effusion, and the patients have recovered with excellent joints.

DR. SHERRILL (closing).—Replying to Dr. Shands' statements, I do not think he quite understood what I said in my paper. The ill effects of infection of the joint are so serious that no one, who has not so perfected his technique to be able to avoid inflammatory reaction, should attempt any surgery about the knee-joint. I do not believe it should be taught in this association, whose members are competent to do surgery of this kind, that any one can invade the knee-joint with safety in all instances. I agree with Dr. Winslow that there is no part of the body more dangerous than the knee-joint in the hands of the unclean. Infection of the knee-joint is by no means as easily taken care of as infection in the abdominal cavity.

The experiments that have been made along the line of arthroplasty are to me very interesting, and if it is possible to get a movable joint at the knee with a good amount of strength I should advise that method. I have always believed, and still believe, that in order to get a firm, strong joint at the knee, or at least a firm, strong knee, and a good useful limb, it is much safer to have fixation without pain than to have a flail joint with the possibility of pain. If we can reach the point of a good, strong, painless knee and mobility, we have an ideal result, and it is possible that these experiments may lead to that end. I have one case in which a girl had fixation and flexion at the hip, and at the knee, following tuberculosis in childhood. At the age of thirteen, osteotomy of the femur with resection at the knee was done.   In this case we obtained a straight limb, and with sufficient motion from the pelvis to be of great usefulness to the girl, so that she could walk without crutch or cane, and without marked limp.   Until we can get a joint which is strong and movable , as well as painless, we should not recommend arthroplasty in the knee.   In the other joints we can get good results, as has been stated by Dr. Whitacre.

MYOSITIS OSSIFICANS TRAUMATICA.

By J. M. T. FINNEY, M.D.,
Baltimore, Maryland.

THE pathological condition which forms the basis of this paper is one the existence of which has been recognized for a long time, but only within a comparatively few years has it attracted any general attention. Recently it has been the subject of several exhaustive articles, the best of which are those by Strauss, Berndt, Cahier, De Witt, Binney, and Bloodgood's reviews in *Progressive Medicine*. Any one wishing a complete literature on the subject can find it by consulting these authors. Including those here reported, over one hundred and fifty cases in all have so far been recorded. This disease is interesting not alone from a clinical standpoint, but from a pathological as well. There is always the danger of mistaking it for a more serious affection, namely, sarcoma. Amputation of the thigh has been performed under the mistaken idea that this condition was a subperiosteal sarcoma (Whitelock). Three of our cases came to us with a provisional diagnosis of sarcoma of the femur. Pathologically, there has been and still exists a considerable difference of opinion as to the manner in which these bony deposits take place and the source from which they come. It is for the purpose of directing your attention to these points, as well as reporting a group of interesting cases, that this communication is submitted.

A number of distinct conditions have been grouped under

the general head of "Myositis Ossificans." These all represent different pathological processes, and can be divided into four main classes:

1. "Myositis ossificans progressiva," where one muscle after another becomes ossified. Practically the whole body, more especially the posterior muscles of the trunk, may become transformed into bone. A marked example is the "ossified man" of circus fame.

2. "Myositis ossificans traumatica," where the bony deposit follows usually as a direct result of a single severe trauma, and is often quite sharply circumscribed.

3. An ossification occurring in some one particular muscle due to repeated slight traumas, the result of some special occupation. For instance, the so-called "rider's," or "drilling," bone.

4. The ossification occurring only in tendons. For instance, the tendo Achillis, a marked example of which was reported by the writer in 1903 (Binnie).

It is our purpose to limit ourselves to a consideration of the traumatic form alone (Group 2), as all the cases here reported save one (Halsted's) represent that variety.

ETIOLOGY. The factor most concerned in the production of this trouble is unquestionably a single severe trauma, for instance, a kick by a horse. Nearly one-half of all the cases are observed in the front of the thigh, involving the quadriceps extensor muscle. This and the flexor muscles of the arm seem to be the most common sites. Strauss has collected 127 genuine cases due to a single trauma. Of these, 43 occurred in the quadriceps femoris, 13 in the adductors of the thigh, 64 in the flexors of the upper arm and the remainder scattered throughout various muscles in different parts of the body. It has been observed with relative frequency in association with dislocation of the elbow. There seems to be no satisfactory explanation of the choice of site or method of production. It has been suggested that it may be due to the force of the blow being exerted always in a tangential direction, due to the thick muscles overlying the bone. It is also a fact worthy of some note that this condition is almost invariably met with in the large muscles and in those whose fibres take origin directly from some rough bony ridge, or which are directly attached to the periosteum without the intervention of much tendinous material (Whitelock).

It has also been observed that while the trauma giving rise to the condition is usually of some severity, still it is rarely seen in connection with very severe injuries to bone, *e. g.*, fractures or crushes. Instances have been reported of this affection developing without trauma or associated with very slight injury. It is a question, however, whether or not they ought properly to be included in this category, although pathologically as well as clinically they cannot be distinguished.

Males are almost invariably the subject of this affection. Only two cases have been so far reported in women. This is in all probability due to difference of occupation, and to the more robust muscular development. It is found much more commonly in young adults; the youngest case reported was a boy, aged twelve years, and the oldest a man, aged fifty-seven years. In Strauss' collection of 43 cases ccurring in the quadriceps femoris, 20 were due to the kick of a horse. In my series, 2 were due to this cause and the remainder to injuries sustained while playing football. Nichols and Richardson, in an interesting study of the injuries sustained by the Harvard football squad, throw some light upon the etiology of this trouble and its close association with this particular sport. They observed the same or a similar condition in two cases following "poop," the term used in football parlance to designate a rupture of some of the fibers of the extensor muscles of the thigh. It may occur as the result of a direct or an indirect injury. It usually follows a traumatism received while the muscle is in a state of tense contraction.

The symptomatology is, as a rule, quite characteristic. Following a severe trauma there may be noticed the usual clinical phenomena, namely, localized swelling, tenderness, ecchymosis, and disturbance of function. These symptoms, however, are not usually present to an exaggerated degree. The patient is not often laid up immediately, but may continue his usual occupation for some days following. Soon, however, pain on motion and more or less serious disturbance of function make their appearance, so much so that the patient is forced to seek medical advice. The objective symptoms are at this time those of an ordinary subcutaneous contusion, and fractures and exfoliations of bone can in most cases be excluded. The swelling, which at first is of only moderate consistency, with the occasional observance of localized fluctuation, gradually becomes harder and harder, as the disability increases. Both active and passive motion of the neighboring joints become limited, but rarely, if ever, entirely arrested. Perhaps the most characteristic symptom at this stage is the pain produced by forced flexion and extension. The tumor itself is somewhat irregular in outline, but on the whole rather fusiform in shape. It may apparently be movable, but is usually firmly adherent to the underlying bone. Tenderness, as a rule, is not pronounced. Any sudden strain or jar, such as stumping the toe, produces great pain. At first the swelling inercases slowly up to a certain point, after which it remains stationary or subsides.

Subjectively, a rather characteristic dull, aching pain is described by most patients, which is rather sharply referred to the region of the injury, but it may involve the whole extremity.

DIAGNOSIS. The diagnosis is ordinarily easy if a careful account is taken of the history and clinical findings. The location of the trouble, on the anterior aspect of the thigh or flexor surface of the arm, or following dislocation of the elbow, the history of a single severe trauma, subsequently the rather slow onset, absence of any very definite local signs at first, with the gradual appearance of the painful swelling in the region of the trauma coincident with increasing limitation of motion, absence of diagnostic signs of other diseases, no elevation of temperature, together with a very constant and characteristic *X*-ray picture, point so strongly to this particular affection that a diagnosis of myositis ossificans traumatica can readily be made. It might be well to add that in interpreting the *X*-ray pictures due attention must be paid to the time, in the course of the disease, when the photograph was taken, as pictures vary according to whether they were taken early or late. Those taken early in the disease may show little or no evidence of the presence of bone formation, while those taken late show unmistakable evidence of its presence.

DIFFERENTIAL DIAGNOSIS. This condition is to be differentiated from ordinary contusion, interstitial hematoma, myositis, periostitis, osteomyelitis, exostosis, gout, lues, and sarcoma. The skiagraph is essential to its proper differentiation from interstitial hematoma and myositis, which are both rather rare conditions and need be little considered. The characteristic night pain of periostitis and osteomyelitis, together with the elevation of temperature and pulse, localized heat and tenderness, and the skiagraphic differences between the two conditions, enables one to distinguish between them with little difficulty. The history and the *x*-ray picture determine at once the presence or absence of exostosis, osteoma, enchondroma, etc. Constitutional conditions, such as lues, can usually be excluded by the history and special tests (therapeutic, Wasserman, etc.). The only really serious difficulty that will be encountered will be in the differentiation of this condition from sarcoma. The age of the patient, the character of the injury, the mode of development, and in some cases even the *x*-ray picture, may correspond to those seen in sarcoma. If, however, the history be carefully considered, it will be observed that sarcomata are more often found near the epiphyseal line, while this condition is more frequently seen on the diaphysis. The growth of sarcoma is steady and progressive, while in this affection it is rather spasmodic and not continuous; later the tumor becomes smaller, which is never the case in sarcoma.

The bony structure in the *x*-ray plates shows out more distinctly, is more normal in appearance, and is more sharply defined than in the case of sarcoma, which is more cellular and less distinct.

Senn reports a case of gouty deposit under the deltoid muscle operated upon by him under the mistaken impression that it was myositis ossificans.

PROGNOSIS. The ultimate prognosis is good. So far as the individual operation is concerned, it depends largely upon the stage in which it is performed. There is always the tendency to recur in those cases operated upon early during the period of activity of the osteoid tissue. Later, cases do not tend to recur, that is, those in which growth of bone has ceased.

PATHOLOGY. The pathology of this interesting condition has given rise to a great deal of discussion, and is as yet not definitely determined. In the main, those who have studied the condition are divided into two groups—(1) those who believe the trouble to be of periosteal origin, and (2) those who would explain it as a transformation of fibrous tissue into bone. The hematic theory and that of aberrant sesamoid bones, mentioned by Cahier, are too fanciful to deserve serious consideration. The idea which was accepted by most of the earlier observers was that of transplanted periosteum. According to this theory, myosteomata are produced by the tearing off of fragments of periosteum or bone covered with periosteum, and the subsequent displacement of these fragments into the surrounding muscles by their contraction and retraction. These portions of misplaced bone and periosteum later proliferate and give rise to new bone formation. This theory has more adherents perhaps than any other, even at the present time, particularly among the French and German schools. It is also capable of experimental proof. Ollier, Berthier, Sultan, and others have transplanted portions of periosteum with or without bone from the tibiæ of rabbits into muscular tissue. Subsequently there developed from these foci bony tumors of considerable size. Clinical evidence also is not wanting to support this contention. It is not rare to observe, as a result of ordinary fractures, the development of bony tumors from layers of periosteum which have been detached by the injury and transplanted into the surrounding tissues. Virchow early called attention to this condition. A very interesting case of a development of bony tumor at the site of a fracture of the humerus has been observed in the Johns Hopkins Hospital, a photograph of which I here present. Not a few cases have been recorded of bony tumors following injuries to bone where portions of periosteum have been detached by cutting instruments or other trauma, with the subsequent development of bony tumors therefrom.

In studying our own cases, there seems to be perhaps two distinct conditions; in the first place, it will be observed that the periosteum was stripped from the bone in a manner similar to that occasionally observed in the newborn, the condition known as cephalhematoma. Beneath the periosteum thus elevated there was to be found a distinct new formation of spongy bone tissue. In addition to this there was noted several times a new formation of bone in the substance of the quadratus muscle. This bony tissue frequently assumes a finger-like shape, one end of which appeared to start from the periosteum, and was directly attached thereto. The other end projected out into the substance of the muscle and was surrounded by an area of fibrous myositis shading off into normal muscle fiber. The picture presented by our cases would bear

out strongly the theory of periosteal origin of those structures.

More recently the theory of those who hold that the
transformation in situ of muscular fibers into osseous
tissue, under the influence of an inflammation of special
nature, has gained ground.   Under this theory there must
be an interstitial inflammation which brings about a disappearance of the original muscular elements and its re-
placement by new bone, and a transformation, first, of muscle
into fibrous tissue, and secondly into bone.   In support of
this theory, attention is called to the production of bone
under the influence of a chronic irritation in various regions
—in the walls of abscesses (Guepin), tuberculous foci
(De Witt) about foreign bodies that have been in the tissues
for some time (Schwartz), atheromatous patches in the
walls of arteries (Bunting), about the scar of an old incision,
(Rixford), etc.   There is evidence, therefore, in the support
of the contention that almost any irritation or inflammation
of connective tissue is capable of ending in bone formation.
This theory is gradually gaining ground, and is supported
by most of the recent observers.   In some of the older
cases a distinct capsule is to be made out.   In the early
cases this cannot be demonstrated.

From a study of our own cases, it seems not impossible
to conceive of both these influences at work at the same
time.   The spongy bone found beneath the periosteum
is certainly of periosteal origin, just as seen in cephalhematoma, where there is no rent in the pericranium, and
where new spongy bone similar to that observed in my
cases is invariably found.   The finger-like formation of
bone projecting out into the muscle, and surrounded by
an area of fibrous myositosis, can readily be explained either
on the ground of periosteal origin from a misplaced shred
or of direct formation from fibrous tissue.   It is interesting
to note that in a number of cases the presence of marrow
cells with the actual formation of bone marrow has been

observed in the new bone. It was present in one of our cases. In Dr. Halsted's and Dr. Fisher's cases there was present a central cyst containing clear serum. These cysts are of relatively frequent occurrence, and are supposed to be due to non-absorption of the contents of a hematoma, or its failure to organize, due to insufficient blood supply, as a result of the early transformation into bone of the surrounding tissues, with the resulting formation of a bony cyst wall.

Cartilage is also found in a considerable number of cases. It was observed in one of ours, and in the sections from this case bone can be seen in the process of formation from the cartilage cells, as well as from the osteoid tissue.

TREATMENT. As prophylactic measures, aspiration and pressure are of somewhat doubtful efficacy, although highly recommended. Early incision with the evacuation of effused blood, the thorough removal of small fragments and spiculæ of bone, with drainage of the affected area, may, in some instances, prevent the formation of the trouble, but of this one can never be quite sure. Massage in the early stages is contra-indicated, as it may affect unfavorably the development of the trouble by stimulating the production of bone. The indications for operation are the presence of the tumor, the disturbance of function, pain, etc. As has already been indicated, there is an unfavorable as well as a favorable time for operation. It should never be recommended early in the development of the bony tumor, even for diagnostic purposes, since if we have to deal with a subperiosteal sarcoma, it is of doubtful efficacy, and in this condition the tendency to recur at this stage is very great. If the operation is left until later, when increase in the size of the tumor is no longer present and its consistency has become harder, the chances of a recurrence are very materially lessened. The operation should consist in a thorough excision, with ample margin, of all the osteoid tissue, including some healthy muscle. The underlying periosteum should be thoroughly excised and the shaft of the bone cleaned off until a smooth surface remains. Cauterization with the actual cautery of the denuded bony surface has been recommended (Pickrel). Operation is not indicated in every case; many of them recover under rest and later massage and active and passive motion. Two of our cases made excellent recoveries without operation.

Aizner, in a recent communication on the subject, recommends the use of fibrolysin, and reports a number of cases with favorable results. He recommends its use early, that is, in the stage of connective tissue induration. He thinks it is of no value after ossification is well established.

In addition to the three cases here reported, I have seen in consultation three others, all of them in football players. One of these cases came to operation. The other two were treated by massage and passive motion. All recovered. It is a very interesting fact that in all three of these cases the provisional diagnosis of subperiosteal sarcoma had been made. The one case operated upon twice recurred, necessitating three operations in all. Amputation at the hip-joint had been recommended and was about to be performed on this case at the time I saw him. It is also a fact of no little interest, and, so far as I am aware, not before observed in this class of cases, that marked blood changes were present. During the period of recurrence and active growth of the bony tumor, a marked anemia was noted, the hemaglobin falling as low as 60 per cent.

After the removal of the tumor marked improvement in the blood condition at once took place.

PATHOLOGICAL REPORT. The tissue received from Dr. Finney is composed of muscle which is extremely firm. The bundles are separated by a slight increase in fibrous tissue, which increases markedly toward the centre, where there is a hard, bony substance. Sections containing the central bony mass and the muscle peripheral to this show microscopically the following picture:

The bands of muscle seem almost entirely to be separated from the tumor mass, and nowhere through the body of the tumor are there any evidences of voluntary muscle fibers. The muscle fibers at the periphery of the mass are separated from each other by a slight infiltration of fibrous tissue in which considerable numbers of small mononuclear cells of the polyblast type are found. The fibers themselves are shrunken; in many places only remnants are seen with their nuclei bunched together. In other areas they show a slight swelling with loss of normal striation, but for the most part the striations are to be made out.

The impression that one obtains, however, is not that the muscle has been pushed away by the developing mass within it, but rather that it has undergone a primary inflammatory stage, for definite muscle bundles run directly into large hyaline masses, where no definite structure is to be made out. These are composed of faint pink strands divided by large spindle-shaped nuclei.

The central mass of the section presents a very complex picture, bone, cartilage, and osteoid tissue alternating in rather indefinite masses. The process which seems to be taking place, however, might be divided into two general classes—(1) the formation of bone from osteoid tissue, and (2) the formation of bone from cartilage.

1. To the inner side of the muscle fibers there is a great proliferation of rather atypical fibrous tissue. The protoplasm stains considerably pinker than normal, and seems to be proportionately larger than normal. It occurs in coarse strands, which become progressively coarser and in which the individual fibers become obliterated. The nuclei become less numerous, and are scattered then through a homogeneous, pink-staining matrix, appearing much like the lacunæ in bone. As these strands become thicker they are lined by a layer of cells on their outer margin, which are cubical, with deep-blue staining protoplasm and rather large dark nuclei. Such lamellæ of bone are formed

throughout the section and tend to project in irregular trabeculæ, forming in places small marrow-like cavities.   These contain a coarse fibrous connective tissue, in which large numbers of bloodvessels are seen.   Some, however, contain numerous round cells which belong to the type of polyblasts described by Maximof, while in others a considerable amount of fatty tissue occurs.   On the inner side of these marrow cavities one sees depressions in the periosteal lining of the bone.   In these large masses of bluish protoplasm many nuclei occur which resemble osteoclasts.

2. In other areas one finds typical masses of cartilage, which show in themselves rapid proliferation of cells, which cells then gradually disappear and the tissue surrounding them becomes calcified.   Such masses are rapidly invaded by a fresh granulation tissue, forming much the same picture in some areas as is found at the epiphysis of growing bone.   The result of this process shows itself in a typical mass of bone trabeculæ, including irregular marrow cavities. Many of the trabeculæ of bone contain within their bodies a few cartilage cells, while others are completely converted into bone with typical lacunæ.   These marrow cavities contain much the same material described in the other areas, but the cell contents varies to a greater extent.   For the most part these cells resemble the wandering round cells of Maximof.   They do not seem to be arranged in any definite order, but lie in the interstitial tissue.   In one area a cell can be seen passing through the capillary wall, and there joining a definite chain of cells in this position.   In one area a single typical marrow giant cell occurs.

I am indebted to Dr. M. C. Winternitz, of the Pathological Department of the Johns Hopkins Hospital, for the above pathological report.

CASE I.—F. S., aged eighteen years, clerk.   Referred by Dr. Louis P. Hamburger.   Admitted to the Union Protestant Infirmary April 2, 1906. Operation April 16, 1906. Complaint, pain in right leg.

Family History. Negative.

Personal History. Typhoid fever four years ago. No complications.

Three months ago, while playing "soccer," the patient was kicked on right thigh. There was not much pain at the time, but the next day it was so painful that he could scarcely walk. Patient went to another hospital, where he was treated with hot compresses and was much relieved. He still has pain in the thigh at times.

The right thigh is somewhat larger than the left. On palpation over the quadriceps there is a hard resistant mass. There is no marked tenderness. Fluctuation just above the knee. Patient cannot flex leg more than 20 degrees.

Operation April 16, 1906. Ether. Incision was made over the tumor. About one-half pint of blood escaped with some force. There was considerable new bone formation around the hematoma, which was removed, the femur being left smooth and in good condition. One protective drain.

The patient made an uneventful recovery and left the hospital April 28, well.

He has been examined recently by Dr. Fisher, and remains well.

Case II.—A. D. McM., aged twenty-five years, medical student. Referred by Dr. W. M. Dabney. Admitted to the Union Protestant Infirmary March 16, 1907. Complaint, swelling and stiffness of right leg.

Family History. Negative.

Personal History. Negative. Pneumonia (?) twice.

Began with injury to right thigh caused from kick just above knee during football game in October, 1906. He finished the game, but was in great pain. The leg began to swell rapidly, and he was unable to walk for ten days. There was very little discoloration, but could not flex leg on thigh. At the end of three weeks patient was getting about pretty well, and played another game of football, during which he was kicked on the same leg several times. It again became swollen, and was very painful, especially at night. In five days he was back again in the game, when for the third time he was hurt. There was swelling and great pain. On December 11, 1906, patient was operated upon by another surgeon. "Some fibrous tissue was broken up and some serum drained off." Has been no better since the operation. He is now able to walk around, and has very little pain, unless he stumps his toe or tries to flex leg on thigh. Since the operation a hard lump has appeared at the site of injury, which he thinks has grown very gradually. It is not especially tender.

On the left anterior portion of the right thigh, beginning about 6 cm. above the knee-joint, there is a hard, firm tumor felt just beneath the skin. It seems to be attached to the bone, and extends pretty well all over the anterior aspect of the thigh, extending up to the middle third. It is not tender on pressure and does not seem to be incapsulated. The leg can be flexed on the thigh about 20 degrees. Flexion causes some pain.

The x-rays of this case have unfortunately been lost, but presented a picture similar to those shown.

Treatment. On account of a pleurisy, the origin of which was suspected to be tuberculous, operation was not advised. Massage and active exercise were recommended. About two years later, when the patient was last seen, there had been no recurrence.

CASE III.—W. G. H., aged forty-three years. Entered the Johns Hopkins Hospital August 10, 1909, in the service of Dr. Halsted. Three months ago the left thigh was injured by a log rolling over him. The only thing noted at the time was bruising and swelling of the anterior surface of left thigh. Patient was able to walk, but thigh was very painful. Full extension at knee not possible. Pain and tenderness

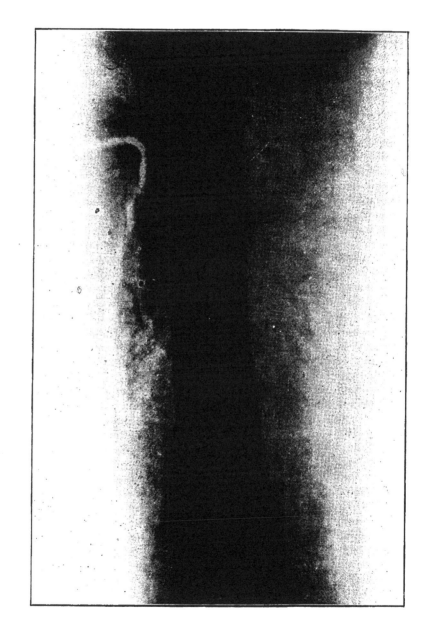

CASE III.

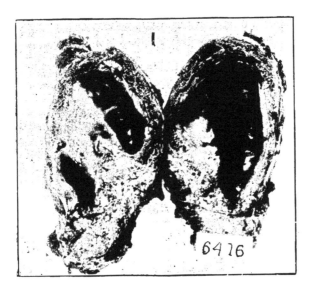

Bony tumor developed at site of fracture
of humerus.

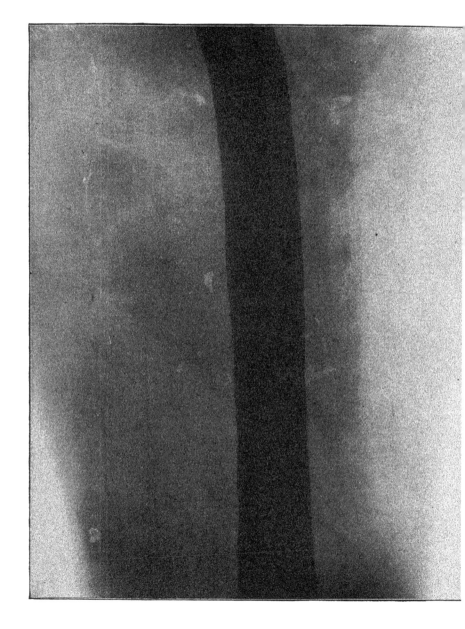

have diminished, but limitation of motion continues. About a month ago he was kicked on the thigh by a horse.

On left thigh, at about junction of middle and lower thirds, and on internal aspect of thigh, there is a palpable tumor which is firmly attached to the shaft of the femur. It is of bony hardness, and shades out indefinitely into the muscles. It is about 10 cm. in diameter. The knee can be completely extended, but cannot be flexed more than 15 degrees on account of tying down of quadriceps extensor muscle.

August 11, operation by one of the internes. Ether. Incision in middle thigh down to periosteum. It was found to be very much thickened and roughened by new-formed bone. Portions of this tissue were removed for examination. Closed without drainage. Discharged August 18, 1909.

Patient reëntered the Johns Hopkins Hospital September 10, 1909. Felt well for two weeks after leaving the Hospital, but during last two weeks thinks general health impaired. The growth in thigh is becoming larger, pains him all the time, dull and constant. Unable to bend knee except to a slight degree.

Condition of thigh similar to that present at former admission.

Operation September 11, 1909, ether. Incision at site of previous scar. As soon as muscle was exposed, it was found to be replaced by a homogenous hard mass of cartilaginous and bony tissue, which was completely excised, exposing the roughened shaft of the femur. This roughened, spongy bone was chiselled away, leaving a smooth normal surface. Muscles closed with catgut, iodoform protective drain.

X-rays show typical picture of this condition.

CASE IV.—H. P., aged thirty years. Admitted to the Johns Hopkins Hospital February 2, 1894, in the service of Dr. Halsted.

No trauma. Pain and swelling three days. Anterior aspect of the thigh swollen, fluctuation. Restriction of motion and pain in knee. First operation (Bloodgood) exploratory. Large cavity filled with blood, 400 c.c., lined by granulation tissue. No bone found. Microscropic sections demonstrated myositis.

Second operation, seven days later (Halsted). Wall of cyst excised. New growth of bone extends to periosteum, which is thickened. Sections, typical ossifying myositis.

In this case, myositis apparently of periosteal origin.

CASE V.—C. D. (colored), aged thirteen years. Admitted to the Johns Hopkins Hospital July 27, 1906, in the service of Dr. Halsted. Traumatism six weeks, fracture of humerus (?). Immediate swelling, which has not disappeared but has become hard. Examination, visible swelling middle of right arm. On palpation, middle shaft of humerus enlarged, swelling of soft parts 6 by 9 cm., almost as hard as bone.

X-rays show thickening of middle shaft of humerus, more like a traumatic periostitis than fracture. A spicule of bone is extending into soft parts. The shadow of the tumor is indistinct, but suggests the early stage of myositis ossificans.

Refused operation, left hospital. The diagnosis in this case is somewhat uncertain. There is a possibility that the swelling may be luetic in origin, as there was a history of this disease.

CASE VI.—A. J., aged thirty years. Admitted to the Johns Hopkins Hospital July 27, 1906, in the service of Dr. Halsted. Trauma to bend of elbow two months ago. Immediate swelling two and one-half weeks, then reduction. Restricted motion. Palpation, bony tumor beneath biceps, above elbow in front of humerus.

Operation (Fisher). Excision of tumor from substance of brachialis anticus. No connection with periosteum. Tumor 4 by 5 cm., composed of bone with central cavity containing serum. Microscopically, myositis ossificans.

X-rays show tumor in bend of elbow.

CASE VII.—I. S., aged eighteen years. Admitted to the Johns Hopkins Hospital December 2, 1907, in the service of Dr. Halsted. Dull aching pain in the right lumbar region six months ago. One month later swelling, increased gradually. Recently pain radiated down leg to knee. Examination, swelling in lumbar region 12 cm. in diameter, fixed to deep structures, does not fluctuate.

Operation. Excision cystic ossifying tumor of right loin; no connection with bone.

Patient returned in a few weeks on account of pain. Exploration revealed nothing.

BIBLIOGRAPHY.

Berndt. Archiv f. klin. Chir., 1902, lxv, 235.

Binnie. Trans. Amer. Surg. Assoc., 1903.

Cahier. Revue de Chir., vol. xxix.

Strauss. Archiv f. klin. Chir., 1906, lxxviii, 111.

Aizner. Münch. med. Wochschr., 1909, lvi, No. 15, p. 757.

De Witt. Amer. Jour. Med. Sci., 1900, cxx, 295.

Bloodgood. Progressive Medicine, December, 1902–1908.

Pickrel. Personal communication.

Bunting. Jour. Exper. Med., 1906, viii, 365.

Whitelock. Sprains and Allied Injuries of Joints (Henry Frowde, London, 1909).

Senn. Annals of Surgery, 1904, xl, 605.

Nichols and Richardson. Boston Med. and Surg. Jour., 1909, clx, 33.

DISCUSSION.

DR. JOSEPH C. BLOODGOOD, of Baltimore.—I shall discuss one point in connection with the subject presented by Dr. Finney, that is the differential diagnosis between a benign lesion and a sarcoma. Let us consider only the cases occurring in the thigh, where we have perhaps more examples of the intermuscular sarcoma, of the ordinary hematoma, and of ossifying myositis. In most of the cases (both benign and malignant) there is a history of trauma, a single trauma, a contusion. Rarely is the injury to the soft parts associated with fracture or dislocation. The contusion to the thigh is followed by swelling; in the majority of cases there is a latent period between the disappearance of the primary swelling and the appearance of the secondary. In some cases, however, the swelling primary after the injury merges into the swelling of the secondary pathological lesion, whatever that may be. Therefore, neither the merging into the secondary condition without the disappearance of the primary swelling, nor the disappearance of the primary swelling followed by the appearance of the secondary, allows us to make a differential diagnosis between the benign and malignant lesion. As to the period of time within which a malignant intermuscular sarcoma may develop—it may do so as quickly as an ossifying myositis. In this latter condition (ossifying myositis) if one waits until bone is formed, the x-ray makes the differential diagnosis. I will speak later of the importance of bone formation in the differentiation between benign and malignant lesions, but in the early period, before bone formation is seen in the x-ray, the differential diagnosis cannot be made from the x-ray, and I do not believe it can be made from the clinical data or other method of examination.   If it is your good fortune to see these patients very early, when the diagnosis is difficult, the differential diagnosis will have to be made at the exploratory incision. The period in which the best results are obtained by removing the sarcoma is one in which the differential diagnosis between sarcoma and the other benign lesions is most difficult.

In this early period it requires great experience to differentiate between an organized encysted hematoma, a myositis with its central hematoma before bone formation, and a sarcoma with a central hematoma.   Even with a rapid frozen section the differential diagnosis is still fraught with difficutly. It is my opinion that in case of doubt an amputation or an operation jeopardizing the function of the limb should not be done, because the prognosis for these very cellular, hemorrhagic sarcomas which are difficult to differentiate from the benign lesions is so desperate that the greatest good can be done to the greatest number by treating these doubtful lesions as benign until it has been proved that they are malignant. The curable sarcoma, solid tumors with considerable fibrous tissue, can be cured by local resection. One, however, must bear in mind that a chronic interstitial non-ossifying myositis might be mistaken for a fibro-spindle-cell sarcoma.

The time limit prevents further discussion of this very interesting and important differential diagnosis.

(I have considered these questions in the following contributions to the literature: "Tumors of the Jaw," *American Practice of Surgery*, Bryant and Buck, vol. vi, p. 813. Importance of the early recognition and operative treatment of malignant tumors, variation of the extent of the operative removal according to the relative malignancy of the tumor, *Jour. Amer. Med. Assoc.*, November 3, 1906, vol. xlvii, p. 1470. *Progressive Medicine*, December 1902, p. 161, 167 and 172. In *Progressive Medicine* for each year since December, 1902, the literature of myositis, sarcoma of the soft parts and sarcoma of bone has been given careful consideration.)

In regard to bone formation in relation to sarcoma and inflammatory diseases I am of the opinion that the term osteosarcoma is frequently incorrectly employed to indicate any sarcoma arising from bone. The term should be restricted to that form of sarcoma in which there is new bone formation, and as a matter of fact such a sarcoma is always of periosteal origin. There are various conditions in which new bone forms. The most frequent are: ossifying myositis, ossifying periostitis, and periosteal osteosarcoma. Bone formation may now and then be seen in benign connective-tissue tumors not connected with bone, and now and then in the connective tissue of the fibroepithelial tumors of the breast and thyroid gland. In that form of ossifying myositis in which there is no communication with the shaft of the neighboring bone there is a clear zone in the x-ray shadow between the bone-forming tumors in the muscle and the shaft of the bone. Such an x-ray picture may be looked upon as pathognomonic of a benign lesion. I have never seen an ossifying sarcoma not connected with bone. When the shadow of the ossifying myositis communicates with the shaft of the bone we must differentiate between the benign lesions—ossifying myositis and periostitis, and the malignant tumor—periosteal osteosarcoma. In my experience up to the present time and in all the illustrations which I have seen in the literature there has been no difficulty in distinguishing the shadow of the bone-forming sarcoma from that of the bone-forming inflammatory lesion of muscle or periosteum. In sarcoma the ray of the bone shadow is perpendicular to the shaft of the bone (*Amer. Practice of Surgery*, vol. vi, p. 825, Fig. 566). There is less bone formation, and the shadow is most dense at the outer rim of the tumor and less so near the shaft of the bone. The shadow of the outer table of the shaft of the bone usually shows areas of erosion and bone absorption. In the ossifying periostitis and myositis this ray-bone formation is never present, the shadow is thickest next to the shaft of the bone and grows lighter toward the periphery of the tumor, and the shadow of the cortical bone itself is either normal or more condensed. Therefore, as I stated before, in the bone-forming period the x-ray makes the differential diagnosis; in the earlier period the differential diagnosis must be made at the exploratory incision, either from the fresh appearance or a frozen section.

DR. JOSEPH RANSOHOFF, of Cincinnati.—In connection with Dr. Finney's paper, I wish to show some x-ray plates of an elbow which had been dislocated for five weeks before the patient came to my service. It was a neglected case. It was an ordinary posterior dislocation of the elbow, and at the time the pictures were taken shadows were seen upon the anterior and posterior surfaces of the arm, flexor and extensor. These shadows indicated the beginning of myositis ossificans, traumatic in character. We attempted to reduce that at once without an open operation, but we did not succeed, so that after waiting a week or ten days I resorted to the open operation and reduced it, and subsequently we had other pictures taken. It appears from what Dr. Finney has stated, that since the second operation the bone masses have grown considerably, particularly the one above the olecranon on the posterior surface; whether because we opened this thing, or whether the growth went on despite that, I cannot tell. In one x-ray plate you will see how much growth has taken place after the reduction of the dislocation.

There is one question I wish Dr. Finney would answer when he closes the discussion, and that is, he did not have cartilage tissue in the cases of myositis ossificans. Unless there were some vestiges left there, which is not likely, at the diaphysis of bone, how can you account for the formation of cartilage? As I understand the pathology of cartilaginous growth, it can only come from pre-existing cartilage. How can we account for the development of true cartilage of the hyaline type in myositis ossificans, unless the injury is near the cartilage line?

Dr. GEORGE W. CRILE, of Cleveland.—I would like to ask Dr. Finney what the clinical course of these cases is if they are allowed to go untreated?

Dr. FINNEY (closing).—There were two points I wanted to emphasize particularly in this paper. The first is the danger of mistaking this condition for a much more serious one, namely, sarcoma. The second is in cases of doubt we should not be in too great a hurry to operate. As has been pointed out by Dr. Bloodgood, in these cases of subperiosteal sarcoma we will mutilate the patient without doing him any good. We have never seen a case of subperiosteal sarcoma of the long bones cured by amputation. I am pessimistic as to our ability to treat subperiosteal sarcoma successfully by amputation. A case has been reported by Whitlock, where amputation of the thigh was done for this condition, under the mistaken idea that it was sarcoma. If this, therefore, is a sarcoma you cannot help the patient by amputation, and if it is not sarcoma, amputation is not necessary.

In answer to the remarks of Dr. Ransohoff as to the presence of cartilage in these cases, undoubted instances of the existence of cartilage in this new-formed tissue are reported. DeWitt's case is unquestionably that, as is also one of our cases. One can see where the cartilage cells unite with the new bone in the process of formation. One of the strongest arguments for the periosteal origin of these cases is that in some of the bony tissue—aberrant, if you will—cartilage cells are present and they are also occasionally found in the periosteum. There may be transformation of the fibrous tissue cells into cartilage cells, but that is not proven.

Dr. Crile's question as to the clinical course of these cases is answered very well in the two cases I had. One of the patients that came to me was a foot-ball player. His case was well developed. He also had at the same time pleurisy, which we thought was of tubercular origin. Therefore, we did not operate on him, and followed him through a rather long course. In these cases massage, if applied early, sometimes stimulates the formation of bone, hence he did not get massage, but the thigh was put at rest in a splint, and was kept as quiet as possible. After six weeks the subjective symptoms all disappeared, and the tumor had grown smaller. Then we began gentle massage and light active motion. After about six months the tumor had not entirely disappeared, but was much smaller and all his symptoms had subsided. Two years afterwards he had an enlargement of the bone at that point, but no subjective symptoms whatsoever.

Other cases of the kind have been reported, so it seems that this affection pursues a rather long chronic course, [which, when subjected to rest treatment and no massage, will eventually recover. One can hasten recovery, I think, materially by operation after the tumor has begun to subside, that is, after the activity of the bone-forming tissue has ceased.

A PLEA FOR THE MORE GENERAL USE OF CHOLECYSTENTEROSTOMY IN CERTAIN CASES OF PANCREATITIS.

By LE GRAND GUERRY, *M.D.*,
Columbia, South Carolina.

I DO not pretend to be offering anything new or novel or original, but rather, out of a purely personal experience, to direct attention to a surgical procedure which, we believe, has a rational foundation and at the same time deserves a more extended field of usefulness. We believe that the operation advocated is thoroughly consistent with the nature of the diseased process, namely, a chronic inflammation of the pancreas, whether the etiological factor be gallstones or infection independent of and apart from stone formation.

From what I have been able to read in books and the current literature, and have observed in actual work of very many large clinics, the operation of cholecystenterostomy in its relation to chronic or interstitial pancreatitis is not as generally in use by surgeons in this country as it should be. There are many and ample descriptions of its technique, but the deficiency lies in the failure to apply the principle of permanent drainage as often as our experience would indicate.

The whole proposition hinges on this point: It appears that quite a number of cases of chronic pancreatitis require more or less permanent drainage to effect a symptomatic and physiological cure; that if the pancreatic inflamma-

tion has progressed to a certain stage the operation of cholecystotomy does not afford drainage of a sufficient length
of time to allow the trouble to subside; indeed, there is a
point reached, in the progress of this malady, in which
the pancreatitis itself is incurable, although the symptoms
due to insufficient bile drainage may be relieved by operation;
in other words, if the pancreatitis which started as interstitial lasts long enough the islands of Langerhans become
involved, and we then have the so-called interacini pancreatitis with its resultant diabetes.

This possibility, it appears to me, is one of the very good
reasons why earlier resort should be had to permanent
drainage. I suppose that at the operating table it would
be impossible to state positively which of the two stages
of the disease was present; it is easy to understand, when
we consider the very small size, comparatively, of the bile
channels, that bile is secreted under very low blood pressure,
and also how slight is the pressure behind to force it on to
the duodenum, that very slight obstruction at the head of the
pancreas would be sufficient to cause its damming back
and consequent absorption.

Gallstones are the most important single cause of pancreatitis, furnishing the causative agent in about two-thirds
of the cases, the remaining third being due to infection
independent of stone formation originating in the stomach,
duodenum, or gall-bladder; the direct mechanical cause
being closure of the ampulla of Vater.

I will briefly relate a case which is typical of quite a number to serve as a concrete illustration. Mr. M., aged thirty-
eight years, married, several years ago had an attack of
pain in the gall-bladder region with very slight jaundice,
pain occasionally radiating under right shoulder, slight
fever, indigestion, etc.; these attacks would occur at infrequent intervals, but there was a gradual weakening and loss
of flesh, no sugar in the urine. Diagnosis: gall-stones or
pancreatitis (chronic), or both. At the operation a slightly

distended gall-bladder with no stones was found; the bladder was full of the characteristic ropy, tarry, black bile, and well-marked colon bacilli odor to it; the pancreatic head was markedly enlarged. Operation consisted in cholecystotomy after the common duct had been thoroughly explored and a probe passed into the duodenum to insure the patency of choledochus; drainage was continued for three months; during this time he not only gained twenty pounds in weight, but was completely restored to health. This is a sentence from a letter received three months after the wound had closed: "Dear Dr. I have just had another attack much worse than any before my operation; what shall I do?" On my advice he returned to the hospital at which time cholecystenterostomy was done, and with the result that he has been permanently relieved from all of his symptoms and is now in perfect health. I notice also that in my list of secondary cholecystenterostomies there are included cases previously operated on by other surgeons of undoubted standing.

The case above reported is simply one out of many; in fact, in my own work there has been such a proportion of cases of interstitial pancreatitis that have failed to remain permanently well after simple cholecystotomy, we feel it safer and more conservative, in the presence of jaundice a dilated and distended gall-bladder and common duct, to institute permanent drainage at the primary operation. I heard a very distinguished surgeon say, not very long ago, while operating on a case of this sort: "If the patient was markedly jaundiced he would do at once permanent drainage, but he stitched the gall-bladder to the fascia of the rectus in order that it could be more readily opened should recurrence take place." This seems to me to be begging the question, and emphasizes the point we are contending for—a more general use of cholecystenterostomy in certain cases of pancreatitis.

We think it most important to try and determine at the

primary operation which cases need permanent drainage and which do not, and not to wait for a recurrence of symptoms to point us to the error of our way, for it is our opinion that this malady is not only a more frequent one, but much more important than the general belief.

The following from Mayo Robson is very much to the point: A simple drainage of the gall-bladder by cholecystotomy is frequently unsatisfactory, and cannot be relied on in well-marked cases of obstruction, as drainage of the bile passages is not sufficiently long continued. This applies especially to the cases in which the interstitial pancreatitis has persisted for some length of time, in which cases, although a cholecystotomy may lead to a disappearance of the jaundice and the digestive symptoms may be alleviated, the metabolic signs found in the urine many months or even years subsequently show that recovery has only been partial."

To my mind it is most important to draw a distinction between chronic pancreatitis due to gallstones and chronic pancreatitis due to infection independent of and apart from the presence of stones; in the first case simple removal of the stones and temporary drainage of the gall-bladder gives permanent relief, because we remove the cause of the disease; in the other case, however, the trouble lies outside of and independent of stone formation, and these cases, within the bounds of our experience at least, are much more likely to require permanent drainage to effect a cure.

"I am impressed with the fact that chronic pancreatitis is not only a much more frequent malady than has been supposed, but a more important one. In looking back over considerable experience in surgery of the gall-bladder and bile tract, I find a number of cases that have failed to make a good recovery—failed because of pancreatic complications. It is certain that a much larger proportion of cases, especially those with a distended gall-bladder and dilated common duct, with or without stones, should be treated by a cholecystenterostomy than has been the practice among American surgeons" (Mayo).

We submit, then, our belief, based on our own individual work, that when operating on cases of chronic pancreatitis, especially that variety of the disease independent of stone formation, in the presence of even very slight jaundice and a dilated and distended gall-bladder and choledochus, with a definite enlargement of the pancreatic head, the application of the principle of permanent drainage not only had its foundation in a rational conception of the pathology of the diseased process, but is entitled to a very much more extended field of usefulness.

PANCREATIC HEMORRHAGE AND ACUTE PANCREATITIS.

WITH A REPORT OF THREE CASES.

By Joseph Ransohoff, *M.D.*, F.R.C.S. Eng.,
Cincinnati, Ohio.

At the thirty-second German Surgical Congress in 1903, Bunge was enabled to record only three successful operations for acute pancreatitis reported by Halsted, Hahn, and Koehler. A fourth case operated on by Henle in Mikulicz's clinic was not included. In Halsted's case only a laparotomy was done. Several years later the patient recovered from a similar attack without operation. Dr. Halsted tells me, in a personal communication, that he saw this patient last about four years ago, and that he was very anemic and weak, and had only a short time to live. Whereas, this shows that an acute hemorrhagic pancreatitis may be recovered from despite laparotomy. Ebner, in his statistics of two years ago, tabulated 20 unoperated cases, with 2 recoveries, and 36 operations, with 17 or 47.2 per cent. recoveries.

Early in 1908 Mayo Robson collected 59 operations, with 23 complete recoveries. He himself had 4 operations, with 2 successes. It is more than likely that a very considerable number of cases have been operated upon, which, because of unfavorable ending, have not been reported. Nor does Mayo Robson, in the valuable contribution referred to, enter upon details as to the nature of the individual cases operated upon. Operations for acute diseases of the pancreas have, after all, been so few in number that at the present writing it may still be worth while to report every case.

Until a year ago no case of this kind came into my surgical service in the Cincinnati Hospital, nor do the records of the institution, where 300 autopsies are made annually, show that, except in one case to be presently reported, death had resulted from acute pancreatic disease. This is particularly interesting in view of the fact that the three cases which I beg to submit all occurred in the West Surgical Service of the house, and were all entered during the month of March of this year. They all had one feature in common. It was that a diagnosis was not made until the operation was well advanced. In one of the cases, which I report through the kindness of Dr. Griess, a perforated ulcer of the stomach or a rupture of the gall-bladder was suspected. In one of my cases a high intestinal obstruction was supposed to account for the fulminating symptoms, and in the third the diagnosis of a perforating appendicitis had been made.

All of the cases were first received in the medical service, and after a varying number of hours referred for operation. If an explanation or apology seems in place for the inaccuracy of the diagnosis, it must be found in the hyperacuity of the onset and progress of the symptoms.

In the last publication of Robson he subdivides the cases of hemorrhagic pancreatitis into acute and the ultra-acute, With the latter all of the cases to be reported may, I think, be properly classified. The desperate strait of the patient precludes the possibility of obtaining an anamnesis, and the many time-consuming laboratory tests, which are indispensable in all less acute conditions, are manifestly out of place. They belong to that fortunately fast decreasing category of cases in which we recognize some great intra-abdominal disaster, the nature of which only an operation or autopsy may reveal. Since the latter possesses only a scientific and, therefore, relative advantage in the concrete case, unless it be moribund, the former has certain unqualified advantages.

Fourteen years ago Thayer believed himself fortunate in having been enabled to follow six cases to the autopsy table. It certainly could not have been less fortunate had they been seen on the operating table before exitus.

CASE I.—Peter F., aged sixty-seven years, hodcarrier. Was admitted to medical service on March 24, 1909. Has no recollection of sickness except an attack of influenza twenty years ago. States that he had a paralytic stroke five years ago, which involved the right side, but from which he recovered. Has had one previous attack of pain in the abdomen, but does not remember when it was. Has had a right inguinal hernia for many years, but had no trouble from it, though it is down most of the time. Uses alcohol moderately. States that on the morning of his admission, while at work, he was taken with excruciating pain in the upper part of the abdomen. States that his bowels have not moved for two days. Patient's temperature, 97; pulse, 108; respirations, 36.

Examination shows him to be a well-developed, fairly well-nourished man, with marked arteriosclerosis. Heart and lungs negative. Urinalysis negative. Complexion sallow, with almost a yellowish tinge. Sclera shows slight tinge. The abdomen is quite tense, slightly distended above the umbilicus, and painful to touch over its entirety, although more markedly so on the right side. There is an old inguinal hernia, which is reducible, but cannot be retained in place.

Treatment. Morphine, $\frac{1}{4}$ grain, hypodermically for pain. A high purgative enema was given without any effect. Calomel was ordered to be given in broken doses and to be followed by saline in the morning.

March 26. Patient vomited a great deal during the night. Much of the vomiting is regurgitant in character. It consists of bile-stained fluid. A second enema of glycerin and olive oil was administered, likewise without results. The patient's general condition rapidly becoming worse, he was referred to the surgical service.

The operation was performed at 4 P.M., twenty hours after his admission to the hospital. Incision above the umbilicus through the right rectus. When the peritoneum was opened, it was found full of free blood, much of which was in large clots. The incision was rapidly enlarged in order to re-move the free blood as quickly as possible and to determine its source. It soon became evident that the bleeding came from under the liver and through the foramen of Winslow. Here a large hematoma was found behind the stomach and evidently in relation with the head of the pancreas. The hematoma was as large as two fists. It was incised through the lesser omentum and clots removed as quickly as possible. While pressure was made upon the sac with one hand, two large tampons of gauze were pressed in from behind. Any-thing like a fat necrosis, if it had been present, would have been seen. The gall-bladder showed many adhesions, but because of the miserable condition of the patient it was not explored. The abdominal wound was closed with drainage. Intravenous stimulation with salt solution was given at 7.30 P.M. At 10.30 P.M. the dressings were changed because they were saturated with blood. Death occurred at 11.40 P.M., eight hours after operation.

Necropsy. (Dr. Hegner.) Hemorrhagic pancreatitis; cholecystitis; cholelithiasis; chronic parenchymatous nephritis; chronic gastritis; chronic catarrhal duodenitis-enteritis; colitis; fatty, cloudy liver; lobular pneumonia; dilatation of heart; arteriosclerosis.

Postmortem rigidity absent; staining slight. Chest emphysematous. Abdomen wound of recent laparotomy to right of right rectus muscle, from which drain protruded. On opening thorax, both pleura free, excepting the right posteriorly, where rather firm adhesions were noted. Right lung, 835, markedly edematous, and showed beginning lobular pneumonia. Left lung, 810, showed similar condition. Heart and pericardium free, 360; aorta at its origin was markedly dilated; same condition obtained throughout;

atheroma was not marked. Aortic ring dilated; valve showed pronounced sclerosis at bases, calcareous deposit being present. Mitral leaflets moderately thickened. Right heart markedly dilated. Myocardium pale, almost bloodless. On opening abdominal cavity, found peritoneal cavity filled with partially coagulated blood. Gauze aprons (2) were present and removed with the coagula. Omentum thickened and contracted and rolled on itself; firmly adherent in region of gall-bladder and spleen. It showed several old, firm scars. On lifting the liver, the gall-bladder showed very firm, extensive, pericystic adhesion to stomach; colon and omentum and head of pancreas tissues all very soft and edematous; turbid fluid noted here. Coagula were much more firm in this region; lesser peritoneal cavity opened and found filled with coagula. Bowels removed were soft and torn very easily. An opening admitting two fingers was found leading to the region of the head of pancreas.

Pancreas: Head firmly adherent to duodenum, gall-bladder under surface of liver was almost completely disorganized and replaced by coagula; the ducts were patulous. Exact point of origin of hemorrhage could not be definitely located, but was in the head of the pancreas. The remaining portion was very soft and edematous and quite small.

Liver: 1465, was small, very pale, friable, and markedly degenerated.

Gall-bladder walls thickened and showed marked pericystic adhesions to surrounding structures; contains turbid fluid similar to that noted above. One mulberry calculus, size of cherry stone, and numerous small yellow calculi. Ducts patulous.

Spleen: 75, small, markedly fibrous capsule, markedly thickened.

Kidneys: Each 185, bloodless; cortex irregular pyramids; fibrous capsule strips moderately; vessels sclerotic.

Bladder and prostate normal.

Stomach distended, mucosa markedly atrophic.

Duodenum showed extremely catarrhal changes; mucosa in relation with pancreas extremely congested throughout entire small and large intestine, most pronounced in duodenum was noted extremely tenacious and abundant pale mucus. In the colon this was very tough and adherent.

Pathological Histology (Dr. Whitacre). Hemorrhagic pancreatitis, chronic nephritis, cloudy and cirrhotic liver, interstitial myocarditis.

Pancreas: Considerable new connective tissue between glandular elements, more in some places than others; the epithelial cells in spots show much cloudy swelling; the bloodvessels are thickened. One part shows extensive hemorrhage, part of which shows much degeneration. The tissues in this region are so changed by hemorrhage as to obliterate evidence of structure.

Kidney shows considerable evidence of connective tissue in places, other places comparatively free; much cloudy swelling, tubules, vessel walls thickened, also Bowman's capsule in places more than others; some glomeruli are obliterated, others comparatively free from connective tissue. Liver shows cloudy swelling and small amount of cirrhosis.

Heart shows increase in interstitial connective tissue.

CASE II.—John D. W., aged thirty-six years, married, patrolman. In care of Dr. Griess. Admitted March 25, 1909. Patient very fleshy man, has been addicted to alcoholic excesses. Has frequently pain in the abdomen, but no attack like the one for which he seeks admission. Has occasionally vomited. The present attack began with excruciatingly severe pain in upper part of abdomen early in the morning. The pain was associated with vomiting. The vomitus was yellowish in color and bitter. On admission, patient was found to be a very large, well-developed male, with a good deal of excess of adipose tissue in the abdomen. The abdomen was distended, rigid, and painful to pressure above the umbilicus and to the right. There were frequent spells of vomiting, the fluid being bile-stained. Temperature on admission was 100°; pulse, 100; respirations, 28. A perforating ulcer of stomach or a ruptured gall-bladder being suspected, the patient was transferred to the West Surgical Service.

Operation performed at 6 A.M., under ether anesthesia. The incision was made to the right of the median line above the umbilicus. On opening the peritoneum a blood-tinged effusion with a considerable number of clots escaped. The effusion could be traced as coming from the foramen of Winslow. A number of areas of fat necrosis were found on the omentum. The gall-bladder and appendix were normal, nor was any trace of ulcer of the stomach found. The operation was completed with tubular and gauze drainage and the abdomen closed.

While the immediate result is noted as having been good, exitus occurred on the third day from peritonitis. A post-mortem was not made.

CASE III.—George S., aged twenty-four years, male. Was admitted on the evening of March 14, 1909, to the medical service. In the receiving ward he was supposed to have had an intestinal grippe. There was no history of any injury at the time; had there been, he would have been referred directly to the surgical service. The patient is a laborer in a dairy, and seems a little lacking in intelligence. Gives no history of an injury on admission, or while in the medical service. While his recovery was in process, and a week or more after the operation, he stated that he had fallen some days before from a hay mow and struck his side. It pained him a great deal, and he had difficulty in getting to the house. For three or four hours before admission the pain was associated with severe vomiting and hiccoughing.

Examination shows a well-developed and well-nourished man. The tongue is coated, breathing regular, with normal breath sounds. Heart sounds normal. The abdomen somewhat rigid and tender to pressure throughout. It seems, however, that the tenderness is most acute in the lower right quadrant. Liver dulness pushed up. Temperature, 99°; pulse, 88; respirations, 26. The pulse is a very good tension and regular. The urine slightly cloudy, acid, 1028, contains albumin, granular and epithelial casts. Extremities negative.

Treatment. Ice cap to abdomen, enema, morphia sulph., ¼ grain, hypodermically for pain.

March 15. Temperature, 99°; pulse, 100 and a little weak. The abdomen is more rigid and tenderness more marked, especially over the right side low down. The patient continues to vomit frequently a greenish fluid.

A probable diagnosis of appendicitis was made and the case referred to the West Surgical Service.

Operation, March 15, 1909. Right pararectal incision three inches in length. When the peritoneum was exposed free blood in large quantities could be seen through it. When the peritoneum was opened a large quantity of dark free blood with a considerable number of large clots flowed from the wound. The escape of blood was so profuse that it looked as though an aneurysm might have ruptured. The head of the bed was immediately lowered and an intravenous salt solution given. The appendix was found normal. The abdominal incision was rapidly lengthened upward and downward, and the bleeding was found to come from beneath the liver. It was packed with gauze temporarily, so that the lower part of the abdominal cavity could be cleansed. It was found intact. There was no trace of any fat necrosis. The gall-bladder seemed normal. Through the lesser omentum and behind the stomach a bogginess was felt, but not interfered with. Attention was then given to the site of the hemorrhage, and the guaze packs, temporarily placed there, were removed. The bleeding was found to come from the foramen of Winslow, and was venous in character.

So far as possible, the under surface of the liver was explored and the pancreas, but no injury of either was found. There was a bogginess easily perceptible behind the stomach and the gastrohepatic omentum.　　Large wide gauze packing was inserted into the foramen, and drainage through the anterior incision provided for.　The great omentum was fixed against the parietal layer, to shut off, so far as possible, the lower part of the general peritoneal cavity.　Except for the drainage, the wound was rapidly closed with interrupted sutures.　The pulse had become very weak and the respirations 30.

March 16.　Patient's temperature was 100.2°; pulse, 142, quite weak.　Still vomiting greenish fluid from time to time. The dressings were saturated, and were therefore reinforced. The Cammidge reaction, repeatedly made, was negative.

March 17.　Vomiting has stopped and the bleeding is evidently at a standstill.　Maximum temperature, 99.5°; pulse, 130.　The last of the packing was removed on March 25.

April 20, 1909, the patient was discharged, with the wound perfectly healed and well in every way.

In considering the cases reported, no question can enter as to the existence of a pancreatitis in the first and second. The third may be open to the view that an injury of the pancreas had existed.　As has already been stated, no history of an injury was given by the patient at the time of admission, for he was referred to the medical service.

When he was well on the road to recovery, he spoke of a fall from a hay loft.　The operation revealed no tear of the pancreas or of the liver, although the former may have existed.　If so, the operation was a life-saving one.

According to Mikulicz, of 13 unoperated cases of sub-parietal rupture of the pancreas, all died; whereas, of 11 operated cases, 7 recovered.　Considering that this case also was one of pancreatic disease, 2 of the 3 cases may justly be called of the ultra-acute type, with the hemorrhage a predominant phenomenon.　Although in these cases the intraperitoneal bleeding was more profuse than one generally sees it in ordinary gunshot injuries, the pulse as one feature of the condition of the patients at the time of the operation was no index of the great gravity of the cases. In the first the pulse was 108 and regular; in the second one, 100; and in the third one, 88. The tension in all of the cases was good. It is difficult to understand this seeming discrepancy between the pulse rate and tension on the one hand and on the other hand the severity of symptoms, which so clearly portray a grave intra-abdominal lesion. The same slow pulse is, as a rule, encountered during the early stages of an acute intestinal obstruction. The great violence of the pain and the persistent vomiting and evidence of shock, other than those of cardiac nature, are common to both conditions.

It has been a question whether the hemorrhage precedes or follows the disorganization of the pancreas, which leads to localized fat necrosis. Two of the above cases appear to establish the fact that in the ultra-acute cases, hemorrhage precedes the fat necrosis, and that even in autopsies, if death follows quickly, fat necrosis may not be found. These are cases of pancreatic apoplexy. They are probably in the beginning, at least, not of an infectious nature. Hlava found both the intraperitoneal effusion and the exudate within the pancreas sterile. If life be continued long enough, infection can easily occur through the channel of the ducts or from the adjacent hollow viscera. If life be prolonged, the disorganization of the gland, consequent on the hemorrhage, sets free its secretion, which in turn causes fat necrosis. The literature of these cases seems to bear this out, since as in cerebral apoplexy most cases of acute hemorrhage from the pancreas have been found in obese individuals and mostly males, in whom the habits or an old syphilis predisposed to arterial lesions and to thrombotic processes in the vessels. Mikulicz very ingeniously believed in a vicious circle, the first factor of which is a lesion of possibly a small vessel. Disorganization of that part of the pancreas takes place and is followed by a localized necrosis of the gland, with the setting free of some of the secretion. Autodigestion ensuing, a larger vessel would be involved and a profuse hemorrhage is the end result.

The relationship which is supposed to exist between gall-stone disease and acute pancreatitis was confirmed in one of the three cases, and might have been suspected from the subicteric tinge of the skin. In this case a possible rupture of the gall-bladder was thought of, but in the absence of a localized jaundice of the umbilicus, which the writer has seen in two cases, was held to be improbable. Free bile in the peritoneal cavity from any cause is likely to show itself first by a tinge of yellow at and about the navel. Severe vomiting of a bile-tinged fluid was present in everyone of the cases and I might state occurs in a preponderance of the cases reported. This is interesting in view of the fact that a mechanical obstruction near the outlet of the common duct or within the diverticulum of Vater is commonly held to be the immediate etiological factor of acute pancreatitis. If this is true, how can the vomiting of bile be explained? The discrepancy can only be explained on the theory that the disease of the pancreas is either an infection or the result of some form of chemical autodigestion due to a primary vascular lesion with hemorrhage.

Whereas, in the ultra-acute cases such as I have described the diagnosis before operation may always remain con-jectural, in the less acute ones, where hemorrhage is less profuse and a localization of the exudates takes place, it is certain that the recognition of acute pancreatitis will be-come more and more simplified. With the development of an abscess, the well-known physical characteristics of pancreatic enlargements, as typified by cysts, are developed, and, as in the latter, the diagnosis must become relatively easy. That where time will permit a most careful examination of the urine and feces should be made goes without further comment.

The writer would here like to protest against the glib manner in which the diagnosis of chronic pancreatitis is sometimes made in the course of an operation for gallstone disease, in which the findings are negative. To make this diagnosis as it so often is made, by the sense of touch alone, appears to me unscientific in the extreme and unwarranted. For example, according to Robson, 113 operations have been performed for chronic pancreatitis, with 8 deaths. It would be interesting to determine, if it were possible, in how many of those that recovered the diagnosis was based on the clinical evidences which we know belong to chronic pancreatic disease, and in what number the diagnosis was made by the sense of touch alone. To anyone made familiar in the mortuary or the operating room with the great variation which normally exists in the density and hardness of the gland, the uncertainty of making a diagnosis during an operation by touch and sight must be at once apparent. Professor Paul Wooley, pathologist of the University of Cincinnati, bears me out in this, with the statement that in all the autopsies he has made he has been enabled in only two instances to make the diagnosis of chronic pancreatitis from the gross findings, cancer excluded.

In regard to the treatment, much has been written regarding the inadvisability of operating the first day or hours of a fulminating hemorrhagic pancreatitis, under the belief that an operation will hasten death. Unfortunately, as Deaver says, a cursory examination of recorded cases will show that in 90 per cent. the correct diagnosis had not been made, before at operation. A year ago Noetzel reported a case, which was not recognized at the first operation, and the second made the condition clear. It is evident that until some more definite early symptoms shall in the future be recognized as belonging to ultra-acute pancreatitis, the discovery of its existence during an operation must yet come to many of us as a disagreeable surprise.

As has already been indicated, shock, as evidenced by the pulse rate and tension, is at times not great enough to make an operation appear extra hazardous. Since the condition is often mistaken for rupture of the biliary ways, of perforating ulcer, and for high intestinal obstruction, conditions in which we recognize immediate operation as imperative, cases of disease under condition will continue to be operated upon as soon as possible.   There can be no question but that, since abscess and gangrenous cases operated upon have shown a more favorable postoperative percentage of recovery, the waiting method would seem a preferable one, where the symptoms are not urgent enough to demand immediate interference.   The history of these cases for the most part excludes them from the ultra-acute type.

When an abscess has formed, it is a relatively simple matter to drain it through the abdominal incision or through an incision in the loin.   Surely, the abdominal incision will continue to be sufficient in most cases.   The drainage of cysts of the pancreas, with which surgeons have long been familiar, has made this certain.   The danger of general peritoneal infection, if it has not already existed at the time of the operation, may be minimized by properly placing gauze tampons and utilizing the omentum before partly closing the incision.

The expediency of operating on the pancreas itself must be considered in each case.   According to Mikulicz, of 41 cases in which the pancreas was not touched, 4 cases recovered. Of 37 cases in which the pancreas was involved in the operative interference, 25 recovered.   Mikulicz himself limits the value of these statistics, and I should not call attention to them at all were it not for a remarkable critique of Eberth, which appeared two years ago, in which he states that the fatalities after operation may largely be ascribed to the incompleteness of the operation in that the pancreas itself was not attacked.   This view, widely circulated in Volkmann's *Klinische Vorträge*, should, I think, be challenged.

While the writer's experience is limited, he believes that the condition of the patient as the operation progresses must guide the operator as to the extent of the operation.   If the grave condition of the patient from hemorrhage limits operative interference, drainage through the foramen of Winslow or through an opening made into the omental bursa, with sequestration of the disease by gauze packing, all of which can be quickly done, will assuredly save many a patient to whom further interference might be disastrous. When a phlegmon of the pancreas is clearly made out, the general surgical principles guiding us in like conditions elsewhere must guide us here as well.

PANCREATO-ENTEROSTOMY AND PANCRE-ATECTOMY.

A PRELIMINARY REPORT.

By Robert C. Coffey, M.D.,
Portland, Oregon.

Food is prepared for appropriation almost exclusively by derivatives of the primitive foregut (the stomach, liver, and pancreas). The upper portion of the primitive foregut lies between the layers of the partition of the primitive body cavity which extends anteroposteriorly. That portion of the partition in front of the foregut is called anterior mesogastrium, while that lying behind the primitive foregut is called posterior mesogastrium. Early in fetal life a bud projects off from the primitive tract between the layers of the anterior mesogastrium and forms the liver and bile tracts. Another bud, which is supplemented by a secondary one, projects from the primitive alimentary tract backward between the layers of the posterior mesogastrium, and after blending form the pancreas and pancreatic ducts, the chief of which empties into the alimentary canal through a common opening with the liver duct. The stomach, representing the upper expanded portion of the primitive foregut, always remains between these two layers of membrane which becomes peritoneum, therefore is surrounded on all sides by a peritoneal coat. The liver with gall-bladder develops between the layers of the anterior mesogastrium, and therefore is always covered with peritoneum. During the process of intestinal rotation which occurs in fetal development, the pancreas and second and third portions of the duodenum are thrown out of the peritoneal cavity.

As surgery becomes a more definite science we are learning that the peritoneum is an essential in almost all abdominal surgery, and in addition to forming a smooth covering and strong support it has another function equally important, namely, that it throws out exudate when injured, which serves a purpose similar to the callus thrown out in the repair of broken bone. This exudate penetrates the adjacent tissues for some distance around. In the course of a few days the exudate or "callus" becomes organized. The bulk of the exudate is soon absorbed, leaving the firmer elements, so that the repair is soon complete and the broken surface covered by a new and smooth peritoneum.

The gall-bladder, which is a part of the hepatic structure ordinarily used for surgical purposes because of its convenience and peritoneal covering, and the stomach have been conquered by the surgeon and brought into the actual and legitimate domain of surgery, while the pancreas remains technically almost a stranger to the surgeon. Many reasons have been given for this, but to the mind of the writer the one most plausible is based on the premise that the fundamental defect in the pancreas, as far as surgical work is concerned, is that it is devoid of peritoneum, and it was with this principle in view that experiments were begun some months ago.

The fat-splitting ferment of the pancreatic juice has been the terror of surgeons up to date, but in a close study of results which have been obtained by experimenters we fail to find any positive evidence that even pancreatic juice will penetrate peritoneum to a serious extent. The fat-splitting ferment seems to travel in the planes of the areolar connective tissues, outside the peritoneum; therefore it proves serious because of the anatomical position of the pancreas, but not so serious as the contents of the intestinal canal would be by escaping in the same neighborhood. So it seems that the principal danger of pancreatic juice in surgery is not that it is so virulent itself, but because it escapes into the retroperitoneal fat. Consequently, the principal problem was to provide unbroken peritoneum with which to surround the part of the pancreas participating in the formation of the operative field. Two methods were considered as being applicable to the situation. First, implantation of the cut end of the remaining pancreas into the intestine, using the peritoneum of the intestinal wall to make the union. Second, a direct implantation of the duct into the intestinal wall and fastening a collar of omentum around the duct and pancreas at the point of intended union. The first method seemed much the better, and was used exclusively in the first series of operations reported below. The first attempt was to implant the cut end of the pancreas into the side of the intestine, which proved to be impractical. The next thought was to invert a cut end of the intestine and implant it there. This was done in two instances, but the postmortem showed that the end was too small, as it constricted the end of the pancreas, causing its death. (There might, however, be conditions in which this would be a suitable method, in which cases it would be ideal). After considering the anatomy of the intestine it was thought feasible to throw the lumen of two intestines into one by using a loop and thus give ample room for implanting the pancreas. The perfected technique resulting from the experience of the two series of operations reported below, and which is recommended for use, is illustrated by Figs. 1 to 12, and may be described as follows:

First, pick up a loop of intestine, preferably jejunum, using care that the mesentery at the point is long enough to reach the pancreas with ease. Clamp both arms of the loop with a rubber-covered stomach clamp, leaving the loop three or four inches long. Suture the intestines together with continuous Lembert suture near the mesenteric edge to a point near the clamp. Grasp the thread with a forceps at this point and hold till all other steps of the operation are complete (Fig. 1, *C*. 1).

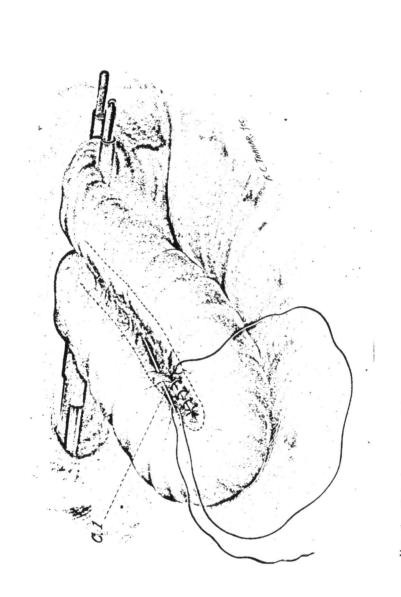

Fig. 1.—Suturing arms of intestinal loop together with primary continuous Lembert suture, C. 1 (dotted line indicates where incision is to be made).

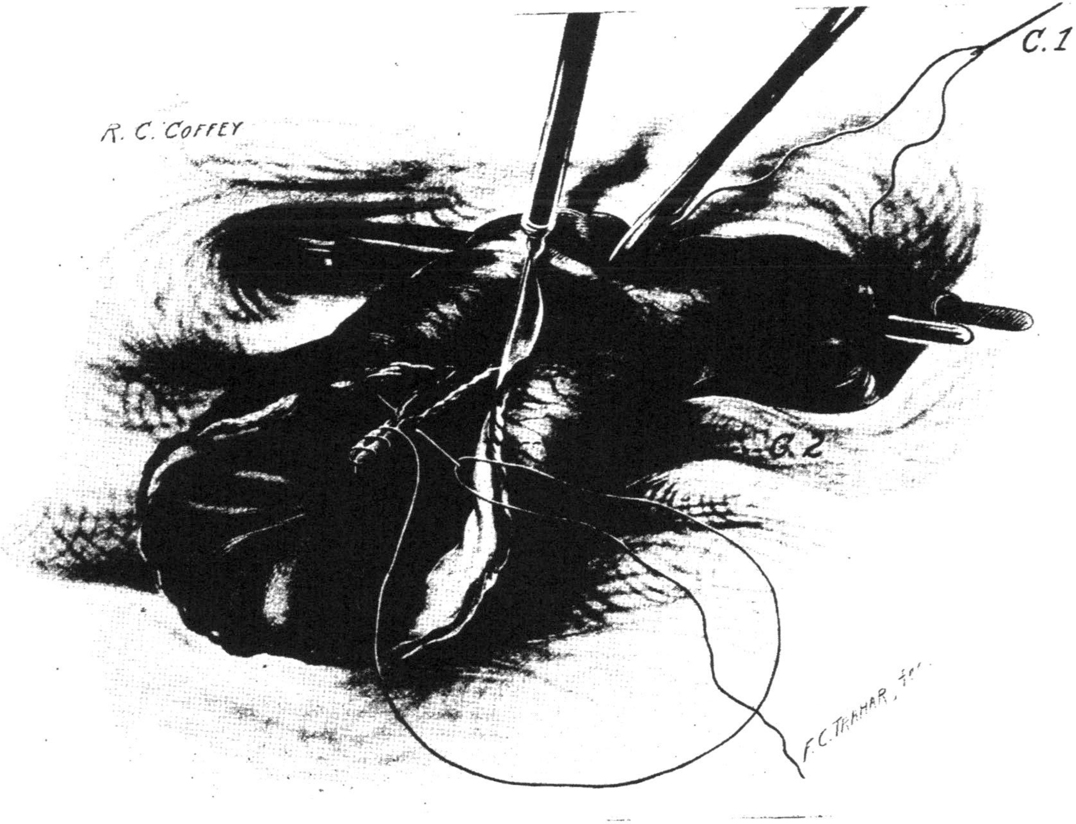

Fig. 2.—Opening intestinal loop and beginning the through-and-through suture, C. 2.

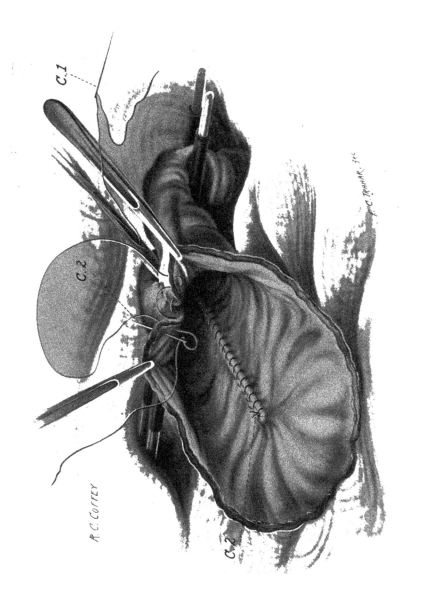

C.1

C.2

C.2

R.C. COFFEY

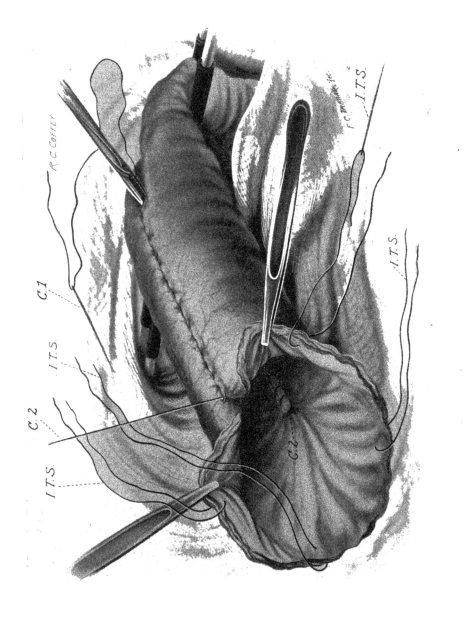

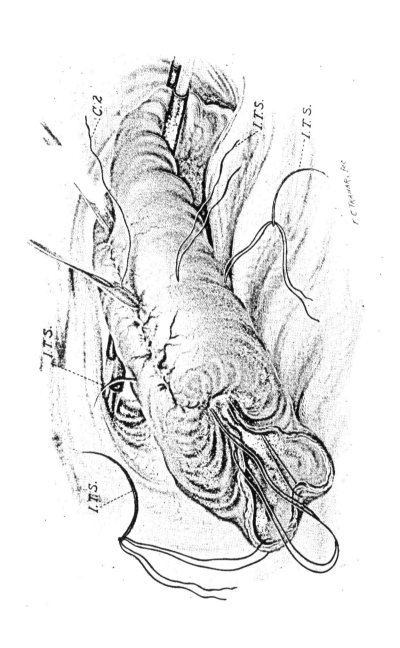

Fig. 5.—Passing intestinal traction sutures (*I.T.S.*) into the lumen and out through the wall of the intestine. *C.* 1, primary continuous Lembert suture. *C.* 2, through-and-through suture used for traction.

R.C.COFFEY

F.C. TRAHAR. fec.

BLOOD VESSELS LIGATED

C.1

I.T.S.

I.T.S.

F.C. TRAHAR. fec.

P.P.S.

P.P.S.

P.S.

P.S.

R.C. COFFEY

P.T.S.

D

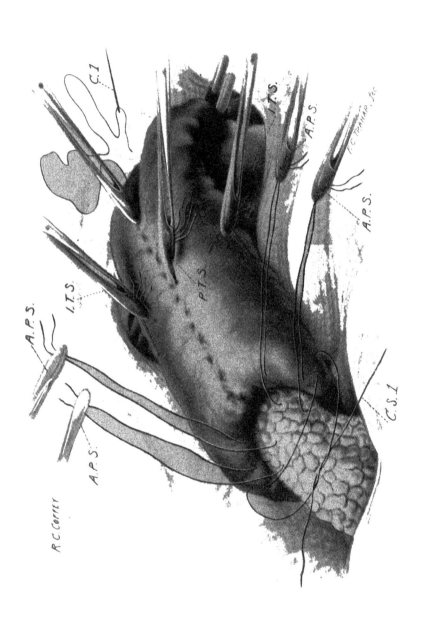

C.1

I.T.S.

A.P.S.

F.C. TRAHAR. fec.

A.P.S.

P.T.S.

I.T.S.

A.P.S.

C.S.1

A.P.S.

R.C. COFFEY

Second, with knife or scissors open the intestine around the loop (Fig. 2) (indicated by dotted line in Fig. 1), one-fourth inch from line of suture, thus cutting the two intestines into one.

Third, with through-and-through continuous suture beginning inside (Fig. 2, *C.* 2) and continuing around (Fig. 3, *C.* 2) close the loop, leaving but a single lumen. Stop when the end resembles the cut end of a single intestine, and tie knot, leaving the suture long (Fig. 4), to be used later as a traction or inversion suture (Fig. 5).

Fourth, pass four or more traction or inversion loops through the edge of the intestine (Fig. 4).

Fifth, thread the two ends of each traction suture, also the single end of *C.* 2, through large-eyed needles, and pass them into the lumen and out through the wall of the intestine one and one-half to two inches back of the cut edge (Fig. 5). By pulling on these sutures the intestine is perfectly inverted when the traction sutures are caught by forceps to maintain inversion, and thus keep a clean field (Fig. 7), while the operation progresses.

Sixth, with the back of a scalpel strip the pancreatic tissue from the duct and vessels, ligate the vessels, split the duct and cut it so as to leave one-quarter to one-half an inch protruding beyond the pancreatic tissue (Figs. 6 and 7).

Seventh, complete the required operation on the pancreas and pass a quilt suture (using a needle on each end of the thread preferably) from each side of the pancreas at a point near the end to be implanted. These sutures are to be used as traction sutures in pulling the pancreas into the lumen of the inverted gut (Fig. 7). Owing to the friability and the seriousness of tearing it during the operation it is necessary to avoid traction on the sutures which are to fasten the pancreas to the peritoneum of the intestine. Therefore it is well to pass four or more sutures, which include a bite of the pancreas and a corresponding bite of the intestine, grasping both ends of each suture with forceps as it is placed, to avoid entanglement (Fig. 7). These sutures are designated posterior pancreatic sutures (*P.P.S.*). Now thread all the pancreatic traction sutures into a large-eyed needle and pass the needle into the lumen well above the inverted edge and out through the intestinal wall near the line of sutures so the final continuous Lembert suture (*C.* 1) will cover the hole. By traction on these sutures draw the end of the pancreas into the lumen until the corresponding points of the pancreas and intestine which are caught by the posterior pancreatic suture are in contact, when the sutures are gently, but firmly tied and cut.

Eighth, pass four or more anterior pancreatic sutures including a bite of pancreas and intestine (Fig. 8, *A. P. S.*) in such a manner that the sutures will form a circular row continuing the posterior pancreatic sutures. Grasp the two ends of each suture with a forceps as soon as it is passed.

Ninth, pick up the intestine on each side of the pancreas with a suture at such a distance as will permit it to be drawn loosely around the pancreas in the form of a collar. Make counter traction on the pancreatic traction sutures (*P.T.S.*) while the collar suture (Fig. 8, *C.S.* 1) is being drawn below the pancreatic sutures. The anterior pancreatic sutures (*A.P.S.*) should now be tied within the collar suture before the collar suture *C.S.* 1, Fig. 8, is completely tied. A second collar suture (Fig. 8, *C.S.* 2) is placed below this one of points which will draw the intestine snugly enough to prevent leakage, but not tight enough to constrict the circulation or duct. This point, of course, must be left to the personal equation of the operator. After these sutures are tied, two or three more sutures are used to close this space. While these remaining sutures are being placed an assistant makes traction on the collar suture with one hand, and on the pancreatic sutures with the other, to avoid tension on the pancreatic sutures till the operation is completed (Fig. 9). Thus, both the anterior and posterior pancreatic sutures are included within the peritoneal collar which has been placed around the pancreas. All traction sutures are now cut short and allowed to drop back into the intestine.

Tenth, continue the primary Lembert suture (*C.* 1), which has been held in the forceps during the operation, around to the pancreas, covering all previous sutures (Fig. 10).

Eleventh, as an additional safeguard (which is possibly an unnecessary refinement), we have wrapped omentum around the point of union and stitched it there.

FIRST SERIES OF EXPERIMENTS.

Our work has all been done on dogs—the dog's bile tracts are practically the same as in man. The pancreas, instead of being a long straight organ, is arranged in the shape of a horseshoe, from which a tail extends back of the stomach to the hilus of the spleen, thus corresponding to the human pancreas. For want of a better name, we have designated this the retrogastric tail. The other tail follows the concavity of the duodenum, lying loosely between the peritoneal folds of the mesentery. In operating on this tail it is necessary to strip off these layers of peritoneum from the pancreas in order to make it conform to the human pancreas, which is largely extraperitoneal. The ducts of the two tails meet at the toe of the horsehoe to form the duct of Wirsung, which is from one-fourth to three-fourths inch in length and empties into the duodenum one to two inches below the opening of the bile duct. The duct of Santorini usually has a common opening with the bile duct. This duct has been present in all of our dogs, and seems to drain an area of the pancreas more or less independent of the greater pancreatic duct, but one or more of its branches connect it directly with the greater duct. The connection seems to be much the same as a canal used to connect the branches of two rivers which flow in opposite directions from the top of a watershed. If a nozzle attached to a fountain syringe filled with methylene blue solution is tied in the

duct of Wirsung and the fluid allowed to run, the pancreas
rapidly becomes stained throughout, but is a more faint blue
toward the surface.   If the pressure is considerable, the fluid
after a time finds its way through the duct of Santorini (Fig.
13, *A*).   If the ends of the tail are cut off, the fluid flows out
without apparent resistance and does not pass through the
duct of Santorini (Fig. 13, *B*).   If the duct of Wirsung is
ligated, and if the pancreatic tissue is scraped off from the
duct of one tail, and if the tip of the other tail is cut off, fluid
introduced into the bared duct of the one tail easily (Fig. 13,
B) passes around and out at the end of the other tail, and
sometimes, in this experiment, the fluid flows through the
duct of Santorini simultaneously with the flow through the
cut tail, while at other times it does not, but in all cases will
begin to flow through the duct of Santorini if the open end
of the cut duct is held with forceps.   These experiments hold
good in both living and dead animals.

   If the tail is implanted into a loop of intestine by the method
we have just described, and if both arms of the loop are
clamped below, so as to shut the loop off from the intestinal canal, fluid introduced into the duct of Wirsung flows
through the duct of the implanted end and extends the loop,
without leaking at the point of anastomosis (Fig. 14, *B*).

   Thus, by the foregoing study, we demonstrate the anatomical possibility of the following procedures: First, the
surgeon can in cases of either malignant or non-malignant
obstruction at the outlet of the pancreatic duct or in the duodenum, remove the head of the pancreas and implant the cut
end of the remaining portion into a loop of intestine—which
operation would exactly correspond to the removal of the
lower end of the bile duct for similar obstructions, with implantation of the remaining cut end into the intestine at
another point; and would also correspond to the removal
of the pylorus with anastomosis of the remainder of the
stomach with the intestine lower down for similar obstruction.
Secondly, in obstructions from whatever cause at the mouth

of the pancreatic duct or in the duodenum which are not to be removed, the pancreas can be drained by implanting the cut end of the tail into a loop of intestine below, which would cause the pancreatic fluid to flow backward in the ducts. This operation would be exactly parallel to cholecystenterostomy for low obstruction in the common bile duct and to gastro-enterostomy for obstruction at or near the pylorus. (Dr. W. J. Mayo in a personal communication has suggested this application of pancreato-enterostomy for clinical use.)

The next question to be solved is: Will these problems work out clinically as well as they do mechanically and anatomically?

From May 15 to July 28, 1909, forty operations were done on dogs with the view to answering this question. Twenty-four of these operations had for their essential feature pancreato-enterostomy, as described above. Three varieties of operations were performed. First, the duodenal tail of the pancreas was stripped of its peritoneum and cut in two and each cut end was implanted into a separate loop of the jejunum (Fig. 15 and 16). Second, the tail was cut off and implantation was made as in class one, but in addition the duct of Wirsung was ligated close to the intestine. Third, pancreatectomy was done in two stages, as follows:

First operation: The common bile duct was transplanted to the duodenum lower down, gastrojejunostomy was performed and the stomach was cut off and ends turned in just above pylorus (Fig. 17).

Second operation, or second stage of operation: The body and duodenal tail of the pancreas and the duodenum were removed and the retrogastric tail of pancreas was planted into a loop of jejunum (Fig. 18).

There were four operative recoveries from which specimens were removed, belonging to the first class of operations. Of these 1 was removed the tenth day, 1 the eighteenth day, 1 the thirtieth day, and 1 the forty-ninth day after operation (postmortem findings of the forty-ninth day dog reported in next class). The specimen from tenth-day dog showed good union, no leakage at anastomosis, no pancreatitis, and no necrosis. The ends protruding into the intestine were still raw and covered with some fibers sloughing away. The mouth of the duct could not be identified at this stage.

The specimen from the eighteenth-day dog showed similar conditions, except that the raw area was smaller and in the end of the isolated tail the slough had disappeared and the duct could be identified.

The thirtieth-day dog, at the time of killing, had entirely recovered, had a splendid appetite and was rapidly gaining in flesh. On opening the abdomen, no adhesions were found except where the omentum had been tacked to the peritoneum of the intestine. At other points the omentum glided easily over the pancreas, indicating that there had been no leakage. The line of union between the pancreas and intestine was as perfect as if it had been between two intestines (Fig. 12). The same condition existed at the point of each implantation. There was no evidence of pancreatitis or degeneration in either the body or in the isolated tail. On opening each loop, as shown in Fig. 12, we were able to locate the duct after carefully wiping away mucus. All of our later tests by methylene-blue solution indicate that this duct leading to the body of the pancreas was probably closed by thin film (Fig. 16), which was wiped off by gauze.

In the second class of operations there were three operative recoveries from which specimens were removed. Of these, one dog died on the twentieth day from intestinal obstruction. One was killed with chloroform on the twentieth day, and one was killed with chloroform on the thirty-fifth day. Both twenty-day specimens showed perfect union between the intestine and pancreas, no adhesions in the neighborhood of the implantation, no pancreatitis or evidence of fat necrosis. In both instances the pancreatic tissue of the retrogastric tail was stripped from the duct and methylene blue solution injected, when it was found that the implanted cut end had closed, and fluid all came out through the papilla of the old duct of Wirsung unobstructedly (Fig. 16). After grasping the papilla of the duct of Wirsung in a pair of forceps, the fluid flowed freely through the duct of Santorini, and we thought it flowed more freely than in the normal dog. When a filiform bougie was inserted into the opening of the duct of Wirsung and passed down the duct of the tail which had been planted, it went easily to where it could be felt and even seen through a translucent covering which had formed over the cut end of the duct (Fig. 16). On laying open the duct it was found that the ligature which had constricted it had been circumvented and the continuity of the duct reëstablished. The blue solution which had been injected had passed down into the implanted duct through the intestinal collar, but had been held by the film which had formed over its end.

The thirty-fifth-day dog is the same dog reported in the first class as a forty-ninth-day dog, the duct having been ligated fourteen days after double pancreato-enterostomy was done. We may here state that in order to make sure of the ligation, in our early cases a probe was introduced from the inside of the duodenum while the ligature was being placed. The same conditions were found that have just been described in the twentieth-day dogs, namely, a perfectly healthy pancreas, perfect union between pancreas and intestine, closure of the duct of the implanted end of pancreas, circumvention of the ligature which had been placed around the duct of Wirsung, and duct wide open, carrying all of the injected blue solution. When the papilla was grasped, the solution immediately flowed through the duct of Santorini. The implanted isolated tail was in this case perfectly healthy, union perfect, and on stripping the pancreatic tissue from its duct and injecting the blue solution into the duct, it was found to pass freely into the intestinal loop. A noticeable feature was that one of the line sutures was hanging in the opening in this case.

In the third class of operations, there were two operative recoveries from which specimens were removed—one eight days and the other thirty-four days after the second step of the operation. The eight-day specimen showed no leakage, no pancreatitis, and no necrosis. Implanted end was still in the raw sloughing state. The thirty-fourth-day dog had the first operation fifteen days before or forty-nine days prior to the time the specimen was removed. The first operation consisted of the transposition of the common bile duct, gastro-enterostomy, and cutting off the stomach as shown in Fig. 17. The thirty-fourth-day specimen showed perfect union, no surrounding adhesions, no pancreatic necrosis, no fat necrosis, but showed evidence of a previous pancreatitis in the form of an induration along the duct which was dilated but not filled with fluid. On stripping the duct and injecting it, the blue solution passed into the loop of intestine by following a thread which had apparently caught the duct at the time of operation and had led the pancreatic fluid through the wall of the intestine by a seton-like action (Fig. 19). The result resembled a hole in the lobe of the ear made for earrings, in that the lining of the duct seemed to be continuous with the mucus side of the intestine. The dog had entirely recovered, had a splendid appetite and was apparently in perfect health. Pancreatitis had subsided and everything in the history of the case pointed to the fact that the duct had been caught in a suture and held until the end had time to heal over, and that during this time the pancreatitis had developed and had subsided as soon as the pancreatic juice began to follow the thread. The common bile duct which had been transplanted at the first operation was as large as a man's finger, while the mouth would admit a lead pencil. The hepatic ducts were distended in the same way well into the liver, but the dog was well and hearty. Five other dogs with the same operation showed the same condition of bile ducts.

From these experiments, it has been learned positively that the cut end of the pancreas may be implanted into a loop of

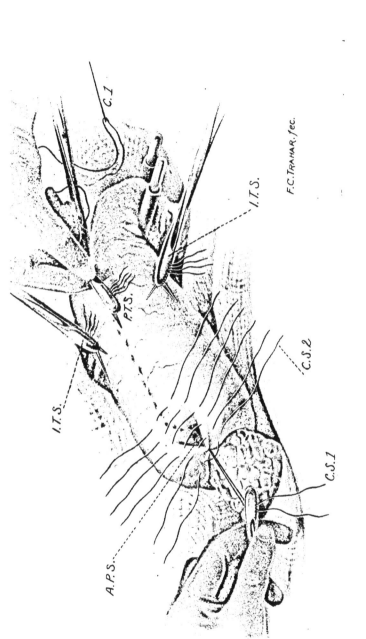

C.1

I.T.S.

P.T.S.

I.T.S.

C.S.2

C.S.1

A.P.S.

F.C.TRAHAR. fec.

FIG. 9.—Completing the collar of intestine around the pancreas, the anterior pancreatic sutures having been tied, A.P.S. Hands indicate traction and counter traction on the collar suture 1, and pancreatic traction sutures while other sutures are being placed. I.T.S., intestinal traction sutures. P.T.S., pancreatic traction sutures. C.S. 1, collar suture 2. C. 1, continuous primary Lembert suture.

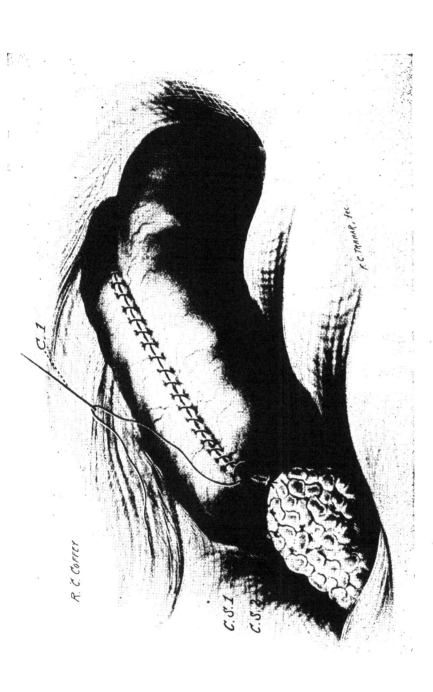

Fig. 10.—Completing operation with the primary continuous Lembert suture.

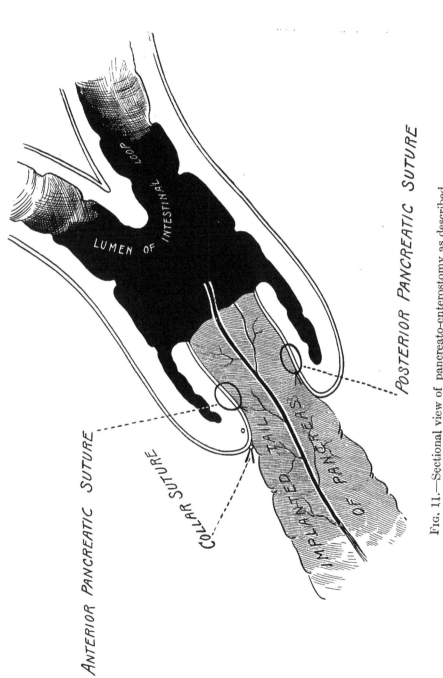

Fig. 11.—Sectional view of pancreato-enterostomy as described.

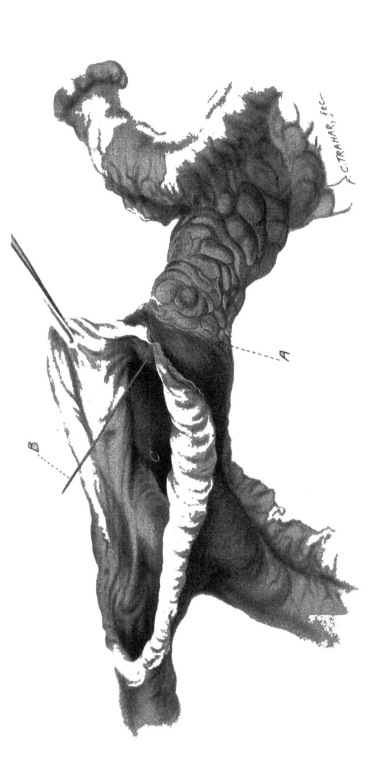

Fig. 12.—Drawing from fresh specimen removed from dog five weeks after operation, showing result of pancreato-enterostomy. A, line of union between pancreas and intestine. B, probe in open end of pancreatic duct. C, intestinal lumen through the loop.

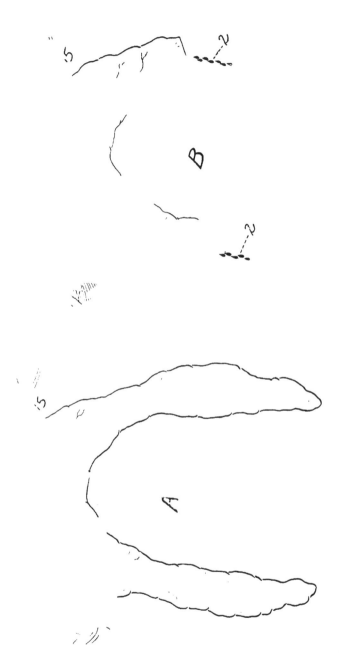

FIG. 13.—Anatomical diagram illustrating relations of ducts in a dog's pancreas. *A* 1 and *B* 1, nozzle carrying methylene blue solution into the duct of Wirsung and filling pancreatic duct. *A* 2, drops of fluid forced out through the duct of Santorini under pressure. *B* 2, drops of fluid dripping from ducts of both pancreatic tails. *B* 4, duct of Santorini. *A* 5 and *B* 5, bile duct.

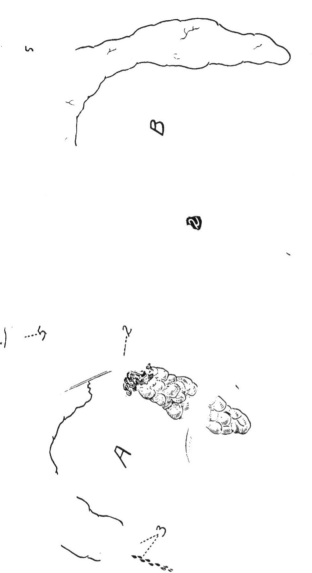

FIG. 14.—Diagram illustrating the surgical anatomy of a dog's pancreatic ducts. *A* 1, duct of Wirsung, ligated. *A* 2, nozzle carrying methylene blue solution inserted into duct of retrogastric tail of pancreas. *A* 3, fluid dropping out of ducts of cut end of duodenal tail. *A* 4, fluid in duct of Santorini not delivered into intestine until duct of duodenal tail is clamped. *B* 1, nozzle carrying methylene blue solution into the duct of Wirsung. *B* 2, intestinal loop distended with methylene blue solution after pancreato-enterostomy. *B* 3, drops of fluid forced out through the duct of Santorini under pressure from distended intestinal loop. *A* 5, and *B* 5, bile duct.

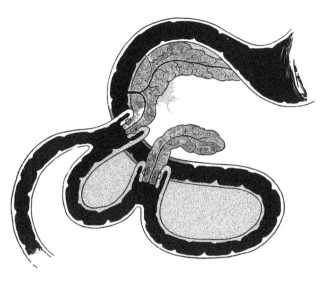

FIG. 15.—Diagram showing double implantation of cut ends of severed tail of pancreas.

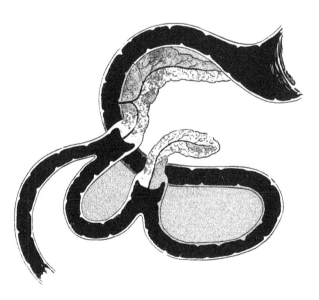

FIG. 16.—Result following double implantation of severed tail of pancreas, showing how isolated tail maintains the opening of its duct while the duct in the other loop heals over. (Diagrammatic.)

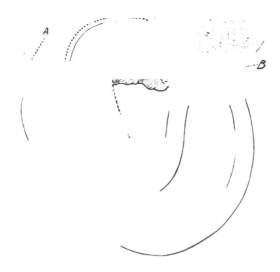

FIG. 17.—First step in two-stage operation for removing the head of the pancreas, as was done in the first series of experiments. *A*, bile duct transplanted to intestine below the pancreas. *B*, posterior gastro-jejunostomy. *C*, stomach cut in two and ends turned in. Dotted line encloses part to be removed at next operation.

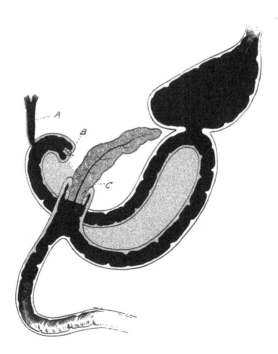

FIG. 18.—Second step in two-stage operation for removing head of the pancreas. *A*, widely distended bile duct which was transplanted at previous operation. *B*, remaining stump of duodenum after removal of duodenum and head of the pancreas. *C*, remaining tail of the pancreas implanted into intestinal loop. (Diagrammatic.)

intestine with practically the same assurance of primary union as could be expected from a gastro-enterostomy. Secondly, the dangers of fat necrosis and pancreatic necrosis in pancreato-enterostomy are apparently no greater than the dangers of sepsis in gastro-enterostomy, except in that pancreato-enterostomy is a much more delicate and technically a more difficult operation. Thirdly, it seems that when the pancreas is cut in two the duct retracts into the pancreatic substance and is covered by the healing process unless it is kept open by a flow of pancreatic juice, which can find no other easy exit. Fourthly, an isolated portion of the pancreas which has been implanted will maintain communication with the intestine, usually through the end of the duct, but there seems to be special tendency to follow out a thread when present instead of the duct if the duct has been cut off even with the pancreatic tissue. Fifthly, ligation of the duct of Wirsung produces no pancreatitis or pancreatic necrosis when pancreato-enterostomy is performed at the same time; while ligation of the duct of Wirsung without pancreato-enterostomy produces serious consequences in many cases, as shown by all experimenters. Sixthly, the duct of Wirsung is the normal exist for the pancreatic fluid, just as the pylorus is the normal exit for the stomach fluids. So, just as the stomach canal circumvents a ligature which has been placed around the pylorus for the purpose of forcing the gastric fluid through a new opening, so the pancreatic juice circumvents a ligature which has been placed around the duct of Wirsung for the purpose of forcing the pancreatic fluid through a new opening. But it is quite probable that the duct of Santorini could be developed into a substitute for the duct of Wirsung in some cases by planting the tail of the pancreas and thus using the upper end of the duct as a safety valve during the process of development of the duct of Santorini to sufficient size to carry all the pancreatic fluid, after which the duct of the implanted tail would probably close. Seventhly, a bile duct which has been transplanted by the direct method, becomes widely dilated and at the same time thickened by intra-intestinal pressure of some kind, which may have a very important bearing on this subject. Eighthly, the persistency with which the cut ends of the ducts tend to heal over leads us to fear the possibility of the eventual cicatricial narrowing of these ducts in some cases unless a special method is used.

SECOND SERIES OF OPERATIONS.

September 13, a second series of operations was begun. These experiments were instituted, first, for the purpose of devising a means of dealing with the pancreatic duct which would prevent the healing pancreatic tissue from covering its end; second, for devising effectual methods of closing the ducts of Wirsung and Santorini simultaneously with the implantation of the tail; third, for devising a physiological operation for implanting the bile duct; fourth, for determining the practibility of implanting the stripped pancreatic duct directly into the intestine by using a reinforcement of omentum.

Beginning September 13, to October 5, 22 operations were done on the bile ducts and pancreas. Of these, 4 were done as follows: The ducts of Wirsung and Santorini were ligated and cut, the intestinal openings of the ducts were turned into the intestine with sutures and the omentum was drawn through the spaces between the pancreas and duodenum to effectually prevent reëstablishment of the ducts (Fig. 20). The end of the duodenal tail was cut off, the duct stripped and the vessels ligated as in Fig. 6, and the cut end of the pancreas, with the duct hanging out, was planted according to the method set forth in Figs. 1 to 12. Two of these dogs were poorly nourished, having evidently been starved for many days, and died—one on the fourth day and one on the eighth day after operation, without having manifested any appetite. No cause could be discovered for their death except inanition. Two of the four were well-nourished, and were operated on September 14. These dogs made an immediate and complete recovery.

On the twenty-fourth day after operation they were killed with chloroform. After stripping the duct of the retrogastric tail which had been left, a needle was inserted into the duct and methylene blue solution injected. The fluid passed unobstructedly into the loop of intestine, but none escaped into the duodenum. Longitudinal section of the pancreas through the duct for its whole length, including its insertion into the intestinal loop, showed that the duct had been maintained at its full size all the way through to a point slightly beyond the pancreatic tissue of the implanted end. Pancreatointestinal union was perfect, as it had been in all the other specimens.

These two specimens effectually remove the defects in our first series of operations, and prove that with the ducts of Wirsung and Santorini effectually closed and the duct of the tail allowed to protrude beyond the pancreatic tissue of the implanted end, the pancreatic juice of the other tail and body is easily delivered backward through the duct of the implanted tail. The experiment, as just described, at once produced the pathology and supplied the remedy for a case of obstruction of the pancreatic duct (from whatever cause) at or near the ampulla of Vater.

PHYSIOLOGICAL IMPLANTATION OF THE BILE DUCT.

Our next defect was in our method of implanting the bile duct. By studying the bile duct of the dog, it is observed to run under the mucous membrane of the duodenum for almost one inch before it opens out into the canal. It is at once seen that this arrangement effectually prevents the intraintestinal pressure from being brought to bear from within the duct, owing to the fact that it is brought to bear along the course of the duct through the mucous membrane, thus effectually making a valve as shown in Fig. 24. The problem then was to duplicate this condition as near as possible. The first thought was to split apart the layers of the intestine with forceps and drag the duct through. This was a cumbersome method until we were reminded of the protrusion of the mucous membrane which occurs after the outer coats of the stomach and intestine have been cut through, during the operation of gastro-enterostomy. The following operation was, therefore, devised for implanting the bile duct.

First, the duct is located and ligated with linen or silk near its point of entrance into the duodenum. It is then cut in two and the edges caught and held with mosquito forceps while one wall of the duct is split down with a pair of scissors, as shown in (Fig. 22 A). A linen suture is now passed through the split end of the duct so as to include about half of it, and tied (Fig. 22, A). The linen thread is then thrown around the other half, and tied (Fig. 22, B). The loose end is then threaded into another needle. By this method, the full strength of the duct is then retained for traction while the opening is maintained by the split (Fig. 22, C). The end of the duct is now wrapped in gauze while the intestine is prepared for its reception, which is done as follows. Pick up the part of the intestine desired and cut down through the peritoneal and muscular coats including the submucous tissue until the mucous membrane pouts out through the incision (Fig. 23, A). This incision should be about one inch long. Second, pass five sutures which pick up the peritoneal and muscular coats, on each side of the incision. Tie the suture at the upper end of the incision. Lift up the three intermediate intestinal sutures on the flat handle of an instrument, as they cross the incision. Make a small stab wound in the mucous membrane near the lower end of the incision. Now bring the intestine close down to the end of the split duct and pass the two needles, carrying the threads on the end of the duct, beneath the three intestinal sutures and into the intestinal lumen through the stab wound in the mucous membrane, and out through the intestinal wall one-half to three-quarters of an inch further along the intestine and one-eighth to one-quarter inch apart (Fig. 23, *B*). By making tension of these threads and at the same time pushing the intestine toward the duct, the bile duct is drawn beneath the intestinal sutures and into the intestinal lumen, through the stab wound, when the two ends of the threads on the duct are tied on the outside, thus anchoring the end of the duct on the inside of the intestine at this point (Fig. 24, *B*). The intestinal sutures are then tied, producing the results shown in Fig. 23, *C*. After this operation the duct lies just beneath the mucous membrane, which has been loosened for approximately three-quarters of an inch of its course, so that the intra-intestinal pressure is brought to bear on the duct along this entire distance, thus counteracting the intra-intestinal pressure which in the direct implantation is brought to bear on the inside of the duct (Fig. 24, *A* and *B*).

Two of the dogs on which this operation was done have been killed for the purpose of recovering specimens; one 14 days and the other 15 days after the implantation. The results were ideal. The end of the duct which had been drawn inside the intestine had apparently been digested down to its junction with the mucous membrane so that it was difficult to locate the opening from the inside of the intestine. The bile ducts were enlarged beyond normal, but in no degree were they so large as fourteen-day specimens seen after the direct implantation of the duct. By incising the duct above, a probe was easily passed into the intestine, after which a knife was passed along the probe splitting the duct, which revealed the fact that healing had taken place in accordance with the operation. In short, the specimens indicated the success of the operation both from a mechanical and functional standpoint. After this paper was sent to press two other dogs were killed two months after the physiological implantation of the bile duct into the duodeum and the valve was found to have acted perfectly—no distention or thickening of the duct which entered the intestine obliquely. In fact the result was perfect. I am now conducting a series of experiments to determine the possibility of implanting the ureter into the bowel in the same way.

DIRECT IMPLANTATION OF THE PANCREATIC DUCT.

During the last series of experiments we have done direct implantation of the pancreatic duct six times. The pancreas was held against the intestine with extra sutures and thoroughly reinforced by wrapping it with omentum which was fixed in place with sutures to the intestine. Of the 6 dogs operated on in this manner, 1 died of shock soon after the operation; 2 died of pancreatic and fat necrosis four and ten days after the operation; 1 died of peritonitis four days after the operation. (It is well to state that in this case no omentum was used to surround the duct, and leakage took place.) One died twelve days after operation, having shown a slight tendency to eat during the time. The postmortem showed no pancreatic or fat necrosis. On dissection of the pancreas the duct was found to be dilated to the size of a lead pencil. The pancreatic duct, after leaving the pancreatic tissue, had entirely disappeared and healed over, so that there was no communication between the pancreatic duct and the intestine. One dog lived until he was killed with chloroform on the twenty-fifth day after operation, and was apparently in good health during this time. The pancreas was hard along the duct, indicating chronic pancreatitis. The duct of the pancreas was stripped and injected with methylene blue solution, which passed out into the intestinal canal. On longitudinal section it was found that the duct was much dilated and terminated outside of the intestine, but a fistula had up to this time been maintained into the intestinal lumen. Of course, we are unable to state whether this would have remained open or would have finally closed. All of the specimens from these six dogs seem to indicate that the pancreatic duct depends very largely upon the adjacent pancreatic tissue for its nutrition; therefore, it can not be transplanted in the same manner as can the bile duct, owing to the fact that it dies as soon as it leaves the end of the pancreas. This suggestion, however, can only be proved by a close histological study of the pancreatic ducts.

While these few experiments are in no way conclusive concerning the second method, we feel safe in predicting that direct implantation of the duct is by no means so safe an operation (if practical at all) as pancreato-enterostomy by the method which we have described. Even if the continuity of the duct could be preserved the anatomical diagrams (Figs. 13 and 14) very clearly indicate that the implantation of one pancreatic duct does not necessarily mean that the other branch ducts will not discharge juice into the neighborhood of the wound. This would be especially true if the tail end of the duct was implanted.

APPLICATION OF PANCREATO-ENTEROSTOMY TO SURGERY OF THE HUMAN PANCREAS.

The foregoing experiments on dogs have been conducted with the primary idea of developing a practical method of reëstablishing communication between the pancreatic duct and the intestine, when such communication has been impeded or destroyed. Such methods have been developed for similar pathology in the stomach and bile tracts. A perfected type of gastro-enterostomy has proved to be the central feature of relief for the stomach, whether the pathology is removed. or short circuited; cholecystenterostomy or choledochenterostomy relief for the bile tracts.

The experiments made clearly indicate, to the mind of the writer at least, that pancreato-enterostomy will fill the same place in pancreatic surgery. The experiments prove that pancreato-enterostomy is entirely possible provided we use unbroken peritoneum to make the union with the pancreas.

Owing to the more complete rotation of the human intestinal tract, certain anatomical differences in the arrangement of the peritoneum exist, therefore a slightly different type of operation is required. For instance, the duodenum of the dog is long and for the most part has a mesentery, and is therefore covered with peritoneum, making it available. Such is not the case with the human. The peritoneum of the omentum of the dog has not blended with the peritoneum of the transverse colon, therefore there is no gastrocolic ligament or omentum as is found in man, and which must be severed to properly deal with the pancreas.

We are at the present time conducting a third series of experiments on dogs with the idea of harmonizing the steps of the operations of pancreato-enterostomy and pancreatectomy on the anatomy of the dog, to the anatomy which we find in the cadaver.

The following steps are recommended for doing pancreatectomy. First, removal of the head of the pancreas, for the description of which step we are indebted to Sauve[1] who calls special attention to three dangers—injury to the portal vein; injury to the superior mesenteric vessels, which is followed by gangrene of the small intestine; injury to the right colic artery, which is followed by gangrene of a part of the colon.

Remove the head of the duodenum and pancreas as follows: A median incision from the ensiform to below the umbilicus. Ligature of the pyloric artery and of the gastroduodenal artery. Section of the pylorus, or duodenum just below the pylorus. Division of the fascia along the right border of the duodenum. Posterior dissection of the second portion of the duodenum and the head of the pancreas.

Section of the duodenum at a point sufficiently far from the superior mesenteric vessels to protect them from injury. The dissection of the duodenum should be carried to a point

---

[1] Revue de Chirurgie, 1908, xxxvii, 113.

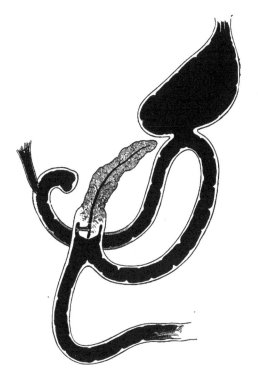

Fig. 19.—Diagram illustrating result following pancreatectomy, in which duct was apparently caught in one of the pancreatic sutures. (Arrow indicates how the pancreatic juice followed out the suture while the end of the duct has healed over.)

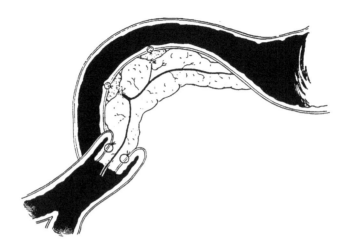

Fig. 20.—Artificial obstruction of the natural pancreatic delivery ducts of a dog's pancreas by ligating and cutting ducts and interposing omentum. Also the relief of the obstruction by pancreato-enterostomy.

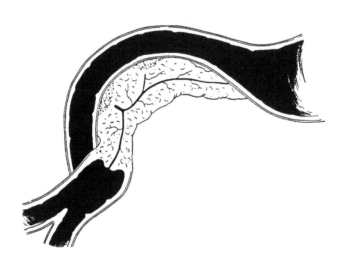

Fig. 21.—Pancreatic juice delivered through implanted duodenal tail. Diagram from specimen 24 days after complete obstruction of ducts of Wirsung and Santorini and simultaneous pancreato-enterostomy.

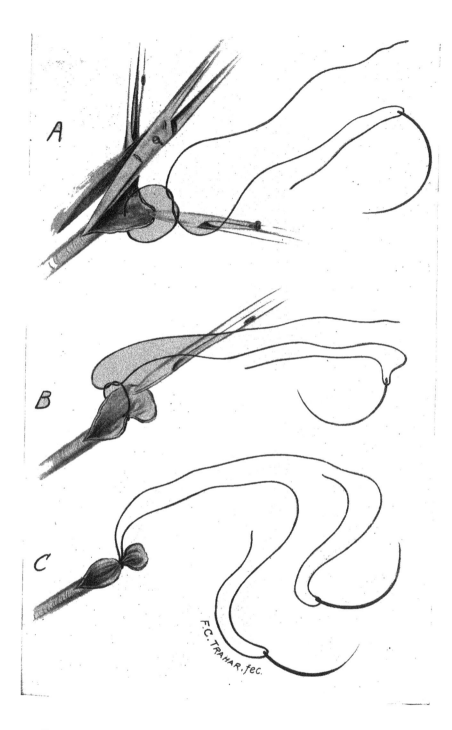

Fig. 22.—Preparing the bile duct for implantation into the intestine.

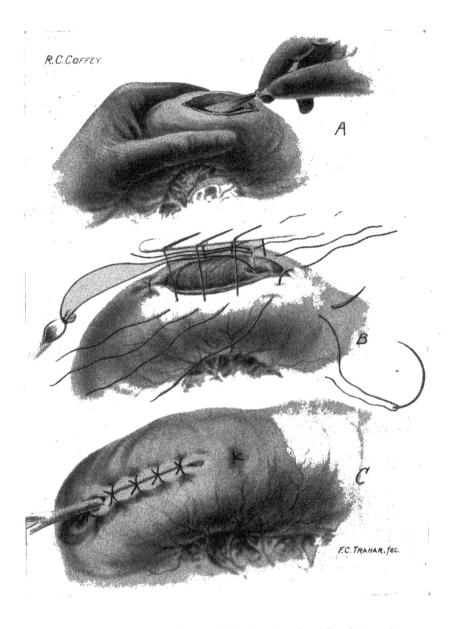

FIG. 23.—Preparing intestine and implanting the bile duct. *A*, separating the outer coats of the intestines from their membrane. *B*, drawing the bile duct into the intestine. *C*, implanting operation complete.

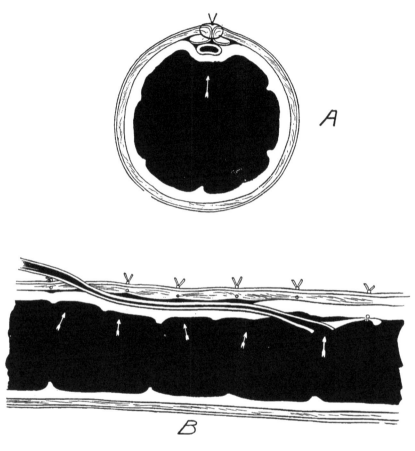

Fig. 24.—Sectional view (diagrammatic) illustrating the relation of the bile duct to the coats of the intestine after physiological implantation of the bile duct. (Arrows indicate the direction of intra-intestinal pressure.) A, cross-section; B, longitudinal section.

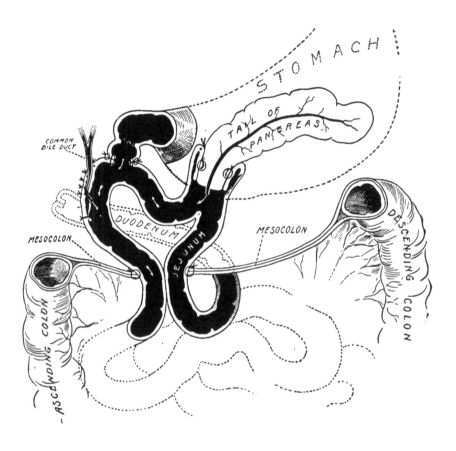

FIG. 25.—Scheme of operation for removal of the head of the pancreas and duodenum

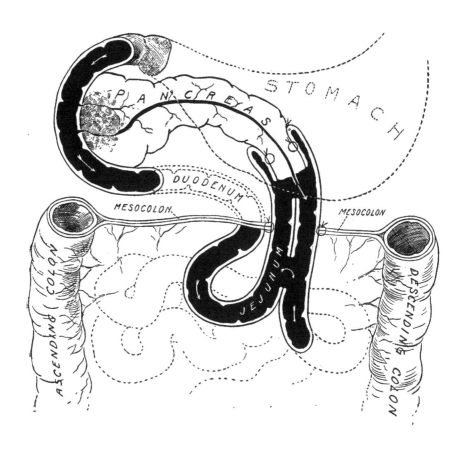

FIG. 26.—Scheme of pancreato-enterostomy, without pancreatectomy.

at which it can be easily separated from the head of the pancreas, but not to the mesenteric vessels. Ligation below of the pancreato-duodenal vessels. Section of the duodenum and suture of its lower end.

Separation of the "lesser" pancreas from the mesenteric vessels which cross in front of this portion.

Separation of the pancreas from the portal vein. Section of the head of the pancreas. Ligation and division of the common bile duct and division of the gastroduodenal artery. and the portions of the duodenum and pancreas are thus removed.

Now the cut end of the bile duct and the cut end of the stomach or duodenum, as the case may be, are held in clamps and the cut end of the pancreas wrapped in gauze awaiting implantation into the loop of the jejunum.

Second step: If the gastrocolic omentum has not already been severed to permit a good exposure for work, it may now be done. An opening is made through the transverse mesocolon near its root, through which a loop of jejunum one or two feet in length is drawn. The pancreas is now implanted into the upper portion of this intestine—lower down the stomach or duodenum is anastomosed, and still lower down the common bile duct is implanted. A few interrupted linen sutures fasten the intestine to the mesocolon as it passes up and down through the slit. These sutures also close the opening and prevent hernia (Fig. 25).

Pancreato-enterostomy without pancreatectomy (Fig. 26) may be done in the human as follows:

First, divide the gastrocolic omentum and loosen the tail of the pancreas by dissection and ligation of vessels.

Secondly, pick up a loop of jejunum as near to the ligament of Treitz as possible, and yet long enough to reach the tail of the pancreas with ease.

Thirdly, entero-enterostomy between the limbs of the loops.

Fourthly, make a hole through the mesocolon well to the

left of the ligament and draw the loop of intestine through the opening.

Fifthly, strip and cut the duct of the tail of the pancreas and plant it into the loop by the method previously described in this paper. Fasten the intestine to the mesocolon where it passes in and down through the opening.

Sixthly, repair the gastrocolic omentum.

DISCUSSION OF THE PAPERS OF DRS. GUERRY, RANSOHOFF, AND COFFEY.

DR. JOSEPH C. BLOODGOOD, of Baltimore.—The statement has been made here, and it is still seen even in recent literature, that the abdomen should not be opened during the stage of peritoneal shock or collapse in acute pancreatitis. Two Viennese surgeons, Guleke and Doberauer, have from a series of experimental investigations demonstrated that the cause of death in acute hemorrhagic pancreatitis is a toxic one, due to the escape of trypsin and, perhaps, other pancreatic ferments into the free peritoneal cavity and into the circulation. These ferments are toxic and are the direct cause. of the so-called peritoneal shock or collapse, and of the fat necroses. The best treatment, therefore, for this shock or collapse is the rapid removal of the peritoneal exudate, which contains the toxins in excess and the drainage of the pancreatic gland to prevent further leakage.

Laboratory research has, therefore, in this disease been of immense practical importance. The question of the operative treatment of acute hemorrhagic pancreatic should be looked upon as settled. I have studied carefully practically every case of acute pancreatitis subjected to operative treatment and find one thing in common—the drainage of the exudate. So that at the present time clinical evidence agrees with the results of laboratory research. I would like to call attention here to a method of exploring the abdominal cavity when the diagnosis is somewhat in doubt. I make the incision in the middle line below the umbilicus; this is rapidly made, and through this opening better than through any other a larger area of the abdomen can be explored. If the condition proves to be one of suppurative peritonitis we can employ this incision for temporary drainage of the abdominal cavity with gauze moistened in salt solution, while the area of local infection is attacked through another incision. In pancreatitis it allows the rapid evacuation of the fluid and the rapid inspection of the omentum for fat necroses. In a recent case of my own the exposure of fat necroses in the omentum through this exploratory incision led to the correct diagnosis, and justified me in making a second incision for exposure and drainage of a small pancreatic hematoma. Had I made the higher incision first, it would have required unusual courage to bore through an immense quantity of fat between the stomach and colon to reach the pancreas, because in this case no further evidence of pancreatic disease was present until the pancreas was exposed deep in its bed of fat. In such cases it is a great comfort to the surgeon to have seen the fat necroses before he attacks the deeply situated pancreas.

There is a second method of exposing the pancreatic region. Withdraw the omentum and transverse colon as is done preliminary to a gastroenterostomy. As a rule one can see shining through the peritoneal coat of the mesotransverse colon fat necroses. In a recent case I found the fat necroses only in this position—there were none in the omentum.

I am particularly interested in the question discussed by Dr. Guerry. It is one to which I have given considerable attention in my paper, because I looked upon it as one of the most important. The question is: When shall we do cholecystenterostomy for chronic pancreatitis? If there is obstructive jaundice, an indurated pancreas and no stones in the common duct, the indications are clear. Whether this induration of the pancreas is inflammatory or malignant, the anastomosis of gall-bladder and intestines will permanently relieve one and temporarily the other. I have discussed in my paper a newer method of making this anastomosis, one in which the jejunum is anastomosed to the gall-bladder through a split in the transverse mesocolon, practically as we do in posterior gastroenterostomy. I have had three cases—two of them successful. One is still living now, one year since the operation; the other—a case of carcinoma—recently died. This patient, however, for four months was relieved of her jaundice and all her discomforts. The third case died of hemorrhage, but the anastomosis was working well before death and the autopsy demonstrated a very successful suture.

The decision when to make this anastomosis in the absence

of jaundice is more difficult.   But, as Dr. Guerry has shown, cases are not always relieved by cholecystostomy.   As soon as the gall-bladder fistula closes or a few months later the abdominal attacks return.   The accumulated experience today of one man with this group is necessarily small, and I trust Dr. Guerry's contribution will stimulate others, so that definite indications for his operation may be formulated.   In one of the cases reported in my paper the patient was not relieved by a cholecystostomy: there was no jaundice at the time of the operation; the recurrent attacks began within two months.

We must also remember that there are a group of cases in which we find and remove stones from the common duct, in which we may even pass an instrument into the duodenum through the common duct, but yet, the symptoms are not relieved, because of the secondary pancreatitis. These cases are not many, but their discomforts are great and the relief is rapid and permanent by a wise selection of cholecystenterostomy.

Diet in pancreatitis is often neglected.   It is a well-known physiological fact that the pancreatic secretion is stimulated chiefly by the passage of the acid chyme from the stomach into the duodenum.   Starvation, therefore, or a restricted diet will diminish pancreatic secretion.

In the cases of acute hemorrhagic pancreatitis, especially in those of a very high mortality, in which death takes place within three days, we usually find that the acute attack began within a few hours after overindulgence in food and drink. There is no question, from my study of the literature, as to this definite etiological relationship.   Patients, therefore, with symptoms suggestive of chronic pancreatitis, or with a history of gallstones, or who suffer from intermittent diabetes, should be informed of the greater danger of overindulgence in food.

After operations for any lesion of the pancreas a pretty strict, almost starvation diet, diminishes the dangers.   This is commented upon in recent literature by a number of observers.   In cases of a pancreatic fistula after drainage of a pancreatic hematoma, abscess or cyst, in which the pancreatic ferments have been found in the secretion of the fistula, it has been demonstrated that coincident with a restricted diet the secretion diminishes and the fistula closes more rapidly.

It is interesting to recall another physiological fact, which should be borne in mind in cases of cholecystostomy.   The bile enters the duodenum only when the food passes from the stomach into the duodenum. There is a sphincter at the end of the bile duct. If one wishes to maintain longer drainage after cholecystostomy the food should be restricted and given at longer intervals. On the other hand, if the indications are to allow the biliary fistula to close rapidly, feed the patient every two hours day and night. Since my attention has been called to this fact some two or three years ago, I have been able to confirm its efficacy in a number of observations.

There is one other point which I think is new and should be borne in mind. It has been referred to in the second case reported with my paper, namely the difficulty of differentiating a hypertrophied Luschka's gland from adenocarcinoma. This case was clinically one of cholecystitis; there was very little jaundice. On exploring the gall-bladder we found it enlarged; on opening the gall-bladder it was seen to contain a material like the white of an egg, but no stones. In passing a spoon for bringing out the stones from the cystic duct, I removed only gelatinous material like that in the gall bladder; it looked like colloid carcinoma of the stomach or of the rectum. Under the microscope dilated and hypertrophied Luschka's glands were demonstrated. Subsequent events in this case demonstrated that there was no carcinoma.

DR. STEPHEN H. WATTS, of Charlottesville, Virginia.—I am very much interested in this subject, as during the present year I have operated upon three cases of acute pancreatitis. These cases presented a good many points of interest and have been the subject of a paper which I have recently written. One of the most striking things in acute pancreatitis is the presence of hemorrhage, and it is still a mooted question as to whether the infection gives rise to the hemorrhage or whether the hemorrhage occurs first and later the hemorrhagic areas become infected. What Dr. Ransohoff says is suggestive, namely, that he has not found infection in his early cases, the cultures having been negative; moreover he has stated that there was marked arteriosclerosis in one of his cases which might easily have led to rupture of one of the pancreatic vessels.

I think that a slight bile staining of the sclerotics may help us in the diagnosis of acute pancreatitis, the jaundice doubtless being due to the swelling of the head of the pancreas and the mucosa of the common duct.

I think the best treatment of acute pancreatitis depends upon the condition of the patient when seen by us. Unfortunately most of these cases come to us in bad condition and often we hardly feel justified in operating,.even after making a diagnosis, though operation probably offers the best prospect of cure. The simplest thing is to make a stab wound in the mid-line above the pubis and thus drain away the blood-stained fluid which Guleke and Doberauer have shown to be quite toxic, the toxicity being due to trypsin. If the case is in better shape we can go a little further, divide the gastrocolic omentum, expose the pancreas and actually make incisions in the pancreas; the latter is important, otherwise we get an extravasation of the enzymes beneath the peritoneum and they have no chance of getting out. If we find gallstones in the gall bladder and the condition of the patient warrants it the stones should be removed and the gall bladder drained. In one of my cases I found a good many adhesions about the gall bladder, apparently indicating a cholecystitis at some previous time. The patient gave a history of a severe attack of typhoid fever some time before, but cultures from the gall-bladder at operation proved to be sterile. It is rather surprising to me that we do not find more cases of acute pancreatitis due to the typhoid bacillus considering the length of time this organism may live in the biliary passages.

DR. ROSWELL PARK, of Buffalo.—I wish to refer briefly to the tragic event which occurred at Buffalo a number of years ago. Of course you are all familiar with the case of President McKinley, who was shot, and in which I was more or less concerned. This is the first time I have referred to that case in any public place.

The remarks of Dr. Bloodgood have prompted me to say this, that at the autopsy on President McKinley there were certain revelations which we had not been led to expect. There was a tremendous amount of interest taken in his case, as you all remember, and after the conclusion of the autopsy I and others were besieged by newspaper reporters for all the information we could give them, and all the explanations which we could furnish. In some respects the findings were unexpected. It was at a time when we did not know much about the surgery of the pancreas, or diseased condition of that organ, or the relation of one to the other. In seeking an explanation for the peculiar necrosis which we found in this case, it was my suggestion, based on the very meagre amount of information which we all of us possessed at that time, that in all probability the wound of the pancreas in his case had to do with the subsequent course of events. I really believe now it had much to do with it, although it had not been discussed at the autopsy. The suggestion was taken up later, and made the basis of a large amount of experimentation by our own pathologist in Buffalo, Professor Herbert Williams, and many others, and that unfortunate instance, I think, attracted surgical attention to this matter in a way nothing else perhaps would have done had it not occurred. That is a little bit of history which it is not too early now to put on record.

DR. CHARLES H. MAYO, of Rochester, Minnesota.—I think this society is to be congratulated on having heard this group of papers presented to it, covering this most important subject. Especially would I compliment Dr. Coffey on the enormous amount of labor, which has proven so successful in his experimental work on the pancreas in dogs.

Last Friday Dr. Coffey at Rochester operated on a dog, using the technique he has described, and on Saturday afternoon the dog was up and about, inmediately showing no effects from the operation.

I was struck with what Dr. Guerry said, namely, that there is no question but what we should more frequently resort to cholecystenterostomy. If there is jaundice present and hardening of the pancreas, with no gallstones, then we would at once think of the advisiability of doing the operation. As to the question of doing this operation in simple inflammatory adhesions, such as cholecystitis, that is something for the future to show, yet it is a possibility. These are not the gall-bladders today that we would excise, but they are the ones that may lead to further operation. If one finds gallstones they expect to get relief, but if we find cholecystitis with a foul-smelling bile, and hardening of the pancreas, drainage which is kept up from ten to fifteen days is not enough to insure success in relieving that condition. We may have a liver which is defective in its excretion, and in the destruction of bacteria passing through it. So it is in that type of case probably that cholecystenterostomy will be done more and more in the future, and it is to be hoped that results of this operation will find a permanent place in that type of work.

Dr. Bloodgood speaks of our inability to diagnose pancreatitis, but at the same time it is becoming more and more evident that we are able to do so. The time was when we did not know when we had the abdomen open, and now we are recognizing it and in a good many instances before operation, so that there has been a most wonderful gain in our ability to diagnose clinically these cases of chronic inflammation of the pancreas and the acute conditions also. Dr. Ransohoff speaks of the inability to pass the hand over the pancreas, and say there is disease of it or not. I think one of the most important things in the abdomen is to be able to explore it with the hand in abdominal operations. Especially in all gall-bladder cases the pancreas should be run over and one should be able to get an idea of what it is like, how it feels, and whether there are any symptoms connected with it or not, and also get a look at the pylorus.

Dr. H. A. Royster, of Raleigh, North Carolina.—I wish to put on record a practical observation, which bears upon the paper of Dr. Guerry.

Two months ago, a man, aged seventy years, came in for operation for gallstones, with a typical history of that disease. He had had jaundice only once, and that had disappeared entirely. Examination of his urine three days before operation showed well-marked reaction to sugar. We opened his gall-bladder, removed one hundred and eighty stones, and simply drained in the usual manner. The head of the pancreas was enlarged. One week after the operation the sugar disappeared entirely from the urine, and has not returned.

Dr. Walter C. G. Kirchner, of St. Louis.—I have been very much interested in Dr. Bloodgood's paper and I consider it a valuable contribution to surgery, as a knowledge of the methods of the treatment of injurious of the pancreas and other conditions which involve resection of the bowel is very important.

I recall a case of gunshot wound of the transverse colon, in which we had a condition similar to that described by Dr. Park. The repair of the colon was satisfactory, and good drainage was established, but later at the autopsy it was found that nearly half of the stomach had been digested, evidently by the pancreatic secretion. If a method similar to the one described by Dr. Coffey had been used in this case I believe a successful result would have been obtained.

Of five cases of pancreatitis I have met with, three of them were of the suppurative type, and resulted fatally. In two of these cases a diagnosis was made, but the conditions were so fulminating that operative procedure did not seem to be indicated, that is, by the time the patient reached the hospital his condition did not warrant an operation.

I was particularly interested also in the hemorrhagic type of pancreatitis, and I have not been certain as to that classification. In one case in which a pathological diagnosis was made out microscopically of hemorrhagic pancreatitis there was no hemorrhage in the abdominal cavity, but the pancreas itself was involved. This patient gave all the acute symptoms of pancreatitis, and at autopsy it was found that an ulcer of the duodenum was present, which seems to have had a direct communication with the head of the pancreas. As I have said before, the findings in this case were those of hemorrhagic pancreatitis.

Last week I was unfortunate enough to have a case more in line with the one described by Dr. Ransohoff. The patient entered the hospital with a diagnosis of cyst of the pancreas. In addition there was dulness in the left flank, indicating splenic tumor. The patient was kept under observation. He was in a critical condition, and was observed for two or three days, when suddenly this tumor disappeared, and there was fluid in the abdomen. The diagnosis was very obscure. At operation fluid was found in the peritoneal cavity. There were also a great many adhesions. The fluid resembled that which we find in cases of ectopic pregnancy. There was a sort of cyst wall in the region of the spleen. The spleen itself was not enlarged, but was more or less friable.. In the lesser peritoneal cavity there was a large collection of fluid and clots, and at the time of the operation the diagnosis was so uncertain and the condition of the patient so critical that this diagnosis was still undecided; I believe, however, that this was one of the cases of the type described by Dr. Ransohoff, and we may speak of it as a condition of "apoplexy" of the pancreas. In this individual case the arteries were sclerotic, and the history given was that of syphilis; but I am not clear in my own mind as to the classification of this hemorrhagic type of pancreatitis.

DR. GEORGE W. CRILE, of Cleveland.—The symposium to which we have listened this afternoon is one of the most important that it has ever been my privilege to hear, and I think the association ought to be congratulated on the amount of material, both clinical and experimental, that has been presented.

The experimental research of Dr. Coffey is inspiring, the work is carefully planned, the facts clearly presented, the illustrations are excellent, the conclusions clear, and the clinical results will be important. Discussing the gall-bladder infections, I have, I think found some benefit from the autogenous vaccines and addition to drainage.

I am inclined to believe that in cases of acute hemorrhagic pancreatitis, in which the surgeon might otherwise be prevented from carrying out the technique indicated because of the poor condition of the patient, the following plan will prove valuable, viz.: Tranfuse a sufficient amount of blood to restore the patient to an operable state, then continue the connection, during the operation, giving blood as needed. I would strongly advise nitrous oxide anesthesia.

Dr. John C. Munro, of Boston.—I cannot let these papers go by without commending the splendid work that is being done here, and I feel grateful to Dr. Guerry for bringing up a point which it seems to me is of great value.

His paper recalls to me a case in which I did a cholecystenterostomy six or eight years ago, for a supposed lesion at the ampulla of Vater, which proved not to be such; it was probably a case of chronic pancreatitis. The diagnosis can be made both in the chronic and in the acute forms in a fair proportion of cases. I have had quite a number of acute cases of pancreatitis, and in a number of them I was able to make the diagnosis beforehand. I think the type of jaundice, both in the acute and chronic forms, is rather significant, although it is not, of course, absolutely to be depended upon.

As for operating upon the very acute cases I should say yes, because I have had two practically moribund cases of acute pancreatitis that have recovered after operation, which I feel convinced would not have been the case if the pancreas had not been drained.

Dr. Bloodgood made an important point with regard to fat necrosis. In making the exploration I have used the same opening between the stomach and colon, and in every case I have found a small or large lesion in the pancreas. Drainage usually brings about recovery. In a few cases I have also drained through the left loin, but I believe anterior drainage is usually sufficient.

I am not inclined to accept Dr. Ransohoff's remarks with reference to our inability to diagnosticate these cases of chronic pancreatitis. I do not believe he is right. For years I have made it a practice in practically all abdominal cases to examine the pancreas, and only in the cases where there has been some concomitant biliary lesion do we find this condition of the pancreas, which I have always supposed to be a chronic pancreatitis. We can tell the condition of the pancreas by touch, and I should dislike to give up my position on that point.

DR. O. H. ELBRECHT, of St. Louis.—These papers on pancreatitis have been so thoroughly instructive and valuable that I am impelled to report a case of pancreatitis that has recently come in my experience that differs somewhat from those reported here, in that it was a form rarely met with.

It was a case of chronic pancreatitis that gave a classical picture of a subacute obstructing gallstone attack, in which the icterus was so profound that it was greenish in hue. It was thought that a gallstone was producing all of the trouble from the severity of the pain in this region, and a very distinct mass could be outlined in the region of the gall-bladder. At operation dense adhesions were found about the gall-bladder and duodenum and the omentum enclosing the entire mass; gall-bladder being immensely distended. It was thought best, owing to the moribund condition of our patient not to invade these adhesions, but to simply content ourselves by gall-bladder drainage. The pancreas at this time was not thought to be the seat of trouble. The patient lived less than twenty-four hours, and at autopsy showed that these adhesions also involved the head of the pancreas and all the adjacent lymphatics. Numerous ulcerations were found along the duct of the pancreas and also in the gland substance itself, which in several places had been excavated to a considerable extent and contained free pus, as did also some of the adjacent lymphatic nodules. The character of the pus was suggestive of tuberculosis, and while the autopsy was still in progress stained specimens of this pus showed tubercle bacilli in abundance. We searched carefully for the seat of the trouble, by examining all the other organs for tuberculous lesions, with a view of establishing the primary focus, but could find none, which forced us to conclude that the pancreas was the organ primarily affected. The bile obstruction was plainly the result of the external pressure brought to bear upon the common duct by the swelling of the surrounding infected structures and adhesions. In going into her history more closely we brought out the fact that she had had repeated attacks, and in only one instance did she have hemorrhage that was known of, but she survived this attack and had a long period of quiescence. Each of these attacks had been treated as gallstone disease.

I mention this for the reason that it would seem that in the chronic form there is apparently no hemorrhage in counterdistinction to the acute cases. The condition seems to be quite rare, and this is my only excuse for bringing it up here, as a careful perusal of the literature at our command only revealed eleven reported cases. The contrast of the picture of this slow inflammatory pancreatitis seems to be very different than those reported in the delightful papers we have just heard.

DR. GUERRY (closing the discussion on his part).—There is practically nothing for me to say, except to thank the members for the discussion, which I think has been a great deal of help to us all.

I would like to mention, in conclusion, one point that was touched on in the paper, and that is the great necessity in the future, if we can, of determining at the time of primary operation those cases that require permanent drainage, and those that do not need permanent drainage. But that is a hard thing to do. Personally, in my experience that has been decided by the patients coming back for a second operation.

Leaving out of consideration the cases collected, and associated with gallstone formation, I think I have had something like twelve or thirteen cases of my own of chronic interstitial pancreatitis independent of stone formation. All of them at the primary operation were simply drained. Out of the twelve or thirteen cases I have had seven come back for permanent drainage, and for a recurrence of the symptoms. That was what led me to write this paper. I have had three cases in addition to those operated on by other men of undoubted reputation and standing, in which temporary cholecystotomy was done, and in these cases I show recurrence occurred. We want to try and save these patients the necessity for a second operation.

DR. RANSOHOFF (closing the discussion on his part).—There

are one or two points I want to refer to. I am very sorry indeed that I, myself, do not stand upon as high a plane as a diagnostician as my friend, Dr. Munro, from Boston. It has been said that 90 per cent, of the cases of acute pancreatitis come as a surprise at the operating table, or at the autopsy. I think for a long time the ultra-acute cases, of which I described two instances, will come in the nature of a surprise. When a man has repeated attacks of gallstone colic; when he has jaundice at the inception of the attack, one would necessarily suspect acute pancreatitis, because a positive diagnosis cannot be made. When the disease has advanced further, when you have an exudate that is circumscribed, the diagnosis can be made with certainty, but these are not the ultra-acute cases to which we called attention.

When Dr. Bloodgood rises to close the discussion I would like to have him explain why it is that in these cases of acute pancreatitis, almost without exception, as found in the literature of the subject, we have vomiting of bile. That is one of the symptoms to which even Fitz originally called attention. Why should we have this, in view of the etiological factor that is always given, namely, obstruction of the common duct, or obstruction within the diverticulum of Vater?

Dr. Mayo tells us that he runs his hand over the pancreas when operating in the abdomen for other pathological conditions. Most of us have done the same thing.. When we have to do an operation on the gall-bladder or stomach we examine these parts, but that does not change the view I expressed that a diagnosis of chronic pancreatitis is often made glibly from a sense of touch alone. The pancreas, like the salivary glands, varies in its density and particularly when it has back of it such a variable basis to lie upon as the vertebral column. There it is difficult from a sense of touch to see that the pancreas is harder than it has a right to be. A diagnosis of chronic pancreatitis is sometimes not made at the operation for suspected gallstone or gall-bladder disease until the biliary ways are found normal. Then there must be something wrong with the pancreas if the surgeon feels over the region of the pancreas and discovers some little hardness. Thus a diagnosis of chronic pancreatitis may be established at the operation. If we have a chronic pancreatitis it shows in some way, clinically, such as an increase or decrease in the hardness of the gland.

Dr. Crile has alluded to the value of transfusion of blood. If perchance he should cut the common carotid artery in an operation, if he could not catch the bleeding vessel with forceps, would there be time to get a donor and to make an anastomosis? Not long ago I had a man come under my observation who was shot through the vena cava.   Would there have been time to get a donor?   Sometimes blood is pumped out of a very large artery or vein a great deal faster than you can possibly pump it in from any donor.

DR. COFFEY (closing the discussion on his part).—I think I omitted one thing that was recommended in Dr. Binnie's surgery, as coming from Desjardin some months ago, in which he recommended (purely from cadaver work) the feasibility of stripping the pancreatic duct and planting it directly into the intestines.   Upon seeing this recommendation I tried it and found it wanting.   Of six dogs in which this method of implantation was tried four died in four days from acute pancreatic necrosis.   One lived ten days and finally the opening closed entirely, leaving a dilated duct larger than a pencil—in fact as large as my little finger, without necrosis, but a pancreas that was cord-like or bone-like.   The sixth case lived for twenty-four days, and was in good health when killed, and it was found there was still not only a communication between the pancreatic ducts and intestines, but through the direct medium of the pancreatic duct.   Our experiments show that the pancreatic duct has a feeble blood supply, except that which it derives possibly direct from its contiguous pancreatic tissue.   This is a feature which it will be interesting to work out.   We can transplant the bile ducts and ureter, and the duct does not die, while in all six cases in which we tried direct implantation the pancreatic duct died.   As soon as we have established an opening sufficiently, this will close up.

DR. BLOODGOOD (closing).—I think we have made it plain to Dr. Coffey that we appreciate the experimental work he has done.   Every meeting of practical surgeons is more or less rejuvenated and the interest greatly increased by experimental papers.   Every year adds further evidence to justify the conclusion that experimental surgery on animals leads to practical surgery on human beings.   The cause of death, as I have mentioned, in acute pancreatitis was worked out in the laboratory, and the results became of immediate practical importance in the surgery of pancreatitis in human beings.

I take the liberty of making two suggestions as to the treatment of the pancreas after resection of its head: The anastomosis of the divided gall-bladder into the duodenum and of the body or tail of the pancreas and the intestine by invagination is a somewhat formidable one.

MacCallum has shown that when the pancreas is separated from the intestine all of its secreting parenchyma undergoes atrophy, except the islands of Langhans, but the animal does well. Therefore, if we resect the head of the pancreas and leave a portion of the tail and head the patient will not develop diabetes. In resecting the pancreas it probably will be necessary in many cases to resect a portion of the duodenum; then one could ligate the common duct, anastomose the gall-bladder into the intestine, and perform posterior gastroenterostomy.

I fear, however, there is not a great future for resection of the pancreas for carcinoma.

In answering the question of Dr. Ransohoff in regard to the vomiting of bile in pancreatitis, I am of the opinion that the presence or absence of bile in the vomitus would not influence the diagnosis. The common duct is not always obstructed, and if there is an obstruction by a stone in the diverticulum of Vater some bile gets into the duodenum. In two autopsies by Opie in which he found stone in the ampulla of Vater, one case operated on by Dr. Halstead and one by me, bile was found in the intestine; so it might have been present in the vomitus. As far as my memory serves me, the presence or absence of bile in the vomitus has not been commented upon in the cases reported in the literature.

In regard to the remarks of Drs. Mayo and Guerry as to the question: When shall we do primary cholecystenterostomy? It seems to me that it would be just as well for us to be conservative for a time. When there is no jaundice at the time of the operation, I do not believe that there is any great risk to try drainage of the gall-bladder first; then keep up this drainage for a considerable period of time, and caution the patient as to diet for some months afterward.

It has been questioned here as to our ability to make a diagnosis of acute hemorrhagic pancreatitis. I have seen but two cases in the very acute stage, and it seemed to me that there was no question as to the imperative indication to open the abdomen within the first twelve hours, but I did not see these cases until after twenty-four hours. Both had been treated with morphia for gallstone colic. I have dwelt upon the differential diagnosis in my paper, but I would like to emphasize here that after a careful study of all the cases in the literature one is thoroughly impressed with the fact that the symptoms in the first twelve to twenty-four hours in the grave forms of pancreatitis are sufficient to justify any surgeon in opening the abdomen. You can make any diagnosis that you wish, provided only you attempt to confirm it at once by exploratory laparotomy. The chief danger is to look upon the condition in the early hours as gallstone colic and to attempt to relieve it with morphia.

We come now to a still more important question: In the literature a large number of patients died within twenty-four hours after the initial pain, others forty-eight hours. If a patient survives three days they usually recover completely or with secondary complications like hematoma or abscess. If the operation is then performed after the third day, the condition must not be looked upon as desperate. But when the abdomen is explored earlier, I am of the opinion that, in addition to removing the peritoneal exudate and draining the region of the pancreas, the patients should be treated along the lines which have been found efficacious in other toxic diseases, like eclampsia; salt solution should be given intravenously, subcutaneously and per rectum; a stomach tube should be passed, the stomach washed out and salt solution left in; in some very critically ill patients, perhaps almost moribund, it would be justifiable to try bleeding from one vein and direct transfusion of blood, according to the method of Crile, at the same time. I have recently had a very successful experience in a very grave case of eclampsia. The patient was in convulsions, comatosed; she had been so for twelve hours; the blood-pressure was 240. During the operation as soon as the diagnosis of pancreatitis has been made, these other therapeutic measures could be started, and it is my opinion that more patients will be saved.

SUTURE OF THE RECURRENT LARYNGEAL NERVE, WITH REPORT OF A CASE.

By J. Shelton Horsley, M.D.,
Richmond, Virginia.

The literature on surgery of the recurrent laryngeal nerve is very scanty. A thorough search of the literature in the library of the Surgeon-General's office, at Washington, has not revealed a single case of suture of this nerve in man. Consequently, the case reported below is apparently unique. There has been some work done along experimental lines, in which the left recurrent laryngeal was divided and its distal end inserted into the vagus higher up. These experiments have been carried out chiefly with a view to the cure of a disease in horses, called "roaring." This peculiar affection is caused by paralysis of the left recurrent laryngeal, which abolished the function of all the intrinsic muscles on the left side of the larynx except the cricothyroid, a muscle supplied by the superior laryngeal. It always occurs on the left side, as the greater length of the left recurrent laryngeal and its course around the aorta render this nerve subject to any lesion that involves the aorta, or to excessive functional strain upon the aorta. So far as the appearance of the larynx is concerned, resection of the left recurrent laryngeal presents conditions identical with those found in a "roaring" horse.

J. Broeckaert's experiments on monkeys (*Annales de la Société de médecine de Gand*, 1904, p. 209) show results similar to those of like experiments on the dog, the rabbit, and the guinea-pig. Resection of a portion of the recurrent laryngeal nerve was followed by decided and progressive atrophy and degeneration of the external thyro-arytenoid muscle, and by less pronounced nutritive changes in the internal thyro-arytenoid and in the posterior and lateral crico-arytenoids. He thinks that similar effects of resection of this nerve are to be expected in the human subject.

E. Cotterell (*Veterinarian*, 1893, p. 357) performed operations on three dogs and one donkey. After division of the left recurrent laryngeal nerve, he found the muscles of the left side of the larynx were paralyzed and placed in a condition similar to that in horses affected with "roaring." The recurrent nerve was cut across and its peripheral end carefully dissected out for about an inch. The left vagus was then found and was divided a little higher than the level of the section of the recurrent laryngeal. The end of the peripheral portion of the left recurrent laryngeal was then sutured along with the peripheral end of the cut vagus into the upper end of the vagus. Two experiments on dogs were failures. The third dog on which this operation was done was examined five months and three weeks later, and the left side of the larynx was seen to be working well, but not quite so well as the right. Cotterell thinks this was due to the fact that the period of time that had elapsed between the operation and the examination was not sufficient for the nerve to regenerate fully. The dog was killed and the dissection showed that the peripheral end of the left recurrent had united to the vagus. The experiment upon the donkey was done January 30, 1892, and laryngeal examination on April 22, 1893, showed that the left side of the larynx worked synchronously with the right side and just as well. The dissection showed that the peripheral end of the left recurrent laryngeal nerve had united with the vagus.

F. Macdonald (*Atti del XI. Congresso medico internazionale*, 1894, ii, 111) performed somewhat similar experiments, taking a section from the left recurrent laryngeal in order to prevent any reunion with the proximal end and grafting the distal portion into the trunk of the vagus. Two years after the operation the result was said to be successful.

These experiments seem to prove that surgery of the recurrent laryngeal nerve has a wider field than has heretofore been supposed. If so much of the nerve has been destroyed as to make a direct suture impossible, its distal end can be grafted into the vagus with hope of eventual restoration of function. We must remember, however, that though many of the experiments quoted were successful, the nervous structure of the human being is more difficult to repair than that of a lower animal. Even in man different individuals often present variations in their readiness of repair of injured nerves, which cannot be accounted for by obvious conditions.

On account of its anatomical position, lesions are more likely to occur in the left recurrent laryngeal than in the right. Affections of the aorta are a frequent cause of paralysis of the left nerve and diseases and injuries of the thyroid gland may involve either of the recurrent laryngeals. They are sometimes injured during operation on the thyroid gland, and in such cases suturing the nerve should give excellent results. Occasionally, paralysis of the left recurrent, resulting from dilatation of the aorta, might be treated by transplantion into the vagus, though, as a rule, the disease of the aorta would contra-indicate operation.

In the following case the left recurrent laryngeal was sutured about three months after injury.

Martha J., colored, aged forty years, married for twenty years, has had three children. Her previous health has been good except for the usual diseases of childhood. There is no history of syphilis or tuberculosis. On June 22, 1908, she was shot by a pistol, the ball entering at the lower border of the chin about the median line and just grazing the bone. It was evidently deflected by the bone, and took a course downward and to the left, just beneath the skin, to the larynx, where it penetrated deeper in the neck. Just above the larynx the bullet so nearly penetrated to the surface that a keloid developed as a result of the injury to the deep layers of the skin. After striking the left side of the thyroid carti-lage the bullet took a deeper course, wounding the left recurrent laryngeal nerve. There was only slight bleeding at the time, but the patient's voice was at once affected and was so hoarse that she could not speak above a whisper. She readily recovered from the immediate effects of the injury, and was referred to me by Dr. J. S. Gale, of Ivor, Virginia, on August 17, 1908. The bullet was located with the x-rays in the left side of the root of the neck, about half way between the clavicle and the outer border of the trapezius muscle. The patient could not speak above a whisper and seemed to have considerable difficulty in breathing. The condition of the larynx is described below in the report of Dr. Miller.

Operation was performed under ether August 20, 1908. The bullet was first removed, and an incision was made along the anterior border of the left sternomastoid muscle. The centre of the incision corresponded to the lower limit of the larynx. The sternomastoid, together with the carotid artery and the jugular vein, was retracted toward the left. The left lobe of the thyroid gland was exposed and was retracted along with the trachea and larynx to the right. The re-current laryngeal nerve was identified, where it runs in the groove between the trachea and esophagus. It was found to be injured just before its entrance into the larynx, and was involved in a small mass of scar tissue where the bullet had evidently grazed the nerve. The diseased portion, about one-third of an inch in length, was excised, leaving a small filament, which was probably the posterior portion of the sheath of the nerve with a few fibers that had escaped direct injury. The proximal part was freely loosened to relieve tension and the nerve was sutured with No. 0 twenty-day chromic catgut in a fine curved needle. Some muscular tissue was drawn over the sutured nerve. The skin was closed with interrupted silkworm gut. The patient had difficulty in breathing before the operation, and seemed to suffer from dyspnœa to such an extent that the anesthesia was begun with some apprehension. However, she stood the anesthetic well and reacted satisfactorily.

August 23, 1908, it was noted that the voice and dyspnea were the same as before the operation. August 29, 1908, the wounds had healed perfectly, but there was no improvement in speech. The patient was discharged August 29, 1908. The dyspnea disappeared before speech improved. On the last examination, November 16, 1909; the patient could breathe without difficulty.

Dr. Clifton M. Miller, professor of rhinology and laryngology in the Medical College of Virginia, and laryngologist to Memorial Hospital and to the City Hospital, examined this patient the day before operation and on two occasions since operation. I am much indebted to him for the examinations and for his reports.

August 18, 1908, the day before operation, he wrote as follows: "I have today examined the patient, Martha Johnson, sent by you for laryngeal examination. Her voice is extremely hoarse and produced with effort. Intralaryngeal examination reveals complete paralysis of the left vocal cord, except such tension as is given it by the action of the left cricothyroid muscle. It lies in the cadaveric position. During phonation the right cord in adduction passes the median line in an effort to approximate the left cord, which remains motionless. The larynx is much congested in the entire supraglottic region. *Diagnosis.* Complete paralysis of the left recurrent laryngeal nerve."

October 26, 1908, Dr. Miller made the following report: "I examined the throat of Martha Johnson on October 20, 1908, and found that there is some very slight movement of the left vocal cord in the part that was motionless at the time of my last examination, and there is less congestion in the larynx than was present at that time."

November 16, 1909, more than a year after his second examination, Dr. Miller wrote the following report: "I examined the colored woman, Martha Johnson, that you sent me for laryngeal examination a few days ago. There is almost perfect motility of her vocal cords, the left one lagging slightly behind the right in adduction, but the action of the laryngeal muscles indicates almost perfect recovery from the wound of the recurrent laryngeal nerve, with practically entire restoration of function. The voice, while entirely changed from the hoarse tone of my former examination, lacks much in volume. This is due to a web-like adhesion between the anterior third of the vocal cords, limiting the size of the column of air which can pass through the rima glottidis, and also the length of cord that can be thrown into vibration for voice production. Section of this web with prevention of adhesion during healing would, in my opinion, entirely restore the voice. The adhesion between the cord is due, I think, to inflammation set up by the passage of the bullet and the long period of loss of function of the left cord. From the standpoint of restoration of function by anastomosis of the severed nerve ends, the case is a perfect success."

DISCUSSION.

DR. EDWARD A. BALLOCH, of Washington, D. C.—I think Dr. Horsley is certainly to be congratulated on the results obtained in this case. As I remember it, it was some time after the injury to the nerve that the case was referred to him, and presumably the nerve was nearly if not quite completely degenerated, and I think to get complete restoration of function in a case like this a considerable period after the injury is decidedly a surgical triumph, and it ought to cause great encouragement in our operations upon the thyroid, where the great bugbear we have confronting us always is the possibility of cutting or injuring this nerve. If it can be sutured successfully and with good prospects of return of function, I certainly think it will help us a great deal in dealing with these thyroid cases.

DR. W. P. CARR, of Washington.—The length of time a nerve has been injured does not make much difference in the results of the operation. This has been clearly shown by Dr. Murphy, of Chicago. For a long time it was the opinion that it was useless to operate on a nerve that had been paralyzed for a number of years; but Murphy has operated on cases of long standing, and obtained good results. A year or two ago Dr. Shands and myself operated on a case in which the ulnar nerve had been paralyzed for a long time, as the result of a fracture, and function was promptly restored.

In operating for cancer of the neck in one case, I excised two inches of the pneumogastric nerve, which was tied up in the cancerous growth. After it was taken out, I found I had two inches of the entire carotid sheath, with the carotid artery, pneumogastric nerve and jugular vein. Yet with the exception of a whisper voice, which lasted for two or three days, there was no symptom from it. But in resection of the recurrent laryngeal nerve the effect on the larynx is more pronounced than after resection of the pneumogastric nerve. The same thing follows extirpation of the spinal accessory nerve. I have extirpated the spinal accessory nerve in cats a great many times. The effect on the larynx is much more pronounced than in resection of the pneumogastric nerve.

We can hardly see why this would be the case unless there is some transmission of nerve force from one nerve fiber to another. I think it is important in uniting nerves, if we do not make an end-to-end anastomosis, to make a free lateral incision, so that there will be no nerve sheath between the nerve fibers of one nerve and the other. A little bit of nerve sheath may block the impulse or prevent the nerve fibers from growing one into the other. If the nerve sheath is widely opened on both nerves the result may be very good. In Dr. Horsley's case the final result was good, and I congratulate him. As I understand, it was nearly a year before restoration of function took place.

DR. HORSLEY.—It was six months.

DR. CARR.—Under normal circumstances, where there is union of nerves, restoration of function is generally more prompt.

DR. HERBERT M. NASH, of Norfolk.—I have not had any experience in cases of this kind from the standpoint of operation, but I have in mind two cases that occurred during the

war between the States, in which I was certain that the
recurrent laryngeal nerve was injured by gunshot wounds.
No attempt was made to operate in any way. The wounds
were properly dressed and the patients were sent to the hospital. One of those men could not speak above a whisper for
eighteen months, and the other for a much longer period,
but both eventually recovered their voices, and I have been
always under the impression that the injury to that nerve
was not final, but that the function of the nerve was restored
itself by Nature, without operation. I wish to say that in
these cases the wounds of the larynx itself rapidly healed, so
that the loss of voice was purely from phonation. I think
that Nature very often, if the injury has not been too extensive in these cases, may restore the function of the muscles
of the voice.

DR. W. L. ROBINSON, of Danville, Virginia.—In a case
on which I operated I was impressed with the fact that the
operation upon the thyroid involves an immense amount of
care. It is not always necessary to bring the ends of the nerve
together to accomplish the end desired, but it is essential
to bring the anatomical structures nearer together, in order
to get the functional effects thereafter, as I can verify in a
case I had in mind to operate on for a cystic goitre. We all
know that cystic goitre can be enucleated, but where we have
the interstitial form there are adhesions everywhere, and we
simply bring the parts together to obviate trouble in the
severance of the nerves.

DR. CHAS. H. MAYO, of Rochester, Minnesota.—This is
an interesting subject to me, because there is no question
but what I have cut or injured in some way the recurrent
laryngeal nerve several times. Kocher says in earlier work
that he injured the laryngeal nerve in about 7 per cent. of
his thyroid cases. The only thing that must be considered
in the restoration of the voice is that there is a variable association of the superior laryngeal nerve with the inferior, so that
when the inferior is injured, or both inferiors are injured and
there is loss of voice for a time, the superior may take up a
good deal of the work; but the patient may develop a low
monotone when both inferiors are injured. When both
inferiors are injured for a time there is crowing respiration,
especially in sleep. I recall one case in which the loss of voice
was complete within a few days after operation, and that

patient crowed like a chicken. In doing thyroid work we should always examine the larynx before operation. It will be found that from 10 to 14 per cent. of these cases with fair sized goitres, or with small hard goitres, have paresis of one vocal cord. If they have paresis, and you remove that part of the thyroid which is producing pressure, within two or three days after the operation the voice may all of a sudden nearly drop out, or be abolished altogether, and may not return for two or three months. Such was the case in the patient just mentioned, who had paretic vocal cords for six months before operation. The traumatism to the vocal cord may show delayed paresis, while if you cut the nerve there is trouble right away. When you have injured one recurrent laryngeal nerve, after a time you will find that sound vocal cords will move freely across the middle line, and take up the work of the one that has been injured.

Dr. HORSLEY (closing).—In regard to the remarks made by Dr. Mayo, as he says, many cases of recurrent laryngeal paralysis occurring after a goitre operation are temporary. This is because the nerve has been injured or bruised, but not completely divided. We often see paralysis, which is apparently complete, follow a slight injury and then clear up in a few weeks. This has been noticed after musculospiral paralysis from pressure. If the nerve is completely divided, however, it is extremely probable that the paralysis will be permanent unless the nerve is sutured.

In regard to the possibility of the superior laryngeal nerve taking up the work of the inferior laryngeal, it is difficult to see how the superior laryngeal, which only supplies the cricothyroid muscle, can assume the functions of the more important inferior laryngeal, which supplies all the rest of the intrinsic muscles of the larynx. We must recall that the anatomical distribution of motor nerves is usually very definite and accurate, and it would be most unusual for one motor nerve to assume the function of another motor nerve without some form of nerve grafting. For instance, when the extensor muscles on the back of the forearm are paralyzed from an injury to the musculospiral, we never expect the intact median or ulnar to assume any part of the function of the musculospiral and supply a single one of the muscles normally controlled by the musculospiral. Similarly, we do not look for paralysis of the muscles of the face, caused by injury to the seventh nerve, to be relieved in any way by an overlapping of the motor nerve from the motor root of the fifth or from the twelfth nerve, which supply the adjoining muscles. It would seem most unlikely, then, that the function of such an important motor nerve as the inferior laryngeal can be assumed in a short space of time by the comparatively unimportant superior laryngeal.

Dr. Mayo has mentioned the tendency of the sound vocal cord to cross the mid-line, and thinks that this may account for an improvement in the voice. Such a tendency for the healthy cord to cross over toward the paralyzed cord was noted by Dr. Miller and mentioned in the report included in my paper. Even when this happened, however, the voice was still hoarse and the patient unable to speak above a whisper.

As to the question of repair of these nerves; if they are injured, as Dr. Nash spoke of, it seems to me we should apply the same rule to surgery of the recurrent laryngeal nerve as we do to nerves elsewhere. If a nerve is severed, by something like a bullet, it is very unlikely that it will regenerate, unless its ends are approximated. But we know that nerve ends if brought close together will regenerate and resume function. The question of operation in these cases would depend upon the permanancy of the injury. If it is demonstrated that there is improvement after a few weeks, operation is unnecessary. If these cases go on for months and no improvement is observed, they should be operated on. The case I have reported was operated on three months after the injury. There was no improvement then, and there was complete paralysis of the muscles supplied by the left recurrent laryngeal nerve.

I was agreeably surprised at the ease with which the operation could be done. The recurrent laryngeals on both sides are easily found, because there is nothing in that neighborhood between the esophagus and trachea except the recurrent laryngeal nerve.

TREATMENT OF WOUNDS OF THE HEART, WITH REPORT OF TWO CASES.

By Walter *C.* G. Kirchner, M.D.,

St. Louis, Missouri.

WOUNDS of the heart have for many ages been considered fatal, and it was not until within recent years that the surgery of this organ has been attempted. While cardiac injuries are comparatively infrequent, they are, however, of such seriousness that prompt surgical interference is demanded. It is for this reason that surgeons should be acquainted with a definite plan of procedure in the treatment of these emergencies.

The first surgical operation on the human heart was performed by Farina, of Rome, in 1896, and since this time the heart has come to be regarded as an organ amenable to surgical procedure, just as the other organs of the body. At the St. Louis City Hospital there have been five cases of cardiorrhaphy.

Two of these cases, in 1901, were operated on by Dr. H. L. Nietert, who was among the first in America to suture the heart. At the same institution Dr. Louis Rassicur, in 1903, had a case of heart suture with recovery, so that during my term of service opportunity was afforded of seeing and treating four cases. Of the five cases operated on, three made successful recoveries.

During the past two years I have operated on two cases of stab wound of the heart. The first case when received was in a critical condition and lived only four hours after the operation. The second case was admitted to the hospital under more favorable conditions, and his recovery was uneventful. The case histories are as follows:

CASE I.—The patient, W. S., a white male, aged thirty-seven years, a roofer by occupation, entered the City Hospital February 11, 1908, at 6.15 P.M., with the history of having been stabbed with a knife while fighting with another man.

Immediate Condition. When received in the emergency room it was evident that the patient was in a state of great shock. He was conscious, but drowsy and restless, and his face bore an anxious expression. He seemed to be suffering, and frequently cried out with pain. The skin and mucous membranes were pale, the body was cold, and he was in profuse perspiration. He complained of great thirst. The pupils were widely dilated and reacted slowly. No abnormal nervous reflexes were noticed. While being undressed the bowels moved voluntarily. The urine upon catheterization was found to be clear, but contained a trace of albumin and hyaline casts. The patient bled from the nose and from wounds in the chest and buttock. He expectorated a bloody mucus. The pulse was irregular, soft, and small, and the rate 86 per minute; respirations, 28 and regular; rectal temperature, 99.8° F.

Examination of Wounds. The patient had a contused and lacerated wound of the nose, which was the probable cause of the epistaxis. On the left side of the chest, in the fifth interspace and one inch external to the mammary line, there was a penetrating stab wound of the chest, which wound when explored with the finger was found to take a direction toward the heart and apparently to involve this organ. In the sixth costal interspace and one and one-half inches external to the wound just described there was a second penetrating stab wound of the chest. These wounds were about one-half inch in length, and the tissue surrounding them was emphysematous. Blood escaped in large quantities from the pleural cavity through these wounds, and over the lower and posterior portion of the chest on the left side the percussion note was flat. There was a third stab wound in the left gluteal region.

Diagnosis and Prognosis. With the pronounced symptoms of shock and hemorrhage and the location and direction of the wound in the chest, the diagnosis of stab wound of the heart was simple. It was also evident that the pleural cavity had been involved and that a traumatic emphysema was developing rapidly. The great degree of shock and hemorrhage combined with the nature of the wounds made the prognosis extremely grave. The only hope for life lay in the immediate control of hemorrhage.

Operation. As soon as the nature of the injury was ascertained the patient was prepared for operation. He was wrapped in hot blankets and heat was applied to the extremities. Ether anesthesia was preceded by a quarter of a grain of morphine. When the patient was well under the anesthetic, the operation was started and the administration of ether discontinued.

An incision through the skin at the outer border of the cardiac area and internal to the left mammary line was made, extending across the fourth and fifth ribs. From either extremity of this incision two other skin incisions were made, directed toward the sternum. With costotome, the fourth and fifth ribs were severed, and the intercostal tissues were readily divided with scissors. An osteoplastic flap was thus formed and by forcible traction the flap was reflected to the right, a hinge being formed near the sternal margin. This gave access to the cardiac region, but, inasmuch as the hemorrhage was profuse and ample room for quick work was needed, the sixth rib was also severed and retracted. The pleural cavity was almost completely filled with liquid blood and blood clots, and the heart was beating but moderately fast. There were two incised wounds in the pericardium, from which blood flowed very freely. The infiltration of blood into the pericardial and fatty tissue altered considerably the normal appearance of the cardiac area. The pericardial sac when opened contained mostly liquid blood. The heart was lifted from the sac, and near the apex of the left ventricle there was an incised wound, three-fourths of an inch long, which bled freely. When the heart was raised the left ventricle emptied itself through this opening and the heart stopped beating. As quickly as possible a silk suture was placed to close the opening. By compression and massage of the heart pulsations of the organ were reëstablished, but the heart beats now became considerably accelerated, and were perhaps from 140 to 160 per minute. This made suture of the wound very difficult. Interrupted silk sutures were used, care being taken not to include the endocardium. The heart was supported in the left hand. Mattress retention sutures were placed to relieve the direct tension on the suture line, and the spurting from the partially sutured wound was so forcible that it was necessary to use eight sutures to effectually close the wound. The heart was inspected and no other source of hemorrhage found. The pericardium having been cleansed, the heart was replaced and the pericardial incision closed with catgut. The ends of two of the heart sutures were left long and were brought through the pericardium and tied. A small gauze drain was placed in the pericardium and dependent drainage of the pleural cavity was established by means of a rubber tube. The wound in the chest wall was closed with catgut for the subcutaneous structures and silkworm gut for the skin.

While the operation was in progress the patient had received hypodermoclysis of saline solution, and this seemed not only to increase the volume of the pulse, but also to improve the heart's action. It was noticed that the lungs were not completely collapsed and that they would expand and contract with the respiratory movements. While suture of the heart was in progress, the patient, who had practically received no anesthetic during the operation, stated that he was thirsty, that he wanted a glass of water, and then asked for a can of beer. Before closure of the pericardium the patient made efforts at coughing, and the lung and heart were forcibly pushed into the wound in the chest. The operation was performed in sixty-five minutes. When the patient was put to bed his pulse was 118, of fair volume, and the respirations were 30 per minute.

He became very restless and ⅛ grain morph. sulph. was given. An hour after the operation the pulse was 96 and respirations 24; two hours later the pulse was imperceptible, respirations 28, shallow and short, and rectal temperature 100° F. The respirations became labored, and the patient died four hours after the operation, apparently from shock and hemorrhage.

At autopsy there was no blood in the pleural cavity or the pericardium. When the heart was carefully examined, a second and much smaller stab wound of the heart was found which had been overlooked at the time of operation. This wound opened into the left ventricle and was through the fatty tissues near the septum. The wound could not readily be detected, and it was all the more remarkable that, inasmuch as the cavity of the ventricle had been penetrated, there was no bleeding from this wound, indicating that the muscular contraction was sufficient to prevent leakage. The cause of death was attributed to shock.

CASE II.—The patient, M. L., a white male, aged twenty-four years, engaged as a mechanic's helper, was admitted to the City Hospital, August 22, 1909, at 12.40 A.M., with the history of having been stabbed in the chest with a knife about a half-hour before entering the institution.

He was well developed and well nourished, weighing one hundred and sixty-four pounds and of medium height. The patient had suffered with pneumonia and occasionally had attacks of bronchitis, but he had mostly been in good health.

When examined in the emergency room he was slightly under the influence of intoxicants. He was conscious, restless, noisy, and somewhat unruly. The skin was pale, the body was cold and in cold perspiration. The pulse was very feeble and irregular and the rate 96 per minute. At times the beats were strong, and then again almost imperceptible. Judging from the character of the pulse, it was evident that the heart was laboring under difficulty.

Examination of the chest showed a stab wound parallel with the fifth intercostal space and two and one-fourth inches below the nipple, the outer extremity being in the mammary line, and the wound extending inward for three-fourths of an inch. The wound was clean-cut, and no other injury was noticed. There was profuse hemorrhage from the wound, and his clothing was saturated with blood. The chest was carefully cleansed, and the wound was examined with the finger. The wound took a direction inward and downward, and the finger, entering the pericardium, detected a wound in the heart. When the finger was removed from the wound, there was a gush of blood which showed that active communication existed between the pericardium and the external surface. There was but little escape of air from the wound, and a pneumothorax did not seem to exist. The respirations, 24 per minute, were shallow, but regular. After the escape of blood from the pericardium the character of the pulse improved markedly. The diagnosis of stab wound of the heart was made and arrangements were made for immediate operation.

Operation. General ether anesthesia preceded by morphin and atropin, was administered. When the patient was thoroughly anesthetized, an incision was made between the fifth and sixth ribs extending from the stab wound to the left sternal border. A second incision was made upward from the outer end of this wound, sufficiently long to include the fifth and fourth ribs. The finger as a guide was introduced into the stab wound and the tissues in the fifth intercostal space divided toward the sternum. The pericardial and pleural attachments were separated with the finger from the ribs, and with the costotome the fifth and fourth ribs were easily divided. The third incision was directed inward along the third interspace, thus making a quadrangular, osteoplastic flap, with the hinge at the left sternal margin. There was no bleeding from the intercostal vessels, and the internal mammary artery was not injured. The opening was sufficiently large for cardiac manipulation, and the pleura was but slightly injured.

The incision in the pericardium was about two inches long, and was enlarged upward and downward. The pericardial sac was freed from blood and blood clots, and the heart lifted forward for inspection. A wound one and three-fourths inch in length was found extending obliquely across the left ventricle, the lower end being about one inch from the apex. Blood escaped very freely from the left ventricle, but the bleeding was controlled by placing the finger in the wound. Small tenaculum forceps were inserted at the lower end of the wound and the heart was thus gently suspended. Its own weight produced sufficient traction to cause the edges of the wound to coapt and to control hemorrhage sufficiently for the placing of the sutures. Three deep, interrupted sutures extending to the endocardium were placed, and hemorrhage now only took place in spurts. Seven intermediate sutures were necessary to completely control the hemorrhage. The line of sutures was reinforced by two mattress stay sutures, the ends of which were left long. The heart was carefully examined for further injury and none found. During the entire procedure the heart's action was regular, and no undue manipulation was made. The pericardial sac was carefully cleansed and the incision sutured with continuous catgut suture, leaving a small opening through which a guttapercha drain was placed. The long ends of the stay sutures were brought through the pericardium and were tied over it, hoping in this way to strengthen the wound in the heart. Fine chromicized catgut was the suture material used.

In the chest cavity old pleural adhesions were found, which not only prevented the lung from collapsing, but also made it difficult for the blood to enter the pleural cavity. Drainage of the cavity was, therefore, not indicated. The osteoplastic flap was put in position and the bones approximated. The pleura and muscular structures were sutured with catgut and the skin with interrupted silkworm-gut sutures. A small guttapercha drain was placed in the stab wound. The anesthetic was discontinued when the operation was started, and was therefore reduced to the minimum amount. The operation was performed in forty-five minutes. When he was placed in bed his pulse was weak but regular. His record showed, pulse, 132; respirations, 22; rectal temperature, 99.8° F.

Postoperative Course. On the day following the operation the temperature rose to 102.4° F, respirations 42, and pulse rate 120. He was restless, and small doses of morphine were given to quiet him. He explained that at the time of admission to the hospital he had a slight cough, and it became evident that a bronchopneumonia had developed in the left lung. The symptoms of pneumonia were present during the first week, but the patient complained of little distress. The drain in the wound had been removed on the second day, the wound itself practically healing by first intention. After the first week the patient felt well and was comfortable. After the second week he was practically well, but was not allowed to leave the bed until the end of the third week. His temperature, pulse, and respirations were normal.

Frequent auscultations of the cardiac area were made, but the heart sounds were always normal. There was also no evidence of pericarditis. Sphygmograms were made, and in each case the tracings were normal. An examination of the skiagraph of the chest shows perfect apposition and union of the severed ribs.

The patient suffers no inconvenience or distress as a result of the operation. He has since been hunting and fishing, and in a recent communication states that he is strong and in good health. (See Fig. 1.)

From a study of these cases and a review of the literature on the subject of surgery of the heart, one must be convinced that injuries to the heart can no longer be considered as invariably fatal, but that the heart may be manipulated and treated surgically just as any other organ of the body. In the treatment of these injuries it is well to bear in mind certain observations that have been made in regard to the nature of the wounds, the process of repair, the method of surgical attack, and the complications that may arise.

The principal injuries to which the heart has been subjected are those which resulted in puncture wounds, stab or incised wounds, gunshot wounds, or lacerated and contused wounds. Small wounds of the heart may prove fatal, but many heal without complication. Sudden death may result from injuries which involve the bundle of His, but the heart may without serious consequences be subjected to a greater degree of injury and manipulation than is usually supposed.

The great danger in injuries of the heart lies in the resulting hemorrhage, which usually proves fatal. If the myocardium alone is involved, the bleeding may be profuse, but it is usually greater when the cavities of the heart have been invaded. Wounds of the auricles bleed more profusely than those of the ventricles, the tendency of the muscular contractures of the ventricles being to close the opening and thus to limit the hemorrhage. With certain incised wounds of the ventricles, where the cavities were penetrated, blood spurted from the wound only near the termination of the systolic contraction. The amount of hemorrhage depends upon the blood pressure, the size of the wound, and the contractile force of the heart muscle.

Small wounds of the heart, even if they involve the ventricles, may heal spontaneously. Healing of heart wounds takes place by cicatrization, and the better the approximation the stronger the wound. Investigations have demonstrated that when the wound is properly approximated a true myocardial regeneration takes place. In wounds that are weak, or in wounds incompletely healed, aneurysm of the heart and rupture are apt to occur, and it is therefore safer and better surgery to suture all serious wounds of the heart than to trust to spontaneous closure.

In wounds of the heart the pericardium often plays an interesting and important part. If the rent in the pericardium is large, the sac may distend but moderately with blood and blood clots, hemorrhage taking place either externally or into the pleural cavity. When the flow from the pericardial sac is impeded, the sac will become distended, and hemopericardium results. Then the intrapericardial tension increases and heart tamponade results. The effect of this tension is felt first on the auricles, whose function is so impaired that the ventricles receive an insufficient supply of blood for the needs of the system. The heart's action becomes irregular, labored, and weak, and may cease entirely. The effect of heart tamponade can easily be detected by the pulse. When, after short duration, the blood or clot in the pericardial sac is removed, the activity and rhythm of the heart is usually restored.

The symptoms of a wound in the heart are usually those of hemorrhage and shock. The patients are, as a rule, not conscious of the wound in the heart, and suffer more from the results of the injury. They are anemic, restless, and anxious, and the body is cold and clammy. If they have lost much blood, they may be semiconscious, and usually complain of thirst. The pupils may be widely dilated. The pulse may be weak, irregular, or imperceptible. If heart tamponade is present, the volume, quality, and rhythm will vary from time to time, giving one the impression that the heart is laboring under great difficulty. The respiration may at first be but little altered, but when the lung has also been injured there is usually bloody expectoration. In stab wounds the diagnosis may frequently be made from the location of the wound and the character of the symptoms. However, in gunshot wounds the diagnosis may be more difficult. When the pleural cavity has been penetrated a pueumothorax results and the air will be forced through the wound. Emphysema of the chest wall may result, and sometimes a portion of the lung itself escapes through the opening in the chest. When the pericardial sac is but partly filled with blood, a splashing sound may sometimes be detected. The presence of blood in the pleural cavity may be detected by the usual signs of fluid in the chest. The diagnosis is confirmed by exploration of the wound with the sterilized finger or by exploratory pericardiotomy. The size of the external wound may be no index of the nature of the wound in the heart.

All wounds of the heart should be considered as serious, and death is due usually to shock and hemorrhage. When the peritoneal cavity has been invaded, and there is injury to abdominal viscera, the prognosis is extremely grave. In a list of 160 tabulated cases, Peck records a total of 102 deaths and 58 recoveries, a mortality of 63.7 per cent. It is to be hoped that with improved methods of technique and a more thorough understanding and appreciation of the nature of wounds of the heart, the mortality rate may be materially reduced.

In the treatment of wounds of the heart we should carefully consider the patient's immediate condition (shock and the effect of hemorrhage), the nature of the operation, the sources of infection, and the remote results. Great stress should be placed on the treatment of shock, which in these injuries is usually accompanied by great hemorrhage. The patient should be wrapped in hot blankets, and if restless he should be given sedatives (morphine) in small doses, repeated if necessary. The nature and extent of the injury should be definitely ascertained by exploration of the wound with the finger. The sense of touch is essential in determining the location and extent of the injury, and the finger serves a better purpose than surgical instruments. In suspected injuries to the heart, it is safer and better to perform exploratory pericardiotomy than to run the risk of a fatal cardiac hemorrhage. It should be remembered that strict asepsis is essential in the treatment of these wounds, and frequently the fate of the individual is sealed by the one who first examines the case. The location of the wound in the heart (auricular or ventricular) should, if possible, be determined so that a definite plan of operation may be decided upon. If heart tamponade exists, the condition should be relieved at once, either by following up the wound into the pericardial sac with the finger and letting out the blood, or by pericardiotomy. With the exploring finger the border of the heart should be located and definite information as to pneumothorax should be ascertained. Direct exposure of the wound in the heart is of great value, and the opening in the chest should expose the heart sufficiently to permit of satisfactory manipulation if necessary. If the wound is mediastinal and the pleural cavity has not been involved, we should be careful to avoid these cavities in opening the chest. The tissues should be carefully pushed from beneath the sternum and ribs with the finger, which should serve as a guide in outlining the flap. If the pleural cavity has been penetrated, less care is demanded inasmuch as a pneumothorax already exists. The nature and position of the wound thus often determines the location and character of the opening to be made in the chest. The pericardial opening should usually be enlarged to permit of easy manipulation and inspection of the heart. Stimulants and intravenous or subcutaneous injections of saline solution should not be given, as a rule, until methods of arresting hemorrhage are made possible. They are of special value when the loss of blood has been great. Time is an important factor in these cases, and the operation should be done as promptly and quickly as possible.

In most cases the operation is complicated by pneumothorax and the respiratory function is greatly impaired.

When the patient is unconscious the operation may be performed without an anesthetic. If a general anesthetic is to be used, ether will be found safer than chloroform, and usually but little anesthesia should be used after the chest has been opened. Local anesthesia is unsatisfactory, and may be dispensed with. By the administration of morphine and atropine a few minutes before the anesthetic is started, the amount of ether is materially reduced and the danger of postanesthetic pulmonary complication is lessened.

The cases are at times so desperate that while under observation or at operation the heart stops beating. When the heart has been arrested for a very short period and other signs of life have apparently disappeared, the heart has been encouraged to resume its contractions by gentle compression and massage of the organ. It seems also that the blood supply to the organ itself, as indicated by blood pressure, and the quality of the blood are of great importance in maintaining and controlling the heart's action. Therefore, artificial respiration should always be combined with heart massage and efforts be made to raise the blood pressure.

At operation it occasionally happens, when the heart is quickly lifted or manipulated, that pulsation suddenly ceases. This happend in Case I, and seemed to indicate that reflex action was an important factor concerned with the heart's action. By gentle compression, however, the heart was encouraged to resume its pulsations. However, in many cases the heart's action appears to be independent of the general nervous control and the heart seems to have the power and stimulus within itself to produce rhythmic contractions. In the treatment of these cases we should, therefore, not forget the value of heart massage as an aid in resuscitation.

The wound in the heart having been located, the method of approach through the chest wall must be determined, and for this purpose a variety of flaps have been used. A wound in the heart has been sutured through a wide intercostal space, but usually this is not possible. The flaps that have been mostly used open to the right or to the left, and are either entirely on the left side of the chest or extend across the sternum. The object should be to so construct the flap that easy access to the wound in the heart may be had with the least damage to the chest wall and the pleural cavities. The flap should be made with the finger in the wound as a guide, and this is especially necessary if the pleural cavities have not been invaded.

When the wounds involve the left pleural cavity, Spangaro's intercostal incision, with extension upward or downward along the margin of the sternum as seems necessary, is the one of choice (Fig. 2). ⸱ This incision is made in the fifth or fourth left intercostal space. By retraction of the ribs a view of the pericardium and pleural cavity may be had. If further space is desired after double ligation of the internal mammary artery, the incision may be extended upward or downward and the cartilages divided with costotome near their sternal attachments. The pericardium may be easily incised and wounds of the right and left ventricles can readily be repaired. If still more space is desired for the suture of wounds of the auricles or vessels at the base of the heart, the sternum may be divided, best with costotome, after separation of the underlying tis ues, and forcibly turned to the right, making a hinge along the right costal attachment. Care must be taken not to enter the right pleural cavity, or else a fatal double pneumothorax may result.

If a mediastinal wound is present and neither pleural cavity has been invaded, a flap involving the sternum with hinge along the right costal attachment is preferred (Fig. 3). This flap is of service in operations at the base of the heart. The underlying structures must be carefully separated from the under surface of the sternum and ribs, so that the pleuræ may not be injured.

A flap with hinge internal involving cartilages and ribs, as used in Case II (see Fig. 1), is of service in those cases in which there has been a preëxisting pleurisy and in which

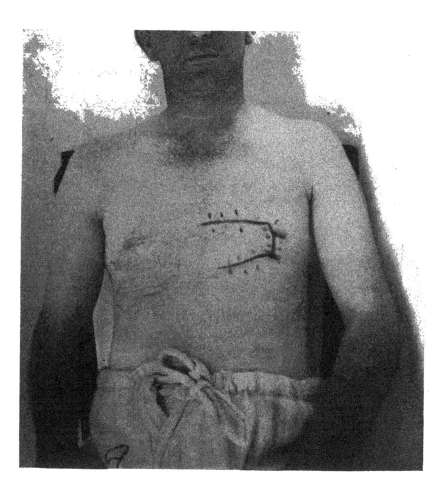

FIG. 1—Penetrating stab wound of the left ventricle of the heart, with recovery of the patient. (Author's case.)

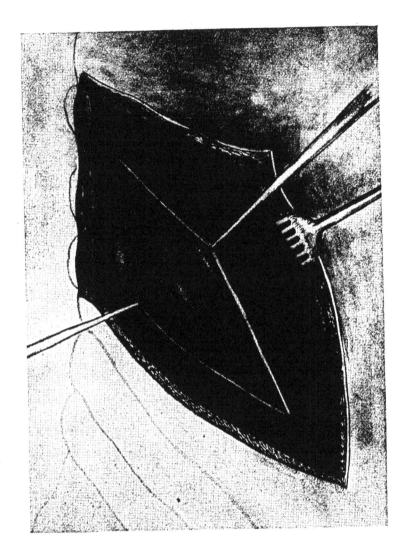

FIG. 2.—Osteoplastic flap made by modification of Spangaro's intercostal incision ving complete access to the heart for operations on the ventricles. Pericardiu ened.

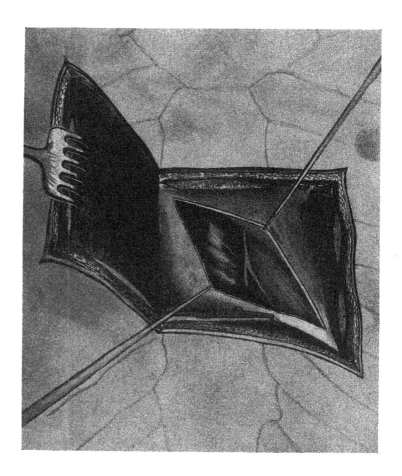

Fig. 3.—Sternal flap used in the interpleural route to expose the mediastinum, and of service in wounds of auricles and vessels at base of heart. Right auricle exposed.

the lung is bound by adhesions. These adhesions prevent collapse of the lung in pneumothorax, and should not be disturbed. This flap gives ample room for manipulation of the heart, but if more space is desired the incision may be extended across the sternum, with hinge at the right costal attachment.

In persons with narrow and long chests the flaps may be somewhat atypical, and in certain of these cases the heart is more centrally located. In these cases it may, therefore, be necessary to use flaps involving the sternum.

The hemorrhage from the wound in the heart is temporarily best on rolled by placing the finger in the wound. In incised wounds, if tenaculum forceps or traction suture be placed at one end of the wound and the heart be permitted to pulsate while thus suspended, the traction and muscular contractions tend to close the wound and limit the hemorrhage. It has been found that by this suspension it is easier to suture the heart wounds than if the heart were held in the hand. Interrupted silk or catgut sutures may be used. The sutures should be deeply placed, but not to include the endocardium. In large wounds, I believe there is an advantage in fastening the pericardium over the wound, as this by adhesion strengthens the wound and may tend to prevent aneurysm or rupture. Before closure of the pericardial sac, a careful search for multiple injuries should be made.

Inasmuch as many cases in which the heart has been sutured die from infection of the pericardium or pleural cavity, the matter of drainage has received special consideration. That this infection may be unavoidable and introduced at the time of injury there can be no doubt. It seems to be a wise plan to consider penetrating wounds as infected wounds and to promote drainage in these cases. Drains that do not drain are harmful, and often a gauze drain serves merely as a plug to enclose infection. Drainage can only be well accomplished when the external wound is kept open so that infectious material may be discharged through it. There must be an avenue of least resistance for the discharge of infection. If drainage is to be instituted, the external wound should be kept open. Rubber tissue as a drain will permit the discharge of infectious material and will not plug the opening. In my own experience I have found it best to drain the dependent portion of the pleural cavity when infection was anticipated. The pleural cavity, especially if the lung is partially collapsed, does not well resist infection, and therefore early drainage is desirable. It seems advisable not to completely close the pericardial sac, so that accumulations of fluid or infections may be discharged and not collected in the sac. It is a wise plan not to close the traumatic wound, but to leave it open for drainage. After all, the matter of drainage is largely a matter of personal experience.

In closing the wound catgut will be found best for the pericardium and muscular structures. It is safer not to close the skin wound too tightly, but to approximate the edges with interrupted sutures, leaving ample opportunity for drainage.

The chief postoperative complications are those associated with shock and hemorrhage, pneumothorax, pneumonia, and infection of the pericardium and pleura. Secondary hemorrhage occasionally takes place, and may prove fatal. Embolism also occurs, but not as frequently as may be supposed.

If the loss of blood has been great and the hemorrhage has been controlled, the extremities should be bandaged to confine the circulation. Saline solution, intravenously, by hypodermoclysis or protoclysis, should be given, or, better, if possible, direct transfusion of blood. One should guard against anemia of the brain, the effects of a lowered blood pressure, and an overdistended heart. Diffusible heart stimulants are indicated, and the restlessness should be controlled by small doses of morphine. The urinary and intestinal tracts should also receive careful attention.

CONCLUSIONS. The heart may be manipulated without serious injury to the organ, and is amenable to surgical interference and procedure.

Hemopericardium with heart tamponade is a serious complication, and demands prompt drainage of the pericardial sac.

In suspected injuries to the heart, the wound in the chest should be carefully explored so that the extent of the injury may be determined, and in cases of doubt, exploratory pericardiotomy is indicated.

Small wounds of the heart may heal spontaneously, but in all cases where hemorrhage from the heart exists, the wound should be promptly sutured.

In operations upon the heart when pulsations suddenly cease, massage of the heart and artificial respiration should be tried as aids in resuscitation.

With a minimum amount of anesthetic the healthy lung is capable of performing its function, though to a less extent, even when the pleural cavity is exposed.

Time is an important factor in injuries to the heart, and an early diagnosis should always be made. The immediate treatment should be directed to the control of hemorrhage and shock. The chief remote complications result from infections of the pericardium and pleura.

In treating injuries to the heart, the surgeon should have in mind a definite plan of attack, and the kind of flap to be used in approaching the heart should be determined by the nature of the wound in the chest.

REFERENCES.

Matas, Rudolph. *Keen's Surgery*, vol. v, 1909.
Ricketts, B. *M*. The Surgery of the Heart and Lungs, 1904.
Vaughan, G. T. Jour. Amer. Med. Assoc., Feb. 6, 1909.
Peck, C. H. Annals of Surgery, July, 1909.

DISCUSSION.

DR. HOWARD A. KELLY, of Baltimore.—I would like to ask Dr. Kirchner why the ligatures were left long in the suturing of the heart?

DR. I. S. STONE, of Washington.—I would like to ask why chromic gut sutures were necessary in this case. It seems to me union ought to take place promptly, and such a suture is a foreign body in fact.

DR. JOHN D. S. DAVIS, of Birmingham, Alabama.— While I have had no personal experience in the treatment of wounds of the heart in human beings, I have done a good deal of experimental work on dogs. All of our gunshot wounds of the heart were fatal. In stab wounds of the lower part or apex of the heart a large percentage of the dogs were saved. I would like to ask the doctor as to the advantages of this larger incision, of which he spoke. We are unable to save any cases where the coronary artery was cut. We found the continuous suture preferable to the interrupted suture. We have had one case of knife wound of heart reported by Dr. Hill, of Alabama, which was sutured with success. I do not recall a case of gunshot wound of the heart successfully sutured. A double or through-and-through wound in the heart is usually fatal. Knife wounds in that part of the heart easily reached are susceptible of relief.

A thing we discovered of great value in our experimental work was the advantage in massaging the heart. After the dog was apparently dead and the heart had ceased beating, massage of the heart would cause it to begin beating again. This led us to utilize massage of the heart in our cases of anesthesia. Sometimes we would kill a dog with chloroform, and after being apparently dead for an hour we could resuscitate the animal by massage or kneading the heart between the finger and thumb. There is another point to which I desire to call attention: in suturing the heart it is difficult to hold the organ, but by picking up the pericardium with forceps, the heart may be lifted up into the opening in the chest and sutured with continuous suture. The continuous suture has the advantage in that it enables you to more quickly close the wound, with less traumatism.

Another point in the treatment of our cases was this, that

we closed with few exceptions without drainage; in the cases we drained we had serious trouble. Of course, this is not applicable in man; where you have infection, drainage is a necessity. Drainage is required in practically all cases in man I would think, and but little was learned from experiments on the dog. I would ask the doctor as to the relative value of the continuous and interrupted sutures. Again, I would ask him why he leaves the ligatures long, and does not cut them short?

DR. JOHN YOUNG BROWN, of St. Louis.—I wish to accentuate that part of the paper that has been brought out by the essayist, namely, the importance of exploring certain wounds of the chest. During my service at the City Hospital in St. Louis we had 536 cases of gunshot and stab wounds of the chest and abdomen, and, as has been pointed out here in the report of these cases, it is not infrequent that wounds of the heart are complicated by other injuries, and neglect to repair these injuries early would lead to fatalities.

One particular point that has been impressed upon me is the frequency with which the chest can be laid wide open, without complicating in any part the operative work. I have had 16 cases in which I have sutured the diaphragm, and in these 16 cases the opening of one side of the chest did not in any way complicate the operative work. A stab wound of the chest may not only injure the heart, but may open the pleura and injure the diaphragm. The same may be said of gunshot wounds of this type. To repair a wound of the heart and neglect a wound of the diaphragm is not good practice, because a penetrating wound of the chest and a penetrating wound of the diaphragm are necessarily penetrating wounds, not only of the chest, but of the abdomen, as I have shown in a number of cases. After repairing the injury to the diaphragm, on investigation we would find visceral perforations, and in these cases we have considered them not only as penetrating wounds of the chest, but penetrating wounds of the abdomen as well.

As to acute pneumothorax, I think the profession is under the impression that it is dangerous to open the chest. I recall one case operated on by Dr. Kirchner, where the chest was laid wide open by a knife wound, the diaphragm cut, the stomach was prolapsed into the pleural cavity, with a wound in the stomach, and the patient took an anesthetic without any trouble. We sewed up the wound in the diaphragm, and during the operation the lung could be seen partially functionating. There was no complication from the opening of the chest. In dealing with these cases (combined injuries of chest and abdomen) it is necessary to open not only the chest, but the abdomen. If we have a stab wound, and it is demonstrated that this wound penetrates the pleura and penetrates the diaphragm, we should assume that something has been perforated in the abdominal cavity and it is necessary not only to explore the chest, but to explore the abdomen. The exploration of the abdomen does not add in any way to the danger, because you already have the pleural cavity filled with air, and if you explore through the abdomen the minute you open the abdomen air will come in the chest through the wound in the diaphragm. In dealing with injuries to the heart and pericardium it is very essential to find out if there are injuries to the diaphragm; then, if there are injuries to the diaphragm, before the work is completed, the abdomen should be opened and an exploration should be made, and the viscera in the upper abdominal cavity, the stomach particularly, should be examined.

I think the subject is an exceedingly important one, and I am convinced from my experience in work of this kind that we hesitate too frequently to make explorations in this type of cases. In injuries of the abdomen explorations are made quite frequently, but not as frequently as they should be. There is a proneness on the part of the profession to wait for symptoms, and in many of these cases symptoms develop late. I have had cases in which there were sixteen or eighteen perforations of the bowel, with practically no shock, because there was no hemorrhage; symptoms in such a case would mean peritonitis, and terminate fatally. I have seen injuries of the diaphragm with prolapse of viscera into the pleural cavity, where the diagnosis was made with the greatest difficulty, and could not be made in time to accomplish anything except by an exploratory operation.

DR. ALBERT VANDER VEER, of Albany.—I have just two thoughts in my mind, one of them a little reminiscence, and the other is, I am profoundly grateful that I have lived long enough to listen to so excellent a paper upon a subject that has been in my mind for many years. Just beyond here (Hot Springs, Virginia) during the Civil War was fought the Battle of the Wilderness. When it was supposed that Meade and Grant had retired to Rappahannock, an order was given by Grant that the Second and Third Corps should advance at 5 A.M., and from that time until 1 P.M. we received 1900 wounded into our First Division hospital. They were brought in and placed along in rows where we had a temporary hospital in the woods, those of us who were at the operating table having assistants who were told to bring in the cases that were bleeding—the cases that required immediate ligation of important arteries or who had chest wounds. I have notes of these cases, and I have a recollection of those chest wounds in which we took care of wounds of the lung most satisfactorily, and the men recovered. I have had a chance to learn since that a number of these old soldiers made good recoveries in caring simply for wounds of the lung itself. Some of the wounded were obliged to wait until we could do the work necessary, and word would come back that such and such a man with a chest wound was dead. He had died of internal hemorrhage. We had a chance to examine some of the cases in which the heart had been wounded. The minnie balls were different missiles from what we see at present. In our First Division hospital service we discussed this subject with a great deal of care and thoroughness, and at the Battle of Gettysburg we had up for discussion the treatment of gunshot wounds of the heart and pericardium. After the war I was called to see a young man who was shot with a number 32 pistol ball, and I made the diagnosis of pistol wound of the pericardium, but very little was done at that time in regard to exploration of the chest. In watching the patient he improved. After twenty-four hours he got better, but he developed all the indications of pus within the pericardium. I aspirated it, and withdrew sixteen ounces of pus. He was comfortable for a week afterward. I wanted to open his chest as we did open the chest in some of our cases of gunshot wounds of the lung, but could not get the consent of his parents. I endeavored to impress upon them that he undoubtedly had pus in the chest. He was the only child, and they were very much attached to him, and would not consent. Matters went on from bad to worse. A second aspiration of the fluid afforded some relief, but shortly afterward he died. At autopsy, which was permitted, I found the bullet lying within the pericadium. We could have operated on that boy, and I believe, with the knowledge we had then of gunshot wounds of the chest, he would have recovered.

About that time my thoughts were turned in another direction, and in the development of abdominal surgery in our section. Wounds that had been inflicted at 1 or 2 A.M. I did not feel like going out to see the patients, and sent my assistant. But in our particular neighborhood I have known of but a few cases of pistol wounds of the pericardium or heart, or stab wound.

Papers like the one to which we have just listened bring us the greatest comfort and satisfaction. It is just along these lines and by the reports of such cases we will reach this kind of surgery.

In regard to opening the chest, I think the doctor has been quite conservative in regard to the size of the wound, and while I have not had any experience in these cases, I believe a good free opening is important.

I think Dr. Davis brought out an excellent point with reference to bringing up the pericardium. Most operators in the course of their experimental work upon the heart adopt a method making use of the continuous suture, which will enable one to get through quicker, and in holding up the pericardium in that way it seems to steady the heart, and you can complete the operation more in comfort.

DR. SAMUEL LLOYD, of New York City.—There is one point Dr. Kirchner made which interested me in this connection, although I have not had any experience with stab wounds of the heart. When he spoke, in the first case, of recovery of function of the lung, it brought out and emphasized some experimental work I have been doing for a good many years, and have been triyng to get my colleagues to take up in connection with surgery of the lung. I agree with everything Dr. Kirchner said in regard to action of the lungs in these cases.

As to the point Dr. Vander Veer makes of having plenty of room, I think we have been deterred from the fear of pneumothorax. My experience is that pneumothorax does not amount to anything. The collapse of the lung is absolutely under the control of the surgeon at the time. It depends entirely upon the degree of anesthesia. If you keep the patient completely under the anesthetic, you do not get as good a response. Take the case of Dr. Kirchner; his patient was only moderately anesthetized. If you keep the patient under mild anesthesia, so that he will respond to irritation of the pleura, you can get the expiratory push of the good lung. It will push out the collapsed one; every time you expand the incision through the pleura, the lung will push out of the opening you have made. There is no risk of pneumothorax. We need have no dread in opening the chest just as freely as we need for any operative procedure. If I may be allowed to wander off into another subject, I would like to say a word or two in speaking of a case of cancer of the lung that I had an opportunity to operate on a year ago last May. This patient had a recurrence of cancer of the breast, and with this recurrence the ribs and pleura were involved. I took out the ribs and pleura, together with the growth, making a flap from the abdomen to cover the opening that I made in the chest. I excised three ribs, and took the pleura with them, comprising an area of three and a half inches square or more. I then discovered that there were two nodules in the lower lobe of the lung each about the size of my thumb-nail, one inch and a quarter apart. I finally decided to remove these, and picking up the lung, grasping its lower lobe in my hand, with scissors I cut out these nodules in one piece, thus making an opening in the lung about the size of the palm of my hand. I controlled the hemorrhage by pressure, keeping the patient under complete anesthesia, so that the lungs would collapse during the operative procedure. I took a lock-stitch, closing the opening closely, and of course the woman had a traumatic pneumonia which lasted for a few days. Two or three weeks later I removed some supraclavicular glands, and now she is well, so far without another recurrence of the disease.

Dr. J. Stanley White, of Washington, D. C.—I was in hopes that some one would say something about the diagnosis. My experience has been limited to three cases. Of these three cases, one had perforation of the ventricle; the other two had a perforation or incisions in the myocardium. The one with a perforation through the ventricle recovered after operation. The other two patients refused operation, and died. These cases emphasize the importance of operation in all cases in which there is a probable diagnosis of injury to the heart. Injury of the pericardium is an indication for operation. There were no adventitious sounds present. One man died after getting out of bed two hours after the injury. The other man died after a trip on a train of forty miles, when, in stepping off the train, he died, following a rupture of the myocardium due to the injury.

The incision for operation should be a large one. After my experience with one operative case, I do not hesitate to advise, and would practise in a case that came to me in the future, a larger incision than the one I resorted to. In the case I operated on I resected two ribs, but I realize now it would be better to have resected four ribs. The danger is not in the operation itself; it is not in the suture of the heart, nor the difficulty of the operation, but it is infection afterward. The danger is from infection almost exclusively, and I question the advisability of drainage.

Regarding the suture, I prefer the interrupted mattress suture, because the continuous suture is likely to pull out. The overlapped mattress suture is better. In those cases which apparently die on the table, I would recommend that the wounds be closed regardless of whether the heart is stabbed or not, and massage practised. Even in a patient who is apparently dead, after operation, with suture of the heart and heart massage, we may perhaps save one case out of a hundred, and if this can be done it is certainly worth while.

Dr. Stephen H. Watts, of Charlottesville, Virginia.— I want to mention a case of stab wound of the heart which I operated upon about a year ago. The patient was a young negro man, who had been stabbed a short time before I saw him, the stab entering the third interspace to the left of the sternum. If I had had the benefit of this paper at that time I would have dealt with the case in a much better manner. I did not turn down a flap, but took out portions of the third and fourth ribs and opened the pleura. I found the pleural cavity and pericardium full of blood and an opening in the base of the pulmonary artery. The wound was small, being less than a centimeter in length. The boy was in bad shape, and I could not feel his pulse when I first saw him, but it improved somewhat after an intravenous infusion of saline. This being my first experience with wounds of the heart, I was rather excited, and I am afraid I sutured the wound too hastily and perhaps not carefully enough. The boy died at the end of a month, and at the autopsy we found the pericardium distended with a blood-stained fluid, with extensive adhesions between the heart and pericardium.

I mention this case to emphasize the importance of listening to papers of this character, because we never know when we will have an opportunity to carry out the technique.

DR. JOSEPH RANSOHOFF, of Cincinnati.—I have but one suggestion to make in regard to overcoming the difficulty of holding the heart. My experience has been limited to one case, and that was a gunshot injury. These injuries are usually more serious than stab wounds. The difficulty of controlling the heart while putting in the suture is entirely eliminated if we do with the heart what we do with the tongue, namely, put a suture through the apex. With a silk suture through the apex of the heart not going deep enough to enter the ventricle, you can throw the heart from one side to the other and get at any part of it without any difficulty. It is simpler than holding the heart through the pericardium. In that case we had no difficulty in getting at and suturing the heart through the two openings, one in front and one behind the ventricle. We sutured the openings, turning the heart from one side to the other to insert the sutures. That patient had a fatal hemorrhage which came from one of the vessels at the root of the lung.

DR. KIRCHNER (closing).—In reply to Dr. Kelly's question as to why the sutures were left long, I was misunderstood. From my knowledge of rupture of the heart after suture and from observations after opening up the wound after a subsequent operation, I think it would be best in such cases to reinforce the line of suture by using a mattress stitch. The wisdom of such a procedure has been illustrated by the case that has just been related, in which, after the patient was discharged, some time later the rupture of the heart took place. The patient on whom I operated has been hunting and fishing in Colorado, and does not seem to be in any way affected by the suture. This reinforcement of the suture line may be made, I think, just as Dr. Kelly recommends, in anchoring the kidney so that the pull is not directly on the line of suture, but on the muscular structure. These sutures having been made in the heart, the ends are left long, and are brought through the pericardium in such a way that when tied the pericardium is in contact with the heart and suture line. This procedure reinforces the line of suture and helps in strengthening the wound. The long ends of the sutures are then cut short. In regard to the suture material, the most successful cases that have been reported are those in which either silk or catgut were used. Fine chromicized catgut would be safer because we cannot always depend upon absorbable catgut. Sometimes the plain catgut absorbs too quickly, and chromicized catgut is preferable.

The second case I saw was one of gunshot wound of the heart, in which the patient made a recovery. I have also seen a specimen of heart in which the organ was penetrated by the bullet. A clot had formed in the pericardial sac, and complete healing of the wound in the heart had taken place. The patient died years after of some intercurrent disease, so that gunshot wounds of the heart are not always fatal, but they are more difficult to handle than incised wounds.

Massage of the heart, I think, is very important, and in cases where the heart stops beating we should not give up until we have given this method a trial. The first case reported illustrated the value of massage. After the sutures were placed the resuscitation was obtained by gentle massage and compression of the heart. It is important, however, that this procedure be accompanied by artificial respiration.

. Infections are the chief complications to be guarded against in these cases, and the treatment by drainage I think is a matter of individual experience. By that I mean that certain operators will drain in such a manner that they will avoid the results of infection. If the infectious material is already present, we ought to get rid of it. If it is not present, drainage should not be instituted in a manner to carry any infection into the wound. Gauze is not a good drainage material to be used in these cases. All we wish to accomplish in the initial stage is to give the infection an opportunity of leaving the body. It is necessary to keep the external wound open, to have an avenue of least resistance, so that infection may come away. The opening for drainage into the pleural cavity in these cases should not be so large that air passes with each inspiration or expiration, but it should be so placed that the fluids may have a chance to drain away.

In regard to Dr. Vander Veer's statement as to gunshot wounds of the chest, Dr. Dalton, of the City Hospital, St. Louis, has emphasized the fact that gunshot wounds of the chest are best treated by confining the chest. But, of course, if the heart is injured we have other complications, and they should be met. The opening in the chest should be as large as possible, and for that reason I think the incision I have mentioned and described should be recommended. By extending the intercostal incision in the Spangaro flap as far back as necessary, and by increasing it upward or downward along the sternum, we have complete access to the pericardium and to the heart, and especially to the right and left ventricles. The intercostal incision may be made very long. Or, if the injury is at the base of the heart, and we wish to suture the vessels there, we can enlarge the opening by cutting across the sternum. It is for this reason that I think Spangaro's modified incision is better than the other. It does less damage to the chest and will by modification give us complete access to the heart.

I am very much interested in Dr. Lloyd's observation, and it is entirely in accord with my own. It is for that reason I mentioned maneuvers of the lung during the anesthetic. The sound lung fills itself, and when the patient is not thoroughly anesthetized the air from the sound lung is forced into the lung complicated with pneumothorax, and we have not those difficulties that are ordinarily mentioned in pneumothorax. For that reason I wish to emphasize the need for a less amount of anesthetic in operations of this sort.

A number of successful cases have been reported in which the continuous suture was used, but certain operators have thought that continuous sutures were not as useful as the interrupted sutures. It was found at autopsy and in certain other cases that these sutures occasionally had sloughed away. If sloughing takes place following the use of the continuous suture, then, of course, union would not be as firm. It was for that reason I felt interrupted sutures were better than continuous sutures.

As to the method of handling or manipulating the heart during the operation, I wish to say that in the first case I had hold of the heart in the hand, and I found it unsatisfactory. The method I describe in the second case, I think, is very much like the one described by Dr. Ransohoff in principle, namely, instead of grasping the apex of the heart I used at once a tenaculum forceps, which resembles in effect a traction suture. The forceps catches the heart wound, and the weight of the heart itself will coapt the edges. The interrupted sutures are then placed and the long ends can be used as handles, thus making manipulation of the heart unnecessary.

SKIN GRAFTING.

By Arthur C. Scott, M.D.,
Temple, Texas.

THE results of skin grafting with large Thiersch and Wolfe grafts are, under favorable conditions, so uniformly good, it would at first appear that the art had reached such a state of perfection that nothing was needed to insure any better results, and yet failures do occasionally occur in the hands of surgeons of large experience. The failure of one or two large grafts may add one or two weeks or more to an already prolonged convalescence, and repeated resort to grafting invariably subjects the patient to much anxiety and discomfort. For these reasons, we have thought worth while to present for your consideration any steps which, though small, may tend to insure a still larger proportion of successes. The chief causes of failure in skin grafting may be summed up in a few words: (1) Suppuration and the presence of sloughing tissue. (2) An excess of blood, lymph or serum. (3) Failure to keep grafts in close contact with the exposed capillary bloodvessels of the wound. (4) Disturbing grafts when they are young and tender.

When, for any reason, time will not permit sufficient preparation to insure against either of the first two causes mentioned, one should not expect too much from large grafts, for the exudates cannot escape freely, and by accumulating between them and the raw surface may prevent sufficient contact to secure union. This is probably the reason some surgeons have better success with small (Reverdin) grafts and continue to give them preference.

PREPARATION OF WOUND. Careful preparation of the wound is of great importance. When the wound is in ideal condition, most any sort of graft will take hold and grow, but it is often difficult to get a wound in an ideal condition. When suppuration exists, it should be reduced as much as possible by removing the sloughing tissue with a scalpel or scissors, and by use of the curette, hot irrigations, and antiseptic applications.

When the time has arrived for grafting, if the surface of the wound is covered with small, healthy granulations, having good capillary circulation, and giving only a slight discharge, it will need no further attention, and the less done for it immediately preceding operation, the better.

If the granulations are large and pale, they should be smoothly excised with a sharp scalpel, leaving no loose pieces of half living or sloughing tissue. The wound should then be rinsed with salt solution and covered with a compress wrung out of salt solution until active oozing has ceased.

CUTTING GRAFTS. When a general anesthetic is not required, local anesthesia may be used on the limbs with considerable satisfaction by injecting $\frac{1}{8}$ to $\frac{1}{4}$ per cent. Schleich's solution, rainbow fashion, with the convexity downward, as shown in Fig. 1. To reach most cutaneous nerves, it should be injected both superficially and deeply into the subcutaneous fat. This procedure does not prevent pain altogether, but moderates it to such an extent that it may be readily tolerated by the average patient. For holding the skin and flattening the surface while cutting grafts, we have found nothing quite so good as the edges of two metal-box lids, or a metal box and its detachable lid. These nickel-plated articles are found discarded about nearly every surgeon's office, and serve a good purpose also for handling the grafts after removal. It matters but little whether the grafts are cut with a razor, amputating knife, or a knife made for the purpose, so long as the instrument is sharp and the operator knows how to use it.

When grafts fail to grow, it is frequently found that they are ballooned up with an excess of pus, blood, or other exudates, completely separating them from the capillaries beneath. To overcome this, we have, for several years, been perforating large grafts for drainage. At first we perforated the skin with an old fashioned scarrifier, having about 16 blades, before the grafts were cut. The scarrifier was difficult to keep clean, and finally got out of order, and we found that we could perforate them very well after they were cut and spread on a sheet of rubber tissue, which was placed on a box lid, with a gauze pad intervening. Holding the rubber tissue on which the graft is spread raw side up, with thumb and finger, a straight, narrow, sharp bistoury is plunged through it, sharp edge up, until the point of the bistoury penetrates the graft, rubber tissue, and gauze pad, and glides on the surface of the box lid (Fig. 2). A dozen or more slits are thus quickly made in each large graft. Wolfe grafts are not easily perforated by this method, and should be incised before being removed.

The perforated Thiersch grafts, spread on rubber tissue, are cut with scissors in sizes and shapes to suit the field to be covered, and when inverted upon the wound permit excessive exudates to escape through the perforations corresponding with those in the rubber tissue, which is often left in contact with them.

As the grafts are being smoothed out upon the wound, it is best to spread them laterally, to widen the slits and insure good drainage (Fig. 3).

DRESSING. The open method of dressing a grafted wound is very good, because of the tendency of the wound to remain dry. However, it is at a disadvantage in the presence of much exudate with nothing to hold the grafts down. Many layers of good absorbent gauze, cut the size of the wound, laid on separately, held in place by narrow strips of adhesive plaster, makes a splendid dressing. When soiled, each layer of gauze can be peeled off in separate

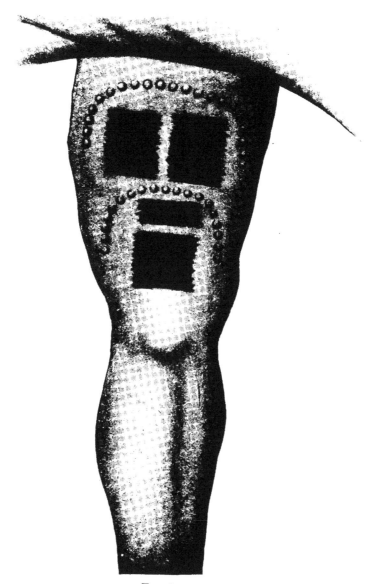

Fig. 1

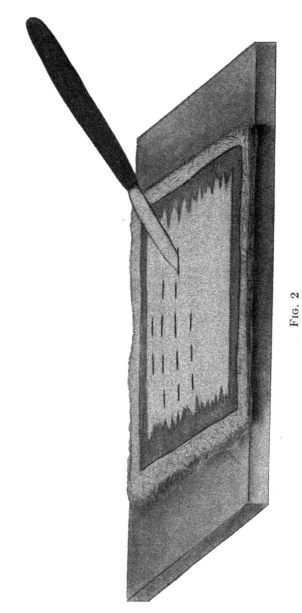

Fig. 2

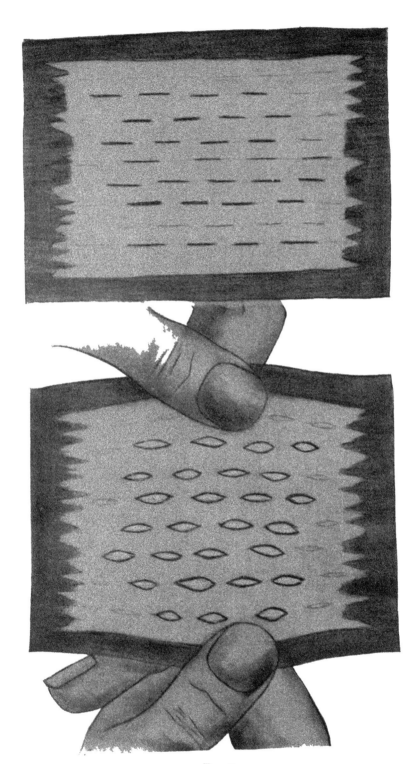

FIG. 3

slips until the last one is reached without disturbing the grafts. The last layer is moistened with salt solution, and left under a wet compress for a few hours, when it readily turns loose. Many strands of horse hair, loosely laid and evenly distributed across the grafted wound before the gauze is applied, will promote drainage to the margins of the wound and facilitate removal of gauze dressing. The same sort of dressing may be applied whether or not the perforated rubber tissue is left in contact with the graft.

DISCUSSION.

DR. JOSEPH PRICE, of Philadelphia.—In the early part of my professional career I studied several specialties. In the University of Pennsylvania I served in the orthopedic department with Dr. Willard for a considerable time, putting on Sayre jackets and treating various deformities. I did many other things. I practised in the alleys and courts of Philadelphia. Unfortunately I got hold of half a dozen bad burns in one winter. About the only places where sound skin remained was beneath the garters, where three or four thicknesses of clothing existed. Large areas of skin were burnt off, so that these patients lost about all their skin. This interesting and valuable paper, to which we have listened, reminds me of some of the early and interesting contributions. I have no doubt whatever that a paper by Richard J. Levis, on the same subject, written a great many years ago, contained many points similar to those mentioned in this paper.. For instance, in his allusion to the preparation of the wound, even the great Levis pointed out the importance of leaving it open to the desiccating influence of the air after placing the grafts. With the exception of a knowledge of salt solution, the practice of skin grafting more than a quarter of a century ago was precisely the same as it is today. In the cases I had I asked for boys and girls to donate skin, and I made a toilet of the extensive wounds and burns with boiled and distilled water. I bought the distilled water at drug stores. As I have said, large areas of skin were burnt off, and some of the patients were not only septic but delirious. I made these simple toilets, and the surfaces looked for all the world like these interesting drawings which you see. For instance, I used a woman's sewing needle and a sharp knife with which to remove the skin grafts. I simply picked them off after shaving and cleansing the areas with soap and water and alcohol, and with other sterilizing agents used at that time. I would sterilize the arm or the leg or the surfaces of those parts donated by boys and girls. Those donated surfaces of skin were carefully sterilized. I picked up these skin grafts with a sewing needle. It was a practice of value to me. I could shave off a delicate skin graft without hemorrhage; then I placed them in rows of one hundred or more. I left them open to the desiccating influences of the air. I protected these skin grafts in various ways, sometimes with medicines and lint. At that time barber's salve and lint were used in surgery. I got beautiful results.

The one suggestion of the use of horsehair is an error, I think, because horsehair is quickly bridged over by granulations, and when you leave them they will cause hemorrhage and injure the wound.

You will find the paper of Richard J. Levis, an early teacher and practitioner of surgery in the old Pennsylvania Hospital and Jefferson Medical College, a very interesting contribution on this subject, which should be read in connection with the paper to which we have listened. I allude to the history of this interesting subject to show you that the advanced thinkers and workers and past masters in surgery have not forgotten the good old things in surgery.

DR. ALBERT VANDER VEER, of Albany.—I want to ask a question of the fellows here present as to what their experience has been in using skin grafts from colored people for white people. A number of years ago my brother-in-law, Dr. N. S. Snow, and I had an extensive burn to deal with, following an explosion of gasoline, in which the face, neck, and both hands were severely involved and required skin grafting. At that time the simplest method was used, one similar to that referred to by Dr. Price, just using Clover's needle and a sharp scalpel to remove the graft. This can be done quickly, and with very little bleeding from the donor. Our students and friends of the patient became tired, because the amount of grafting was so extensive. We got a colored boy, who was willing to part with some of his skin, and we had no knowledge as to the effect it might produce. The injured man afterward became a prominent citizen. We used three hundred and fifty grafts from the colored boy. It was interesting to watch them. They would grow quickly as colored grafts for two weeks, then the pigmentation would disappear, and one could not tell the difference in the white grafts from the colored grafts. I speak of this, as I would like to know whether anyone else has had a similar experience.

DR. RANDOLPH WINSLOW, of Baltimore.—I have not had any personal experience in this matter, but in a book on surgery, written by Mr. Thomas Bryant, of Guy's Hospital, London, which was in vogue in the eighties, there is mentioned the case of a white man in Guy's Hospital who had ulcer on the leg. There was also a negro patient in the ward, and Mr. Bryant took grafts from the negro and placed them upon the ulcerated surface of the white man, and they grew, but the grafts from the negro remained pigmented, so that, as he says, there was a bond of union between the two persons subsequently. That is mentioned in Mr. Thomas Bryant's book on *Practice of Surgery*, which is not well known to the men less young than some of us.

DR. F. GREGORY CONNELL, of Oshkosh, Wis. — With reference to the grafting of extensive surfaces, I wish to offer a suggestion in regard to the source of the material. Considerable skin may, without difficulty, be removed from the abdomen during the course of the ordinary laparotomy. I have recently utilized such material for grafting, and found it to be very satisfactory and practicable.

DR. J. M. T. FINNEY, of Baltimore.—I am very much interested in this subject of skin grafting, because I have had frequent opportunity to make use of skin grafts in the class of injuries that have been described. I do not know of any one particular maneuver in surgery which is more time saving, and which gives greater satisfaction to the patient, than the question of skin grafting.

Dr. J. Staige Davis, of Baltimore, has been making some interesting observations along the line of skin grafting. He has already published one or two articles on the subject, and in a forthcoming contribution will make some additional observations which will help to answer the question that Dr. Vander Veer asked. I have had the opportunity of seeing a number of interesting cases of my own, which have been grafted by

Dr. Davis. He has made quite an extended series of grafts from colored skin, and transferred them to white patients; he has also taken the skin of white patients and transferred the grafts to colored people, and he finds that in a comparatively short time, varying a little in different individuals, and also somewhat with reference to the thickness of the grafts, the pigment disappears in those grafts that are grafted on white people, and that where white skin is grafted upon colored individuals the pigment appears.

We have used for many years the silver foil tissue, first employed by Dr. Halstead for these cases. I know of no dressing which gives as much satisfaction as this.

DR. JOSEPH RANSOHOFF, of Cincinnati.—I simply rise to say with reference to grafting the entire thickness of the skin, that it was first done by Wolfe. A flap of the entire skin transplanted is by very many people called the Krause flap. Of course, it is said that the Germans claim everything, and this flap is called the Krause flap, not only in Germany, but in France. Once in a while you will see in the literature a concession made, and it is called the Wolfe-Krause flap. In reality, it was made some forty or forty-five years ago, for the first time, by an ophthalmic surgeon in Edinburgh.

I have used the dry method almost altogether, and recently I had one case in which a very large epithelioma involved the parotid region and the ear, so that when excision was made it was rather a superficial epithelioma, following tuberculosis or lupus. The lupus had continued for years, and became epitheliomatous. We resorted to excision, and part of the parotid as large as my hand, involving the lower part of the ear, was removed, and skin grafted over the entire surface and dressed by the dry method. We used a cage or frame after the manner described by Dr. Finney, and the patient made a very excellent recovery. This cage was not a comfortable thing for the patient to lie upon.

I do believe that there is something new in the perforating of large grafts, as recommended by the essayist, and I can see where the Wolfe graft would have a decided place.

Experiments similar to those referred to by Dr. Finney were made many years ago by a surgeon who had a large number of colored people in his hospital service. We had twenty-five years ago results that are now being found so interesting at the Johns Hopkins, namely, white grafts placed upon colored people, and colored grafts placed upon whites. These experiments are among the primitive ones which one would naturally be inclined to make with skin grafting by the Reverdin graft.

DR. J. SHELTON HORSLEY, of Richmond, Virginia.—My experience has been that Thiersch skin grafts upon burns or deformities following burns may take and permit the surface to heal, but contraction reappears. In these cases I believe the grafting of the whole thickness of the skin alone prevents contraction. We cannot use a Krause graft or a Wolfe graft in large quantities, because of the fact that the whole skin requires a large amount of nourishment; whereas a Thiersch graft is very thin, and but a very small amount of nourishment is needed to sustain a considerable area covered with these grafts.

DR. GEORGE W. CRILE, of Cleveland.—About two years ago I accidentally noted in several cases the impossibility of making successful isodermic grafts upon cases of cancer in which the cancer had not been entirely removed. That is to say, given a case of cancer of the breast, with a very large wound to cover, isodermic grafts would not grow, provided there was metastases in other parts of the body. I placed isodermic grafts alongside autodermic grafts, and observed death of the isodermic grafts and active growth of the autodermic. In some instances there has been a temporary growth followed by dermatolysis.

DR. THOMAS S. CULLEN, of Baltimore.—Dr. Connell's experience prompts me to say that recently while doing an Emmet operation at the Johns Hopkins Hospital, the assistants asked me to preserve the strips of vaginal mucosa. These pieces, which vary from 2 to 5 mm. in breadth and from 5 to 8 cm. in length are now regularly saved and turned over to the general surgical department to be used as skin grafts.

DR. SCOTT (closing).—Relative to the matter of preparing the field of operation, as suggested by Dr. Price, I beg to say that no originality was claimed. In fact, I claim very little originality for any of the steps mentioned in my paper, except for perforating skin grafts for drainage. However, the method of anesthetizing the skin from which grafts are to be taken without a general anesthetic we have not seen used by anyone else, and we feel that it is of real value where a general anesthetic is not required.

Judging from the question asked by Dr. Ransohoff, I do not think the method of using local anesthesia is clearly understood. The drawing on this side (referring to diagram) does not show plainly, but it is intended to represent an inverted half-circle, which is designed to be so located that the cutaneous nerves, which are distributed from above downward, shall be reached, and carefully anesthetizing the skin, first getting little white blebs all along and then going over the field a second time, making injections of the anesthetic fluid rather deeply. By using a very weak solution a large quantity may be used. In that way, a large area below may be sufficiently anesthetized that the skin grafts may be removed without very much pain.

With reference to perforations, we are not sure, but we think we are original in that, because we have not known of anyone who used perforations deliberately for the purpose of draining grafts before we read a paper upon this subject before the State Medical Association of Texas four or five years ago. Since we adopted that step we have found great improvement in our results, because we believe by that means we have been successful in keeping the grafts in contact with the raw surfaces underneath, which is rather essential for success.

Dr. Price raised some objection to the use of horsehair. I wish to call attention to the fact that we have not recommended small Reverdin grafts at all, and we would not think of using horsehair in a case where Reverdin grafts were used. It is only where large Thiersch grafts or Wolfe-Krause grafts are used that horsehair is of any real value. The horsehair may be laid smoothly across the wound and a dressing applied on top of that, and the horsehair may be lifted out readily so long as the grafts practically cover the entire field. Horsehair can be lifted out without disturbing the grafts at all, and its presence will prevent the gauze from sticking very closely.

Those who attended the meeting of the American Surgical Association, held at Baltimore, in 1901, will remember the beautiful illustrations that were given showing the method of skin grafting following amputation of the breast, as done by Dr. Halstead, and I shall never forget how I was impressed by the beauty of those silver foil layers as they were rapidly placed upon the grafted wound. As soon as I returned home I had an opportunity to try that method, and it seemed to work well. At first, I got fairly good results; but I noticed that when wounds were discharging more than they should to be in an ideal condition for grafts, I found the discharge would lift up the silver foil in great chunks. That was not altogether satisfactory, but I continued to use silver foil in a number of cases. Finally, I ran across a case in which I did a breast amputation, laid the chest wall absolutely bare, and the intercostal muscles were showing very plainly, and the fibers were prominent in places, and when I used silver foil in that case I found weeks and weeks afterward great chunks of silver foil caught in the meshes between these intercostal muscles. I had a very hard time in getting that wound to heal. From that day to this I have not used silver foil. I have had better results from perforated rubber tissue or tissue in narrow strips and dressings as described in the paper.

I have not made any special observation with regard to the matter of grafting cancer cases, as alluded to by Dr. Crile. It reminds me, however, of one case of grafting which I think is of some value to mention in this connection, and that is, grafting upon the pleura. In one case in which I did a very extensive Schede operation, where, after the chest wall had collapsed, there was a strip of pleura two inches wide and no less than seven or eight inches long, which terminated above in a large sinus extending up into the axillary space, and it seemed impossible to get the wound to heal over. Finally, I used grafts in accordance with the method I have described, and succeeded in covering the pleura very nicely with large perforated grafts, and the patient soon made a complete recovery.

CIRCUMSCRIBED SEROUS MENINGITIS OF THE CORD.

By John C. Munro, M.D.,
Boston, Massachusetts.

An interesting paper on this subject by Spiller, that appeared in the *American Journal of the Medical Sciences* for January, 1909, explained a condition which I had observed a number of times at operation, and for which I had previously obtained no satisfactory explanation. At the time of my earlier cases (1897) I reported the findings to pathologists who not only gave me no light on the subject, but even questioned the existence of the lesion. In a small collection of cases of laminectomy reported at the American Medical Association, in 1904, I called attention to one with syringomyelia and to another diagnosticated as subacute fracture dislocation in which I found a "collection of clear fluid under a distinct arachnoid membrane," in which "the removal of this fluid produced marked amelioration in the pressure symptoms." This phenomenon and the relief that followed the removal of a soft extradural myeloma in another case led me to say that "there is a something that produces grave paralysis that is demonstrated clinically, which appears totally inadequate and for which we have no corresponding experimental nor postmortem explanation."

That the lesion had been observed by Krause and a few others was unknown to me at the time. A clinical lecture by Horsley appearing soon after Spiller's paper has stimulated me to report my own cases in detail and to examine the scant literature upon the subject in the hope of arousing surgical interest in a class of patients that otherwise would be condemned to a slow, inevitable, and distressing death.

Von Bruns, in 1908, said that "in more recent times operation has shown that there is a form of disease difficult of interpretation, but which can mimic in a most classical manner tumors of the dura—a meningitis serosa circumscripta." In February, 1909, in a most valuable clinical lecture published in the *British Medical Journal,* based on an experience with twenty-one cases of this type—valuable because it gives general conclusions founded on a broad experience and because it is not a tedious analysis of cases—Horsley says that "many cases of so-called acute myelitis are meningeal in origin, and a laminectomy may arrest the whole process and later injury to the cord."

The disease when it comes to operation is almost invariably considered to be tumor. At present there seems to be no sharp line in diagnosis between the various types of subdural lesions, but greater familiarity with the signs and symptoms of serous meningitis will probably enable the diagnostician to detect it with reasonable accuracy.

No writer has reported a large experience with this form of lesion. As mentioned above, Horsley has seen 21 cases; Krause, in 1907, reported 6 out of 22 operations for supposed tumor. Other writers (Oppenheim, v. Bruns, Mendel and Adler, De Montet, etc.) report one or two cases each.

The lesion is found more frequently in the middle decades of life. Horsley had one patient under the age of puberty, v. Bruns one sixteen years old, and my youngest patient was fourteen. Horsley's oldest patient was sixty.

The earliest mention of this type of disease that I have found is by Schlesinger, who reported, in 1898, a case of hydrops meningeus dying from intercurrent disease, in which he found an intradural cyst adherent to the dura and compressing the cord. The symptoms were typical as we know them now. Undoubtedly other cases had been reported earlier than Schlesinger's, but the important point is that the significance of the lesion was not properly recognized until about 1900 by Horsley, Krause, and a few others.

The case reported in 1903 by Spiller, Musser and Martin is the first one mentioned in American literature so far as I can discover.

The pathology has been demonstrated better in the living than in the dead. But few autopsies are recorded, and then rarely in connection with the symptoms. Schmorl demonstrated a mid-dorsal cyst removed post mortem, full of fluid and compressing the cord. Of two fatal cases mentioned by Horsley, in neither were the nerve roots much affected "so that it is easy to understand that there may be independent paraplegia and yet no absolute anesthesia anywhere." One of his cases died of cardiac syphilis and the other, unoperated, died of a meningogliosis (sclerosis).

In typical cases one finds at operation a tense dura probably not pulsating. When this is opened a small quantity of cerebrospinal fluid escapes under slight pressure, while immediately the dural slit is filled by a thin, more or less opaque pial membrane that bulges forth under tension of the contained fluid. This fluid is clear and spurts forth as soon as the membrane is opened, when the latter flaps back and forth as a definite curtain, attached to the dura and cord and more or less to the nerve roots. This membrane can be dissected out in great part, as in one of my cases, or it may be removed intact without being opened, as in Schmidt's case, when it appeared as a sausage-shaped cyst 7.5 by 1.5 cm., with blunt boss-like projections. The wall in his case was found to consist of dense connective tissue lined on the inner surface with a single layer of flattened epithelium. The membrane has been described as similar to the loose subcutaneous tissue that forms in Schleich's infiltration anesthesia, a "milk-like opacity," as it were.

In a few reported cases this definite membrane formation has not existed as such or else has been overlooked. In all of my cases it was distinctively present. When not reported or not identified there seems to be a localized collection of fluid under abnormal pressure. De Montet examined the fluid and found only lymphocytes and leukocytes and some large mononuclear cells like large phagocytes. He found no plasma cells nor bacteria. The cerebrospinal fluid drawn by lumbar puncture from Case I of my series was sterile.

The extent of adhesions apparently varies, and it is not always clear why the fluid tension should be so localized. In some cases a probe can be passed beneath the pia in one direction without obstruction, while in the opposite direction it is blocked by light adhesions. In other instances a true cyst is found. The cord is reported as flattened in some, while in others it is not obviously narrowed.

No causation definite and common to all cases is known. A case reported by Oppenheim and operated upon by Lexer and one of v. Bruns' cases was secondary possibly to a spinal caries. In Case VII of my series there was a healed spinal tuberculosis. Mendel and Adler's patient had well-marked apical tuberculosis. Syphilis has been present in several cases, including one and possibly two of my own. In this respect it is important to bear in mind that in no case of this sort has antisyphilitic treatment been of any value; rather has it been harmful. In the postmortem examination of a syphilitic case by Schwartz there was found diffuse cervical and dorsal meningitis, with adhesions of the dura, degeneration of the cord, and destruction of the posterior roots. The anterior columns were compressed by a meningeal cyst. In the anterior horns were cavities without gliosis.

Ströbe showed a postmortem specimen of serous meningitis in a case dying of chronic leptomeningitis. He suggests some inflammation in the cord, meninges, or bony spine, or a gliosis, as a cause. Furthermore, an extensive degeneration of the columns or a syphilitic meningitis may serve as a primary cause. At the autopsy of my case dying of operative septic meningitis no primary cause could be found for the serous meningitis.

In several cases, among them that of v. Bruns, no local or general cause could be demonstrated. Schlesinger found a serous cyst in a case dying of multiple cerebrospinal sclerosis, and the lesion has been found in a patient dying of typhus (spotted fever).

Krause has reported at great length a case following gunshot wound of the spine, with subsequent necrosis and abscess. Unfortunately he did not open the dura sufficiently to demonstrate the pial membrane, and the case, in spite of his findings, is not thoroughly convincing. To be sure he punctured the very thick opaque dura, evacuating clear fluid under abnormal pressure, but relief to symptoms had already followed evacuation of an epidural abscess, much as I have seen it follow the evacuation of a soft myeloma pressing or rather resting on the outer surface of the dura. On the other hand, a strong argument that a neighboring infection may act as a cause is seen in the localized serous cerebral meningitis secondary to middle-ear infection (Quincke), and which clears up as soon as the primary cause is eliminated.

Serous meningitis may be found in glioma and syringomyelia whatever the interrelation of the two conditions may be.

Horsley speaks of influenza as a cause, and De Montet's case followed a bad cold (coryza). The former also mentions the fact that a gonorrhea occurred relatively near the onset of symptoms in some of his cases.

That trauma with and without serious damage to the cord may be an exciting cause is shown in Bliss' case and in two of my cases. Oppenheim says, however, that serous meningitis of this type is not a sequela to concussion or to railway spine.

Joachim believes that the condition may be primary in the pia, as shown in a postmortem examination where there was thickening of the pia and of the dura, the latter apparently being secondary. Krause maintains that "disease of the arachnoid leads not only to the formation of adhesions and increased exudation, but the power of absorption at the diseased area, if not wholly impaired, is at least diminished."

Finally, whatever the cause or causes may be, it is important for us to remember that conditions of this sort do exist; that they closely imitate the conditions produced by tumor, and that the outlook under early surgical interference is good, while the outlook under a policy of non-interference is fatal.

The results from operation where no grave primary lesion exists are very good. Improvement may be relatively rapid or quite slow, according to the duration of the lesion and the extent of the damage inflicted upon the cord and nerve roots. Recovery may be aided by electricity, massage, and passive motion, as emphatically demonstrated in one of my cases. Spiller, Musser and Martin's case was well in two months after operation, Mendel and Adler's in five months, while a case of v. Bruns', with returning function two weeks from operation, required twenty months to bring about recovery that was almost complete.

Oppenheim reports a case dying on the table from the shock of a long operation, and one of my cases died within a few days from operative septic meningitis.

A patient of Horsley's operated upon in 1899 is well now. My cases operated upon in 1902 and 1906, both without attendant deep lesion of the cord, are well at the present time.

With recovery certain minor symptoms or signs may persist without impairing the patient's usefulness. Such are localized atrophies, increased reflexes, lack of complete joint extension, etc.

There seems to be but little reaction from operation in the average case. Spiller, Musser and Martin's case exhibited clonic spasms, with evacuation of the subpial fluid. A similar phenomenon I have not seen reported elsewhere, nor have I encountered it in any of my own spinal work. All authorities agree that spontaneous recovery does not take place, and

Horsley is convinced that he has not infrequently found a localized meningitis as the essential if not the sole cause of the paralytic symptoms.

A sufficient number of cases have not been reported to enable me to venture upon the question of differential diagnosis. To quote briefly some neurological authorities will be sufficient here. Oppenheim states that in gliosis we find wanting the cramp-like muscular spasms which are so frequent in tumor and which appear so early in pressure of the cord. In syringomyelia we look for trophic disturbances in the bones and joints, with bowing of the spine and a slow, dragging course with remissions. According to Joachim, "decision on the differentiation between tumor and an inflammatory process depends whether we can establish a propagation of the process upward." Horsley speaks of the unilateral origin in most cases, a condition that must be recognized at the outset. It will be well to take up the symptoms individually as recorded by the various reporters.

Pain. This symptom is practically always present. It may affect the back, the neck, the scapula, or the extremities. It may shoot into the breasts or may appear lower down in the trunk as a typical girdle pain. All patients, however, do not complain of the latter, and exceptionally when present it will be increased on coughing or be relieved on change of position. Pain often starts and is treated as a lumbago. One patient complained of unilateral pain in the penis and scrotum at coitus.

When in the extremities it is described as tearing, burning, or crawling, and according to Horsley it is in the limb substance itself. One of my cases described his sensations as though his thighs were immersed in boiling oil.

Horsley calls attention to the diffuse area of pain as an important diagnostic guide, the pain area in tumor being referred rather to one nerve root.

Paralysis and Paresis. Paralysis often begins as a weakness of the lower extremities or a weakness and stiffness that is unequal on the two sides. Some patients with scarcely any premonitory symptoms suddenly fall down while walking or rising from a chair, and from that time become more or less paraplegic. Spasticity generally co-exists, often appears early, and patients will exhibit a paretic-ataxic gait. A light form of unilateral paresis may be found, or a paraplegia or paraparesis may be complete except in one toe or a foot. As in one of my cases, the paralysis may be spastic at one time and flaccid at others.

Incontinence of the urine and feces singly or combined may or may not be present. Loss of power in emptying the bladder or rectum may be due to a paralysis of the abdominal muscles. When the lesion is in the upper spine the upper extremities may suffer more or less paralysis. In my third case the paralysis of the upper extremity was associated with marked atrophy, while a corresponding degree of atrophy did not exist in the paralyzed lower limbs. The dorsal spine seems to be the region most frequently involved, however.

Spasmodic involuntary muscular spasm is frequently seen, and it may be worse at night. A spasm may be precipitated by light stroking or rubbing of the skin, and sometimes it affects the flexor, sometimes the extensor muscles. In one of my cases the adductor spasm of the thighs was so great that it was almost impossible to separate the knees by main force.

The *reflex phenomena* vary very much in individuals. They may be normal, absent, or generally increased. At times a Babinski will be present on one or both sides, sometimes absent on both sides, or it may fluctuate in the same individual. Patellar clonus may be present on one or both sides, while the ankle clonus is absent. In Case I of my series the ankle clonus was present on one side, slight on the other, while the knee-jerks were increased on both sides, while in Case IV, in which there was complete anesthesia, the knee-jerks were present, but the ankle clonus and plantar reflexes were absent. In Case VI the knee-jerk and the ankle clonus were exaggerated on one side and absent on the opposite side. The Achilles reflex may be absent or present. So with the abdominal reflexes. In short, the presence or absence of the various reflexes varies greatly judging from the reported cases, and individually the different signs may vary during the progress of the disease.

Sensation. We may find normal sensation; anesthesia of the involved area; anesthesia of one area, such as the trunk, and hyperesthesia of another area, as the lower extremities. Anesthesia may be present but irregularly distributed on the two sides. Horsley states that anesthesia may be absolute, always relative, and sometimes only slight, though distributed over a large area. He also points to the parallelism that exists between tactile anesthesia and the deficiency of the secretory system, as shown by the administration of pilocarpine.

Patients often complain of numbness as one of the earliest symptoms, appearing about the same time as the initial weakness or paraparesis. Hypalgesia may be followed by hypanesthesia, and thermal hyperesthesia may be found.

A sharply defined border of sensation may change from time to time, and De Montet states that the behavior of sensation at different examinations is possibly characteristic of the disease. "Hyperesthesia over a large area speaks against tumor where there may be a marked zone at the upper limit of anesthesia or an area corresponding to the nerve root or roots on which the tumor is situated" (Horsley). Occasionally there is hypersensation in some localized area. Trophic lesions are absent and atrophy may be. Two of my cases with trophic lesions had deep lesions of the cord, glioma or crush.

Myosis, astereognosis, irregular temperature (Schmidt), and coitus without ejaculation are rarely present. Horsley has seen herpes but once. Vasomotor symptoms are absent.

We may find tenderness on pressure over one or more spinous processes, but this tenderness is not increased on motion.

The onset of symptoms may be short or long (three and a half years in Joachim's case and almost nine years in my Case V), and any patient may exhibit an abeyance of symptoms for quite a period.

There is no way to estimate except roughly the time that elapses between the onset of the primary cause and the formation of the pial membrane. In my case of longest onset, nine years, the membrane may have existed from the beginning or it may have formed about two years before operation when the acute symptoms arose. On the other hand, the membrane was definitely formed at the longest sixteen days after the causative trauma in Case IV, while in Case III (traumatic) it could have formed nine weeks before operation.

There is no evidence that family history has any bearing on the disease.

Treatment consists in early laminectomy. Nearly every writer condemns lumbar or local puncture as a therapeutic measure or even as an aid to diagnosis except negatively. Early operation would probably relieve most if not all cases suffering from serous meningitis. Mere evacuation of the subpial fluid with or without excision of the pial membrane, with or without drainage, has brought relief in one case or another. Horsley irrigates the canal with bichloride solution, exceptionally using a solution as strong as 1 to 1000 or 1 to 500. He closes the wound without external drainage, and after healing advises mercurial inunction over the wound area as an absorbent. Whether this is always necessary is doubtful; it, however, can do no harm.

A very brief consideration of my cases is in order before concluding.

Case I, as autopsy showed, was one of glioma and syringomyelia, there being a dilated central cavity in addition to local lateral cavities in the cord. The abscesses in the cord were evidently secondary to the bedsores. The latter probably accounted for the chills and irregular temperature.

In spite of the fatal central lesions. I think it fair to assume that some benefit followed evacuation of the local collection of serum.

Case II was clinically diagnosticated as syringomyelia, but in the absence of trophic and joint manifestations I am inclined to the diagnosis of glioma. It is unfortunate that at the second operation I did not open the canal above rather than below the original opening. I believe more relief would have been obtained thereby.

Case III demonstrated that a serous meningitis may be secondary to trauma. In view of his recovery, which was complete except for slight atrophy of the forearm, I think it fair to assume that there was no serious cord injury at any time, while Case IV demonstrates that an irreparable crush of the cord may co-exist and will prevent a complete recovery after operation for a serous meningitis.

Case V was most unfortunate in every way. Had he not been infected at operation there is every reason to believe that recovery would have been complete. In searching for the origin of this and other cases of infection in our clinic at that time, we found that the 70 per cent. alcohol used in disinfecting the operative field and the hands, taken from the original container, gave positive cultures. Since then we have discarded the use of alcohol in our preparations.

Case VI has been a most satisfactory one when his paralytic condition is considered, but his final recovery must be credited in great part to the tireless after-treatment. I could not explain the profuse hemorrhage that took place at the first operation. No pial nor dural vessels were injured; the hemorrhage seemed at the time to come as a result of sudden relief of tension, as is occasionally seen in the abdomen and other cavities tensely distended.

CASE I.—Robert McV., aged thirty-two years, entered Dr. G. W. Gay's service at the Boston City Hospital on November 12, 1897. The history is as follows:

Gonorrhea nine years ago. Denies syphilis. Moderate

use of alcohol. Was strong and healthy up to one year ago, when he began to have neuralgic pains in his head and shoulders lasting for ten weeks and then moving downward to the middle of the back. The pain was constant, but worse at night, sharp and spasmodic at times, or dull and aching. He had girdle pain, and complained of formication and numbness in his feet and legs. At first he walked with a cane, later with crutches, and finally, two months before entrance he became bedridden.

For six months there had been dribbling of urine and some fecal incontinence. At entrance there was no control over bladder or rectum, and the paralysis of the lower limbs was nearly complete.

Dr. W. N. Bullard examined him at this time and made the following notes: Diminished sensation below the fifth interspace in mammary line reaching back to the sixth on the right and the eighth on the left. Diminished sensation in lower extremities. Subjective numbness in both legs, ankle clonus present on the left, slight on the right, knee-jerks increased.

In addition it was noted that there was general weakness of both lower extremities without absolute paralysis except in dorsal flexion of the left foot. No muscular spasm. Slight patellar clonus on right side. Plantar reflexes good; cremasteric reflexes present, but diminished. Abdominal and epigastric reflexes absent. Pupils equal and reacting to light and accommodation. Arm reflexes not increased.

Lumbar puncture gave sterile fluid. Smears negative.

A few days later Dr. Bullard made a second examination, and reported that the sensation to touch and pain at about the level of the fifth ribs in the mammary line and at the sixth dorsal spine was diminished about equally on both sides. This diminution in sensation involved the entire trunk, where it was well marked. Sensation reappeared at the right groin and somewhat over the entire right lower extremity, though it was probably somewhat diminished in places over the right leg. In the left lower extremity sensation was markedly diminished over the patella and along the crest of the tibia, and apparently somewhat so along the inner surface of the thigh and leg. On the whole, it was less good in the left than in the right, though over both lower extremities it was apparently delayed, and the patient did not always know how to answer.

Operation was arranged for November 29, but the patient became suddenly ill with chill and high temperature, rapid pulse, and vomiting. On November 30 I operated, my notes stating that at the time there was cystitis, and bedsores, and that he had had occasional chills for some time.

Under ether I removed the fourth to seventh dorsal laminæ inclusive, and opened the dura the entire length of this space. At first there was escape of considerable clear fluid. The dorsal vein of the cord appeared a little more distended than normal. In the lower half of the incision there was a thin, opaque, white film apparently in the pia and slightly adherent to both the cord and to the under surface of the dura. A probe passed in all directions failed to disclose any tumor. The upper three fourths of the dura was closed with catgut and the external wound closed with silkworm gut, allowing for a temporary rubber tissue drain at the lower angle. The wound was previously flushed out with bichloride solution and salt solution. There was no shock.

December 2. Patient not as well as on first day, both temperature and pulse being elevated.

4th. Stitch abscess. Stitches removed. Bedsores over sacrum and left trochanter. Patient feels a puckering sensation in skin of legs below knees. Has gained control of the bladder. Some subjective improvement in motion and sensation of legs.

8th. Worse. Much pain, requiring morphine. Has chills and most exhausting sweats. Is very weak. Wound looks well.

16th. Improvement lately. Wound clean.

23d. Much improved. Has very little pain and can move his toes a little.

January 2. Very comfortable. No pain. Has been on an air bed, and the bedsores are better.

12th. Chilly sensations, with temperature varying from 100° to 105°.

20th. About the same. After this he rapidly grew worse and died January 29. At autopsy only the spine was allowed to be opened. Report by Dr. F. B. Mallory. After describing the wound and external parts it says: Spinal canal completly filled by distended dura. On slitting up the dura in situ the cord was found to be enlarged and closely applied to the dura, which was adherent to it over the dorsal and lumbar regions. The pia in this part of the cord much thickened, fibrous, and œdematous. The enlargement of the cord began about 7 cm. above the cauda equina, and extended upward as far as the cord could be removed in the cervical region. Section of the cord in the cervical region showed two cavities each several centimeters in diameter, occupying apparently that part of the cord where the gray matter ordinarily belongs. At the lower end of the cord there seemed to be swelling and edema around the central canal for an area of 2 or 3 mm. The cord was hardened and numerous sections were made, the concluding diagnosis being syringomyelia, glioma, and streptococcic abscess of cord.

CASE II.—Charles A. B., astronomer, aged thirty-seven years, was seen in consultation with Drs. B. Tenny and W. N. Bullard on July 29, 1898. Patient first noticed weakness in his lower extremities about two years before the time of my visit. As the weakness increased he was obliged to use crutches, but for the last year paralysis had been nearly complete. He suffered intense pain, describing it as though his thighs were immersed in boiling oil. He had taken morphine regularly for this pain.

Dr. Bullard's notes on examination are as follows:

Spinal muscles in lower back tense. The seventh dorsal

spine is tender to pressure at times. Knee-jerks much increased. Ankle clonus marked on both sides. Paraplegia of both lower extremities, though he can stand with the help of a chair. Sensation to touch and pain is not impaired. Heat and cold cannot be felt well below the level of about the seventh nerve. Galvanic sensation is diminished at a little higher level (fifth or sixth nerve in front and back). No reaction of flexor cruris to galvanism. All superficial reflexes of abdomen and cremasteric reflex absent. Plantar reflex not tested on account of the spasm.

Diagnosis of tumor of cord in upper dorsal region or of syringomyelia was made.

On August 3 I operated, and found the sixth and seventh dorsal laminæ quite hard and ivory like, no opening between the two being found. The fourth to seventh laminæ inclusive were removed. The dura appeared to be normal, and on being opened a normal quantity of serum escaped. Pressing up through the opening was a translucent pial membrane, the pulsation of which and of the cord was less than normal. On opening this sac a large quantity of clear fluid spurted forth under considerable pressure and continued to flow until quite an amount escaped. As the fluid escaped pulsation of the cord returned, and the pial membrane floated back and forth on the wave of serum with respiration. In the pia on the left side were two veins in addition to that on the median line. The cord looked and felt normal. A probe carried upward and downward detected nothing abnormal. Fluid escaped from both the upper and lower ends. There was no evidence of pressure beneath the ankylosed laminæ. The dura was left open and a gauze drain carried outward at the lower angle of the wound, which was closed with silkworm gut.

During the first night the patient was quite uncomfortable, but the pain in the lower extremities, except at the ankle, began to diminish and the spasms began to lessen. He emptied his bladder voluntarily, which he could not do before operation, and the girdle pain moved downward about an inch.

Nine days after operation improvement continued in the way of less pain and the ability to sleep all night and to have long naps in the daytime without morphine, a thing that he had not been able to do for about two years. He could make use of his abdominal muscles in defecation, and the girdle sensation moved downward.

He continued to improve, the improvement lasting for about five months, when the symptoms returned as bad as ever, and in June of the following year (1899) he returned for re-operation in the hope of receiving temporary respite at least. He complained of constant sensitiveness in the lower sacral and coccygeal regions, the clonic spasms had returned, and the left arm and shoulder exhibited tingling pain at times. There were attacks of spasm in the spinal muscles and moderate spasm in the lower extremities.

He was seen by another neurologist at this time, who suspected a tumor at the conus, and with considerable hesitation I consented to operate at a lower level. I removed the two last dorsal and two upper lumbar laminæ, and found a similar condition as at the first operation—a tense dura, through the opening of which bulged a distinct pial membrane full of fluid under pressure. No tumor of the cord or of the cauda equina was found. A probe could be passed upward to the level of the scar without meeting any resistance. The dura was not sutured and the wound was closed with silk-worm gut. The symptoms were benefited less by this operation, but his general condition improved somewhat.

CASE III.—Henry K., aged fourteen years, a professional acrobat, slipped in turning a back somersault nine weeks before entrance to the Boston City Hospital, landing on the back of his neck. He rose immediately to his knees, but was unable to rise any further, and since the accident he had been unable to walk. He remembered that he was positively unable to move his legs the day after the accident, and that he used his hands awkwardly while eating. He was taken to a hospital in Virginia and electricity was given. He had some pain at the seat of injury immediately after the accident, but had had none since. He was catheterized after the injury and had incontinence since, but he had been able to control his rectum. He said that his forearms and hands had "grown thin." Temperature at admission, 99°; pulse slightly irregular, 84. Examination of abdomen negative. He lay relaxed on his back in bed.

Dr. W. N. Bullard examined him, and his notes are as follows: Head: pupils, etc., normal. Upper extremity: extreme atrophy of flexors of the forearm and less of the other muscles, though the atrophy is marked, nevertheless. The hands are claw-shaped. All motions in the upper extremity are possible but very weak, except opposition and abduction of the thumbs. The wrist is extended on flexion of the fingers. Diminution of sensation is not marked over the left upper extremity; in the right upper extremity it is normal.

Sensation is diminished below the iliac crests. Total paraplegia, but apparently no atrophy. Cremasteric reflexes present. Knee-jerks increased, no clonus. Babinski present. Some rigidity of lower extremities on passive motion.

In addition to this the following notes are recorded:

Stereognostic, pain, tactile and thermal sensation normal in hands, legs, and forearms. Flexion and extension of forearms strong. Cannot rise in bed without strong assistance. No obvious atrophy of the muscles of the back. Paralysis of the limbs is at times flaccid, at times spastic. There is a suggestion of Kernig's sign until the thigh has been held flexed for several seconds, and then the muscles relax, allowing complete extension of the lower leg on the flexed thigh. The skin is normal. There is no scoliosis.

On August 19 I removed the seventh cervical and first dorsal laminæ under ether. The dura was translucent, not pulsating. On being opened a small quantity of fluid escaped. Pressing against the dura was a pial sac containing much fluid under pressure. The pia was attached to the dura and laterally to the cord and nerve roots, so that in freeing it fresh bleeding took place. The pia was freed within the reach of a probe. The pia and dura were not closed. The external wound was closed with silkworm gut, allowing for rubber tissue drain. No shock.

August 23. Has had a good deal of pain in the neck, requiring morphine. Has been on a Bradford frame since operation.

27th. Primary union. General condition improyed.

31st. Much improved. Can move head freely without pain. No control over legs.

September 4. Sitting up in bed.

14th. Condition of arms improved. Can raise his body from a chair with his arms. No change in the paralysis of the legs.

18th. Discharged to his home.

In May following operation, that is, nine months later, the boy ran to meet me on the street, and all that I could find that he complained of was a slight atrophy of the back of one forearm. Since then I am told that he returned to his profession as an acrobat.

CASE IV.—Michael J. D., aged forty-four years, fell, May 6, 1903, from a load of leather, striking his head and shoulders on the pavement. He was paralyzed at once in his lower extremities and was taken to the Boston City Hospital Relief Station. Examination then showed equal pupils, complete anesthesia below the nipples, knee-jerk present on both sides, no ankle clonus, no plantar reflex, no bony deformity, distended abdomen, and an approach to priapism. He was later transferred to the main hospital, and on the 10th it is recorded that the temperature had slowly risen to 100°, but the pulse remained slow. There was complete paralysis of the legs, thighs, forearms, and muscles of the abdomen. The anesthesia remained as noted. The knee-jerks and plantar reflexes were absent. Retention of urine.

May 14. Normal temperature. Pulse 60. Dr. P. C. Knapp saw him in consultation, and made a diagnosis of crush of cord at first dorsal segment.

·On May 22 I operated. Soon after starting anesthesia the patient choked and became cyanotic, requiring artificial respiration, quickly recovering. The sixth and seventh cervical laminæ were removed. In the muscles were evidences of old hemorrhage and laceration. No fracture was found. On opening the dura a small amount of fluid escaped. Pushing up against the dura was a firm pial membrane, beneath which a large amount of clear fluid was contained. The cord appeared to be normal. The wound was closed allowing for a temporary rubber tissue drain. No shock. On the afternoon of the operation the temperature rose to 102.4°, but soon dropped to normal. Considerable fluid drained out. Wound clean.

June 4. Temperature irregularly elevated recently.

Beginning motion in forearms, but no change in anesthesia. Respirations shallow, apparently without use of intercostal muscles.

11*th*. Incontinence. Can flex and extend forearms slowly, but has no control of hands. Bedsores beginning over sacrum.

16*th*. Wound firmly healed. Incontinence of urine and feces.

20*th*. Necrosis in all prominent parts of body.

24th. Worse. Delirious. Temperature rising, pulse 120.

6*th*. Worse. Almost constant motion of both arms. Irregular temperature, bad pulse.

9*th*. Died. No autopsy.

CASE V.—Edward C. B., aged thirty-eight years, entered the Carney Hospital on May 9, 1906. He had a primary lesion ten years before, followed by typical secondary manifestations, for which he was carefully treated.

Dr. L. P. O'Donnell, assistant neurologist, examined him carefully, and from his notes I quote freely. About nine years ago patient noticed slowly increasing weakness of his legs and undue fatigue after moderate exertion. He had been able, however, to attend to his work as a commercial traveller up to the present time, although for the last year and a half he had used a cane.

Two years ago there was a sudden onset of numbness and hemiplegia lasting for two or three days, but he does not recall which side was affected. For two years he has not had full control of his sphincters, and for a year and a half he has used a catheter. During this time he has had a dull ache and feeling of weariness in the sacral and perineal regions. He has had no sharp pain or girdle sensation. Mentally he is clear.

He walks without ataxia, does not sway with his eyes open. Very slight Romberg is present. Cranial nerves and special senses normal. Pupils show slight myosis, but react normally to light and accommodation. At a later examination the pupils were unequal, the left being dilated. Supinator and triceps reflexes are sharp, but within normal limits and equal on both sides.

Reflexes of the lower extremities are exaggerated. There is slight ankle clonus on both sides and Babinski on both sides. The muscles of the lower extremities are well nourished, but spastic in a high degree. No disturbance of sensation to touch and pain. No line of hyperesthesia. There is, however, a well-marked zone of muscular and cutaneous irritability corresponding to the distribution of the lumbar and sacral nerves, and throughout this zone slight irritation of the skin or tapping of the muscles produces muscular contractions with a large degree of spasticity. The strength of the legs is not markedly diminished. There is tenderness on pressure over the spinous processes of the last dorsal and first lumbar vertebræ.

The diagnosis of a late syphilitic manifestation with cerebrospinal distribution in islets was made, with probably a well-marked and localized meningomyelitis involving probably the first and second lumbar segments of the cord.

Operation May 15, under ether. The three lowest dorsal or two dorsal and first lumbar laminæ were removed. There was considerable hemorrhage from large epidural veins, so much so that it was thought best to pack and delay opening the dura for forty-eight hours. Increased spastic contraction and pain from the packing, with rise of pulse and temperature, followed this procedure, so on May 17 I opened the dura. Beneath it the pia was distended as a definite membrane, slightly opaque and thickened. Clear fluid was evacuated and the cord appeared normal, without evidence of tumor or thickening. The posterior roots looked normal. Some of the pial membrane was removed, and the dura was closed with catgut. Exploration upward and downward inside the pia failed to show any tumor. The wound was closed with silkworm gut, allowing for a capillary drain to the dura at the lower angle.

The patient reacted well from the operation, but within twelve hours the pulse rose to 120, with nausea and vomiting. He spent a poor night, with increasing vomiting, a temperature of 105.5°, and pulse 130. Lavage was tried, but he rapidly failed, and died about thirty-six hours after the second operation.

Autopsy showed septic meningitis in cervical region as cause of death. Sections of the cord showed no tumor, glioma, or other primary lesion.

CASE VI.—Gilbert N. S., aged thirty-seven years, architect, was seen in consultation with Dr. Alice M. Gray and Dr. John Jenks Thomas, in the latter part of July, 1906. In 1894 he had trouble with his right upper arm, that was diagnosticated and treated as rheumatism for three years. An x-ray then showed it to be osteomyelitis, and from that time until 1903 he had many operations, finally losing the arm at the shoulder-joint.

In December, 1905, he began to suffer from severe "lumbago" pains, stiffness, and numbness of the lower extremities. While on jury duty at about this time he became greatly fatigued, and one day while rising from a chair he fell suddenly, and from that time was practically bedridden.

Four or five months before I operated upon him he had a right middle-ear abscess, which cleared up without any after effects. Within a month or so after operation deafness started in the left ear, and has slowly increased until now it is practically complete.

Dr. Thomas saw him shortly before my visit, and he has kindly allowed me the use of the following notes: In December, 1904, the patient had pain in his hip, and soon afterward noticed that the right leg felt weak and that the knees would give way. While in bed the knees would flex.[1] Stooping caused pain, and he had to give up work, in December, 1905. He noticed that the right side of his body would sweat, but not the left side. In July, 1906, he had cramps in his legs, with flexion and abduction. Numbness was less marked at this time than before. There was no trouble in controlling the bladder nor the rectum, though he suffered from constipation, requiring a suppository daily. Examination showed the patient lying in the dorsal position with the thighs drawn up nearly to a right angle with the body and the legs acutely flexed on the thighs. The legs were in condition of spastic paralysis with marked adductor spasm, which, however, relaxed at times. The spasmodic contractions were for the most part in the thigh muscles, particularly the adductors and recti femoris, and in the abdominal muscles. Handling the muscles and passive movements of the legs brought on a spasm, and practically there was no voluntary control over the lower extremities.

Sensation to touch, pain, and temperature was almost normal in the feet and legs. In the thighs and abdomen the prick of a pin started up a muscular contraction. In the trunk, at the level of the eighth or ninth thoracic root, the prick of a pin was felt as a burning sensation.

[1] This was preceded by a period of spasmodic extension and scissors-like action.—J. C. M.

The patellar reflexes could not be tested. There was double ankle clonus and Babinski's sign. The abdominal and epigastric reflexes could not be tested. Reaction of the leg muscles to the faradic current was good.

The lower thoracic region of the spine was rather rigid on passive motion, while the movements of the lumbar spine was much better. There was slight diffuse tenderness to percussion in the lower thoracic region. No deformity of the spine.

In one of my own examinations I found the knee-jerk increased on the right, slight or absent on the left, with a similar variation in the ankle clonus. There were no bed-sores. No history or evidence of syphilis.

At operation, on August 2, I removed, under ether, the sixth, seventh, and eighth dorsal laminæ, and through a second incision removed the second lumbar lamina. The dura in the upper wound was opened and a considerable quantity of serum escaped under moderate pressure. This fluid was clear at first, and then became more and more bloody, until finally there was a steady outpour of venous blood, which apparently came from below the level of the incision and from between the dura and pia. The dura appeared thickened and opaque on the inner surface. The field could not be dried long enough to obtain a clear look at the cord. The dura in the lower incision was pricked and serum, followed by blood, escaped. Both wounds were closed with silkworm gut, allowing for a capillary drain to the dura. He recovered well from this operation, and in ten days the pain in the legs had ceased. By making an effort he could straighten the knees to about 130 degrees, and there was some general improvement with respect to the spasticity of the legs and abdomen. Otherwise he was the same as before operation, and was discharged August 15.

Two months later (October 8) I again saw him with Dr. Gray and Dr. Thomas, and the latter's notes state that after the operation he could move better and had less spasm, but that within the last two weeks the spasm had increased. At no time had he lost control of the bladder. Examination showed paralysis and spasm the same as before. Sensation for touch and pain was not lost in the feet, legs, or trunk, but was much diminished from below the level of the tenth thoracic segment area. Tenderness to pressure was at this time most marked at the tenth thoracic spinous process. I noted that the ankle clonus on the right was less marked than formerly and that the Babinski sign was present on both sides.

On October 16 I operated again, removing the twelfth dorsal and first and second lumbar laminæ. There was no pulsation of the dura and no growth between dura and spine. On opening the dura a well-marked, definite, bluish-white membrane in the pia-arachnoid bulged forth into the dural slit, there being no fluid between it and the dura.

This membrane formed a definite sac, apparently open below, but at least partly closed at the upper end, which lay under the lower portion of the upper scar. Clear serum escaped from the pial sac, exposing the conus and the upper portion of the cauda. The pial sac was cut away and the dura closed with catgut. Nothing abnormal was seen in the cord and nothing abnormal was felt by a probe passed upward and downward. The wound was closed in layers with catgut, allowing for a cigarette drain to the epidural fat on account of oozing from the diploë of a lamina.

On the following day the patient could straighten his legs somewhat and was free from the painful spasms. In twelve days he was sitting up, the wound being firmly healed, and the legs did not flex spasmodically when he put his feet to the floor, as happened before operation. He had no pain in his legs, and if the skin were rubbed or stroked no spasm was produced. He went home October 29.

When seen November, 1909 (three years after the second operation), he was well, able to do a hard day's work as inspector of buildings that required climbing stairs and ladders. As he walked the knees did not fully extend and the legs were slightly adducted, more than is seen in the average individual, but unless one were critically observing his gait it is doubtful if anything abnormal would be noticed. He had normal sensation and normal knee-jerks. On full extension at the knee the hamstrings were slightly tenser than normal. When overtired he would unconsciously in his sleep forcibly extend the legs. He had no pain.

. He stated that by Christmas following operation he could stand up with assistance, and in the following June he walked with a cane. By July he was able to take a long car ride, and in the autumn of 1907 he was doing a full day's work.

After the patient's return home from the second operation Dr. Gray's treatment played so important a role in his recovery that I shall quote freely from her notes, which she has kindly loaned me. She says: "As soon as the patient returned from the hospital I found the spastic condition still present to some extent, but the clonic spasm could not be excited. The thighs and legs were still held firmly by the contracted flexor and adductor tendons. At the end of two weeks I advised light massage and passive motions for the thighs and legs, leaving the back and abdomen entirely alone. Two weeks later the patient felt a return of the violent spasms of the abdominal muscles, and was discouraged. I discontinued massage as soon as I felt that the patient had grounds for his suspicions and prescribed $\frac{1}{100}$ gr. of corrosive sublimate with 7 gr. of iodide of potassium, three times a day.

"There was no more complaint of the spasm, and again, two weeks later, I returned to the medical gymnastic treatment, giving it myself in order to watch the result better. The internal treatment was continued.

"Slowly and tentatively I began with massage and passive motion, stretching the tendons very slightly beyond their voluntary limit. As the spastic condition grew less, and only the mechanical contractions of the tendons remained to be overcome, I increased the number and strength of the treatments, which by this time consisted of violent and continuous stretching of the contracted tendons. Manual force and resistive exercises, both manual and with apparatus, for the muscles, antagonizing the contracted groups, were employed, and at the end of six months the patient was walking with the aid of a cane and crutch. Up to this time and several times later an acute swelling appeared occasionally in the left knee, apparently following a decrease in the drug treatment and always disappearing soon after the medicine was re-administered. The medical gymnastic treatment was continued for a year with steady and, toward the end, rapid improvement, the adductor tendons being the last to yield. The medical treatment has not been given for nearly two years."

The behavior of the joint swelling to mercury and the late progressive deafness, which, however, did not yield to drug treatment, suggest a specific cause for the spinal lesion. No treatment before operation had any influence on the paralytic phenomena, but this would be expected from what we know of the experience of others. As stated in the beginning, no history or evidence of a recent or an acquired syphilis could be obtained.

BIBLIOGRAPHY.

Schlesinger. Beit. z. *K*ennt. d. Rückenm. und Wirbeltumoren, Jena, 1898.

Quincke. Volkmann's Samml. klin. Vortr., 1893.

Spiller, *M*usser and *M*artin. Univ. Penn., Bull., 1903.

Schultze. Mittheil. aus. d. Grezgeb., 1903, p. 153.

v. Malaisé. *D*eut. Arch. f. klin. Med., 1904, p. 143.

Schmidt. *D*eut. Zeitschr. f. Nervenheilk., 1904, p. 318.

Joachim. *D*eut. Arch. f. klin. Med., 1906, p. 259.

Oppenheim. Mittheil. aus d. Grenzgeb., 1906, p. 607.

Oppenheim. Verhandl. d. Gesell. deut. Naturf., 1906, II Theil, p. 194.

Oppenheim. Beit. z. *D*iag. und Therap. d. Geschw. d. Central nerv. System, Berlin, 1907.

*K*rause. Verhandl. d. Gesell. deut. Naturf., 1906, II Theil, p. 194.

*K*rause. Berl. klin. Wochenschrift, 1906, p. 827.

*K*rause. Verhandl. d. deut. Gesell. f. *C*hir., 1907, 11 Theil, p. 598.

Krause. Deut. Zeitschr. f. Nervenheilk., 1908.

Placzek and Krause. Berl. klin. Wochenschrift, 1907, No. 29.

Mendel and Adler. Berl. klin. Wochnschrift, 1908, p. 1596.

v. Bruns. Die Geschwülste des Nevrensystems., Berl., 1908.

v. Burns. Berl. klin. Wochnschrift, 1908, p. 1753.

de Montet. Cor. Bl. f. Schweiz. Aerzte, 1908, p. 698.

Stertz. Monatsschr. f. Psychol. und Neurol., Band xx.

Spiller. Amer. Jour. Med. Sci., January, 1909.

Horsley. Brit. Med. Jour., February, 1909.

Bliss. Jour. Amer. Med. Assoc., March, 1909.

DISCUSSION.

DR. W. L. ROBINSON, of Danville, Virginia.—I would like to ask Dr. Munro whether trauma, as a rule, is a preceding cause of this trouble?

DR. MUNRO: It has been known to occur from trauma, but there are very few cases reported in the literature. In the early literature some of the cases were incidentally found at autopsy. I report the case of a man who was said to have broken his neck. He was treated at a hospital for some weeks; paralysis came on at once, and nine weeks after the injury, expecting to find crushing of the cord, we found the patient with localized meningitis, which cleared up completely, so that he has gone back to his profession as an acrobat.

DR. ROBINSON.—If it is due to pressure, then the relief of pressure should relieve the case. If it is an infection, then we should strive to ascertain the cause of it. I ask these questions for information. If we resort to lumbar puncture, remove the pressure, and give some form of formaldehyde or urotropin in large doses, why should we not get results such as we do now?

DR. WALTER C. G. KIRCHNER, of St. Louis.—I would like to ask Dr. Munro how one is to differentiate this condition from hemorrhage, especially in cases of trauma?

With reference to meningitis of the epidemic type, I had one interesting case, in which there was a circumscribed spinal meningitis. We knew from the lumbar puncture the exact origin of this condition. The patient was given the Flexner treatment, but the effects of this were not noticed. The outcome was fatal. At the autopsy the cord was carefully examined, and a circumscribed area was found showing that circumscribed meningitis was present. In this case infection was an etiological factor. The chief point to be gained from the standpoint of treatment of meningitis in this case was that while we did not get results from lumbar puncture, it is advisable to puncture the ventricle and administer the fluid in that way. This I have done with this one case of circumscribed meningitis before me as an example.

DR. CHAS. H. MAYO, of Rochester, Minnesota.—I always feel greatly indebted to Dr. Munro whenever he presents a paper. After having a conversation with him some time ago in regard to these cases, I was led to communicate with one patient whom I had turned down for operation. Brain surgery years ago was in the same condition, in that we wanted to be perfectly sure of just what we were going to accomplish before we undertook any work on the brain. It did not make much difference; in the abdomen the same incision uncovered them all, so that in proportion as we have advanced in operative work we have made progress in our methods of diagnosis. People who have an injury or a disease affecting the spinal cord should have the benefit of a doubt of the condition present, which may be relieved surgically, but which would doubtless prove fatal if left alone, and if nothing more can be accomplished than the relief of pressure of an injured cord and the relief of bedsores, it is a sufficient indication for operation. Horsley, in his efforts to relieve tumors of the brain, afterward found that these patients did not become blind, although they might live for many years. So it is a sufficient indication to relieve pressure upon the brain by making an exploration or a decompression. If these individuals cannot be helped from any other standpoint than that of the relief of pressure, preventing them from becoming blind, while they live, and if the tumor does not kill them, an operation is worthy of consideration, and so Dr. Munro is always a few years in advance of the time.

DR. MUNRO (closing).—With reference to what has been said regarding lumbar puncture, I will say that the good it does is doubtful. There is one case reported by Krause, which he cured by laminectomy and puncture of the dura. Personally, I have questioned whether this was really one of the cases in the class under discussion. It does no good to resort to lumbar puncture. It gives no clew to the diagnosis. Lumbar punctures have been made, and in one case reported in addition to one of mine the fluid was absolutely sterile. There is nothing in the fluid that is at all characteristic, and the lining membrane gives us no clew as to the cause of the disease.

As to the differentiation of this condition from that produced by hemorrhage, I am not enough of a neurologist to go into it; but following hemorrhage inside the cord you get trophic lesions. These cases of meningitis are usually diagnosticated as cases of tumor, because there is irritation of the meninges in one case, as well as in the other. I had a case recently in which I was almost sure it was one of serous meningitis, except that the patient did not have acute hypersensitiveness. I operated on her and found a simple cyst of the central canal of the cord, not a syringomyelia. Pathologists have over-looked this condition in autopsies. They find what they have described as edema of the pia arachnoid, and they have not differentiated this distinct membrane.

ABDOMINAL CESAREAN SECTION FOR PUERPERAL ECLAMPSIA.

By LANE MULLALY, *M.D.*,
Charleston, South Carolina.

FOUR cases of puerperal eclampsia in four weeks, with a comparison of the treatment in each, accounts for my presenting this paper to this Association.

The first two cases were brought into the Roper Hospital with the usual history of eclampsia, each having had convulsions for about six hours before being admitted. The first case was delivered under anesthesia by dilatation, instrumental and manual, and high forceps, the second case by similar dilatation and version, each case occupying from one to two hours. In the first case convulsions continued for twelve hours, when the patient died. The second case had several convulsions after delivery, and recovered. Each of these were about seven months pregnant; the child of the first was dead at birth, the child of the second lived a few hours. The third case, a multipara with considerable scar tissue in the cervix, was anesthetized, and an hour or more uselessly spent in attempted dilatation. The external os was soft enough, but the internal os was like a steel band, the rigidity being so great.

Finding it impossible to dilate the cervix, I determined upon abdominal Cesarean section, preferring this to vaginal Cesarean section, and delivered the child in seven minutes, the whole operation, when completed, occupying twenty-seven minutes. The case was a six months' pregnancy, and the child was dead when delivered; in fact, was dead before the operation began. Convulsions continued in this case after the operation, and the patient died. I believe, however, recovery would have taken place had the patient not been subjected to the prolonged shock incurred by attempting dilatation.

The fourth case, a full term pregnancy, entered the Hospital at midnight with a history of having had convulsions every fifteen minutes since 8 A.M. of the same day.

I determined in this case to do an abdominal Cesarean section at once. Chloroform was administered and the child delivered in six minutes, the wound closed, and the patient returned to the ward in twenty-six minutes from the time the operation began. She had after the operation seven convulsions; the convulsions then ceased, and she developed puerperal mania; this lasted three days, when the mania suddenly disappeared, and she went on to an uninterrupted recovery. The child in this case died before delivery, due no doubt to maternal toxemia and eclamptic seizures.

My object in presenting this subject is to call attention to the advantages offered by abdominal Cesarean section, both for mother and child, over other methods of rapid evacuation of the uterus, and to assist in bringing into notice an operation which ten years ago was undertaken with fear and trepidation and as a last resort. Both maternal and fetal mortality in eclampsia must be lowered. Too many women and unborn children die from neglect and lack of attention in the various toxemias. Too long have obstetricians held in awe Cesarean section, probably on account of the high mortality at first attending it.

Bounaire says that during the hundred years prior to 1876 every woman operated on in Paris for Cesarean section died. With such a mortality it is easy to understand the prejudice against the operation.

Recently Cesarean section with the perfect technique

of the present day has materially lowered the maternal mortality, and the operation is selected not only on this account, but also for the reason that it offers better advantages in saving the life of the child than many of the intrapelvic methods of delivery. In this day of advanced surgical technique the operation is far less dangerous than high forceps version and I believe vaginal Cesarean section. A great deal has been written about the pathology and etiology of puerperal eclampsia; in fact, as has been tersely stated, "there is probably no obstetrical complication about which more has been written and less really understood than the condition known as eclampsia."

The chief reason why we have as yet found no satisfactory treatment is because we do not know the cause. The innumerable drugs and methods of treatment recommended show that we are as yet in the dark as regards a satisfactory treatment. The pathological findings of Dr. J. E. Welch in a recent article in the *Journal of the American Medical Association* are valuable and to the point; the question arises, however, are they not the result of toxemia, and not the immediate cause of eclampsia? That fetal metabolism has extended to such a point that the various organs of elimination can no longer withstand the strain put upon them, they become, as it were, waterlogged, and the overflow produces convulsions.

Fry says: "If the lesions pass beyond the reparative stage before the termination of pregnancy death will necessarily result.

"There is no way to determine the progress of these lesions. They may have passed the reparative stage before the onset of convulsions, but ordinarily this is not the case until after a number of convulsions have taken place. Having no means at our command of ascertaining when the lesions began, and to what extent they have progressed, the only safe rule to make is to terminate the pregnancy as soon as possible after the first convulsion." In other words, cut short fetal metabolism by delivering the child, and you stop the supply of poison. Further, not only is the life of the mother endangered by delay, but also the life of the child, for the child suffers death from maternal toxemia and eclamptic seizures. Be the cause of eclampsia what it may, one thing stands out so plainly that it admits of no discussion, viz., ruerperal eclampsia never occurs without pregnancy. Whatever may be the immediate cause, certainly pregnancy is the primary cause, and all must agree that emptying of the uterus must be accomplished to cut short the disease, and as each convulsion tends to lessen the woman's chance of recovery, as well as that of the child, the uterus must be emptied as soon as possible after the onset of eclampsia.

In 1896 the International Congress at Geneva decided that, according to the best authorities, the uterus should be emptied as quickly as possible after the onset of eclampsia.

Edgar says that careful observation seems to show that danger is essentially passed in 90 per cent. of cases immediately after the uterus is emptied.

Davis says the most important indication in treatment is to secure elimination, and the next is emptying the uterus. He had much better have reversed this and said empty the uterus and then secure elimination.

Williams says: "When convulsions have occurred during pregnancy or labor I believe that delivery should be effected as soon as is consistent with the safety of the patient."

Hirst says it seems logical to evacuate the uterus as the first step in the treatment of eclampsia.

McPherson says: "Until we have a more tangible knowledge of the actual cause of these toxemic convulsions, the only feasible treatment for the condition of eclampsia is immediate evacuation of the uterine contents, followed by proper eliminative care in the puerperium."

Fry, in a paper read before the American Medical Association, entitled "A Plea for the Prompt Evacuation of the

Uterus in Eclampsia," presents a conclusive argument. In concluding he submitted this statement: "According to the Bureau of Statistics in the Census Department, about 2,606,860 babies are born annually in the United States. Making due allowance for the usual proportion of plural births, this would represent 2,592,378 labors. Estimating one case of eclampsia to every 400 labors would give 6480 cases of eclampsia every year. Under the expectant plan of treatment the mortality is placed at 25 per cent., and under prompt evacuation of the uterus 10 per cent., a saving of 15 per cent. This means that by radical treatment instead of the expectant, the lives of 972 mothers will be saved each year in the United States.

Granting rapid evacuation to be the rational treatment, what is the best means of rapid evacuation of the uterus that will cause least injury to the mother and child.

I contend that this is best accomplished by abdominal Cesarean section, and why?

To begin with, time is an important element both for mother and child. The entire time consumed in performing abdominal Cesarean section in the hands of any operator need not occupy more than thirty minutes. On the other hand, dilatation of the cervix alone consumes anywhere from forty minutes to one and one-half hours. Added to this is the time consumed in the application of forceps and delivery, or version and delivery, the shock from Cesarean section must be admitted to be far less than the prolonged anesthesia and manipulation necessary with forceps or version.

Besides, Davis says: "In my experience the rapid removal of the fetus through the abdomen sometimes brings about a remarkable improvement in the circulation, with improved secretion and consciousness."

I cannot see why the shock should be any greater than an ordinary laparotomy. Reynolds says most obstetricians agree that difficult high forceps or versions are more severe than Cesarean section.

Warren says difficult high forceps or late podalic version is more dangerous to mother and child than laparotomy. Reddy considers the operation much simpler than many appendectomies or accouchement forcé.

Allen says: "In those virulent cases of eclampsia when immediate delivery is demanded, abdominal section will empty the uterus more quickly and safely than any other operation."

Davis says: "If eclampsia is to be treated by rapid delivery, abdominal section can certainly compete with rapid dilatation and extraction of the fetus."

Among the indications put down for Cesarean section are eclampsia in women with rigid cervices and when prompt interference is demanded. Valuable time is certainly lost in ascertaining a rigid cervix, and the danger of shock is thereby increased. Edgar says: "The cervix uteri is composed of constricting and dilating muscle, and while it is true that the first convulsion usually induces labor, still the resulting asphyxia exerts a marked constricting action upon the body of the uterus and cervix, which is especially marked at the internal ring of the os. Therefore, any method of rapid manual dilatation of the os that is undertaken before the internal os has been made, partially at least, to disappear, is attended with great danger of uterine rupture. We believe a warning should be sounded against the careless undertaking of rapid manual dilatations of the os, particularly in eclampsia. Moreover, undue shock has resulted from the dragging of a fetus through an imperfectly dilated os, to say nothing of the loss of the child."

Added to these dangers we have the risk of sepsis in high forceps, which is greater than abdominal Cesarean section. In the morbidity following Cesarean section may be mentioned adhesions to the anterior abdominal wall and hernia, neither of which are important.

Let me now mention some of the objections to vaginal Cesarean section, which has many strong supporters, and which appears to be the chief rival of abdominal Cesarean section.

In vaginal Cesarean section there is greater danger of sepsis, for we must all admit that it is most difficult, if not impossible, to render the vagina thoroughly aseptic. There is danger, too, of the incision extending up into the peritoneal cavity, rupturing the broad ligaments and causing extensive hemorrhage; also danger of injury to the bladder and rectum. Oftimes there is great difficulty in pulling down the cervix, which makes it almost impossible to make your incision by sight, hence it must be done by touch, which is not surgical; and in sewing up the incision the same difficulty is encountered in putting in the stitches in the upper angle. No one can gainsay that vaginal Cesarean section should not be allowed to be performed except by those who have had a large experience in gynecological work. On the other hand, abdominal Cesarean section can be performed in less than thirty minutes and by any obstetrician. The field of operation can be thoroughly and quickly prepared in an aseptic manner, the operation is performed with everything in full view, and the danger of hemorrhage is slight and the danger to the child *nil*.

In conclusion, I wish to say that I have reiterated the fact that in all cases of puerperal eclampsia rapid evacuation of the uterus is the rational treatment. Also, that this being the case, it should be done in a way that will cause as little injury to mother and child as possible. I have endeavored to prove that this can best be accomplished by abdominal Cesarean section.

DISCUSSION.

DR. W. L. ROBINSON, of Danville, Virginia.—In considering the paper which has been presented to us, a good deal depends upon the selection of cases. We wish elimination; we wish exemption from the convulsions in these cases of puerperal eclampsia. Where we have septic conditions to contend with, independent of pus tubes, gonorrheal infection, malformation, etc., then Cesarean section obtains justly and properly; but so far as efforts at elimination are concerned, I believe we can secure results just as well by the old method of free abstraction of blood by opening a vessel or vein, relaxing the whole system, so that a natural delivery can be effected by forceps. By the free abstraction of blood we get rid of the toxic effect, and, if necessary, we can follow this by saline infusion; and by making use of these measures I think we can accomplish our object as well as by resorting to Cesarean section. It is a question of determining in each individual case as to what is the best course to pursue.

DR. REUBEN PETERSON, of Ann Arbor, Michigan.—I agree with the essayist that in antepartum eclampsia the best results are obtained by emptying the uterus quickly. However, I would take issue with him regarding his choice of operation and for several reasons. In the first place I have always contended that an obstetric operation, to be of any particular value must be of such a nature as to allow of its performance by the general practitioner. The obstetrics of the country are performed by him, only a comparatively few obstetrical operations being performed in hospitals.

The general practitioner is not in the habit of entering the peritoneal cavity, and for this reason alone abdominal Cesarean section would give a high mortality in his hands, especially since in eclampsia attempts are usually made to deliver from below before Cesarean section is considered. Vaginal Cesarean section is a preferable operation for the practitioner, since the peritoneal cavity need not be invaded.

I am in accord with the essayist in his condemnation of manual dilatation in cases of rigid cervices, but we should remember that a rigid cervix is a comparatively rare condition. For easily dilatable cervices manual dilatation will give far better results in eclampsia than either abdominal or vaginal Cesarean section. The latter should be reserved for cases of rigid cervices where manual dilatation could not be accomplished short of an hour or two. Abdominal Cesarean section for eclampsia should be reserved for those rare cases where immediate delivery is called for in the presence of a contracted pelvis. Here the abdominal route will mean added safety to the mother and a chance for the child.

Vaginal Cesarean section is not a particularly difficult operation, if one be familiar with the technique. The bladder is easily pushed out of the way, the cervix split in the median line, and the operation completed in a very short time, in my experience much quicker than by the abdominal route. Even the general practitioner will do far better by both mother and child in eclampsia where the cervix is rigid by doing vaginal Cesarean section, than he will by hours of brutal attempts at manual dilatation.

DR. I. S. STONE, of Washington.—I regret very much that Dr. Fry and Dr. Moran, of Washington, are not here to take part in the discussion of this admirable paper by Dr. Mullally, as they are thoroughly familiar with the subject from the standpoint of operating vaginally or abdominally.

I am glad Dr. Peterson has said what he has, and I merely rise to discuss the subject from that side. I believe, in view of what has been done, in cases of early operation, where, for instance, a patient is supposed to have a pelvis which will permit the extraction of the child at eight and a half months in a case of eclampsia, the vaginal operation seems to be the one most advisable, for the reason that, in the first place, there are a number of men who ought to do the operation more safely from below than from above. Abdominal Cesarean section is certainly the proper thing in certain hands, and there are some men who do not know how and who have never learned to do vaginal surgery, although they are gynecologists, strange as this may appear. These men are accustomed to the abdominal route, and they do better operations from above on that account. On the contrary, there are a number of men in every locality who are capable of doing the vaginal operation, as suggested by Dr. Peterson, that is, making a division of the cervix uteri, or so-called vaginal Cesarean section. It ought to be called "hysterotomy." The practitioner can do this operation with less danger than he can a long and tedious manual dilatation, and especially by the so-called Bossi dilator, or by any one of the mechanical methods other than the hand. My friend, Dr. Nash, who is sitting by me, says that he can dilate his cases easily with the hand. I must take issue with him when he says that he can dilate these cases with his hand. He can dilate some of them with the hand, undoubtedly, but not the class of cases we are discussing, as these need a cutting operation. But certainly in the absence of that possibility, it is much better to make a clean incision in the median line anteriorly, or anteroposteriorly, if necessary, and extract the child. This can be accomplished in a short time and perhaps in less time than it takes to do the abdominal operation. There are some men who favor Cesarean section in every instance when there is any complication about labor. Just as sure as the time comes when that practice is adopted by the profession, our women will have one or two children, and stop right there. They are not going to be willing to subject themselves to repeated operations through the abdomen for the extraction of the child. They will stop having children, and we will no longer have families with twelve or fifteen children; that will be a thing of the past. I look upon this matter from an economic standpoint, as well as artistic or scientific point of view, and believe it is very desirable to let women have children as normally as possible. They know something about operation at the present time, and how many of them will elect to have an abdominal operation in preference to delivery in the usual way? Many would consent to operations through the vagina who would not consent to undergo the abdominal operation.

DR. JOSEPH PRICE, of Philadelphia.—Dr. Stone is surely in error in regard to intelligent women not consenting to the abdominal operation in these cases of puerperal eclampsia. Take the wife of an intelligent physician, or dentist, or merchant, who has reached the age of thirty or thirty-five, having married late; in the midst of our conventional modes of living that woman will accept the wise presentation of a method of operating, because it is well known that late conceptions are favorable to eclampsia and also to surgery. The argument that has been advanced of not favoring race suicide in any way is a good one, and should be carefully considered. Race suicide is due to many things, which I will not stop to enumerate.

The Trendelenburg position gave expert operators a clear view of the field of operation, and it was really a blessing from that standpoint to the profession. If the country doctor, the village doctor, or the cross-roads doctor near the cotton gin and sawmills possessed that refinement of knowledge of vaginal surgery that Pryor possessed—a man who could use the Trendelenburg position and expose everything to view, and do thirty-five vaginal sections for puerperal infection, open up the vaults, the infected lymph zones, free bowel adhesions, and remove pathological conditions beneath the infected zones, resort to the use of large iodoform gauze drainage, and save 34 out of 35 patients, then, I should say, it would be safe for the general practitioner to adopt the vaginal route in those cases. But the distinguished teacher, who advocated the vaginal route, knows perfectly well that these attacks on eclamptics by men of little experience and little judgment are a variety of criminal assaults.

Again, there are some men who attempt forcible dilatation of the cervix so as to permit the high application of forceps, and what do we find? Read the last issue of *Martin's Surgical Journal*, published in Chicago, and you will find there an account of three mutilations of urethras, with attempts having been made to repair them, but with failure to do so. I do not believe we have enough surgeons, general and special, in America at the present time to do the surgical work that ought to be done. There is enough work to keep all the surgeons in this country busy for one year repairing the mutilations of our women incident to parturition. These patients come to me from the sugar zones and the rice zones without a semblance of urethra. I can stand off and view the urine trickling from both ureters, and I am asked to make urethras for these women, and then put a base in the bladder. It is such work that makes me an old man, and sometimes I am sorry that I was ever born, and almost sorry that my cord was tied.

We know that wonderfully good work can be done by vaginal Cesarean section. Let us take the vaginal operators of this country, the men who have served apprenticeships in extirpations of uteri, in the repair of accidents incident to parturition, and they are capable of doing good vaginal work. They are men of varied experience and with good schooling in practical obstetrics. I would trust any one of those men to go in by the anterior or posterior route and do a safe procedure.

Dr. MULLALY (closing).—It is hardly necessary for me to consume much of your time in closing the discussion on my paper. I wish to say this, however, that I think Dr. Peterson will agree with me in saying that in a short time abdominal Cesarean section will be considered the easiest, quickest, and best route, not only for the experienced man like himself, but for the country obstetrician. I may be a little bit ahead of the times, but I really think if women knew how easily they can be delivered by abdominal Cesarean section, they would favor it under certain conditions.

ANATOMICAL, PATHOLOGICAL, AND CLINICAL STUDIES OF LESIONS INVOLVING THE APPENDIX AND RIGHT URETER.

WITH SPECIAL REFERENCE TO DIAGNOSIS AND OPERATIVE TREATMENT.

By John Young Brown, *M.D.*, William Englebach, *M.D.*,

AND

R. D. Carman, *M.D.*,
St. Louis, Missouri.

In two decades the brilliant work of American surgery has developed the disease of appendicitis from a practically unknown to a well-established clinical entity. In fact, this disease has become so popular that it is now credited with almost every symptom referable to the right lower quadrant of the abdomen. For this reason many a normal appendix has been unnecessarily removed, and many other lesions in this region simulating appendicitis have been overlooked. During the past two years a clinical analysis made upon cases before operation, compared with the lesions found during operation has demonstrated to the authors the many difficulties which present themselves in the diagnosis of some of the lesions of this quadrant. This applies particularly to those cases of combined lesions of the appendix and right ureter, appendicitis simulating genito-urinary disease, urinary calculi simulating appendicitis, and lesions of other organs in this region usually mistaken for appendiceal or ureteral disease.

In order to attempt to definitely determine the cause of confusing clinical findings (such as hematuria, and skiagraphic shadows occurring with lesions of the appendix), and to simplify the diagnosis and treatment of these atypical cases, anatomical and skiagraphic studies of the relations of the appendix and ureter were made.

ANATOMY AND PATHOLOGY. The many varied relations of the appendix to the right ureter is best illustrated by anatomical and stereoscopic skiagraphs made upon bodies, the appendix injected with mercury and stylets in the ureters, as shown in the series of accompanying illustrations. The most important relation of these two organs is that which is found at the brim of the pelvis, just anterior to the right sacroiliac synchondrosis. With the cecum in the normal position, this point corresponds to the base of the appendix and the location at which the ureter crosses the iliopectineal line (Fig. 1). This point of the appendix is more or less fixed, and consequently is separated from the ureter by the peritoneum only. When the appendix lies retrocecal, or hangs down into the pelvis, more or less of the whole appendix has this relationship to the ureter, as shown in Fig. 2. The relation of the distal portion of the appendix, and even that of the base to the ureter, will necessarily depend upon the position of the appendix, as shown in Figs. 2 and 3. These illustrate the maximum distance of the appendix from the ureter, and they will probably account for the absence of urinary findings referable to the ureter in the majority of cases of appendicitis. In making the above anatomical investigations of the course of the ureters through the pelvis, we found that in the pelvis of three male subjects it did not correspond to that given in most texts on anatomy. Instead of describing a semicircle with the convexity posterior extending from the brim of the pelvis to the symphysis, it was found that in these bodies the course of the ureters lay practically in the same plane, from a point just anterior to the base of the sacro-iliac synchondrosis to another located at the superior portion of the prostate gland. This is shown in Fig. 4 by a line drawn from these two points, with the green line forming the course of the ureters. It is also demonstrated by stereoscopic skiagraphs, with the sound placed in this plane in the median line of the pelvis, as shown in Figs. 1 and 3. In this plane they traverse along the lateral wall of the pelvis, describing a slight curve with its convexity outward. Reference is made to these anatomical points at this place on account of the bearing which they will have upon the location of the skiagraphic shadows in the pelvis under the paragraph on diagnosis.

It is easy to conceive how a lesion at the base of the appendix or one of a retrocecal or pelvic appendix which has extended to the peritoneum can involve the ureter by contiguity. If this is true, it justifies the conclusion that the erythrocytes, leukocytes, and albumin found in the urine accompanying appendicitis are produced by contiguous inflammation of the ureter. This local ureteritis, however, will not account for casts in the urine. Consequently, it is probable that their production is dependent upon a toxemia usually present in the acute and more fulminating types of appendicitis. The practical diagnostic deductions from the above is that a lesion of the appendix in proximity to the ureter could account for a simple hematuria, pyuria, albuminuria, or the combined findings of any of these elements in the urine. On the contrary, casts with these elements in the urine would indicate probably not this contiguous ureteritis, but a more marked lesion of an appendix, producing considerable absorption of toxins. These latter cases usually present no difficulties in diagnosis on account of having pregnant objective signs of peritoneal irritation referred to the anterior abdominal wall, whereas the former location of lesions of the appendix having a mild, subacute nature present only indefinite subjective symptoms, such as deep-seated tenderness.

This relationship in these positions of the appendix (retrocecal and pelvic) will also help to explain the cause of the peculiar type of pain transmitted down the ureter and the retraction of the testicle present in some cases of appendicitis. It will also show how concretions in the appendix may have the same locations in skiagraphs as ureteral calculi, and *vice versa*.

Clinical Cases Demonstrating the Pathological Relationship of the Appendix and Ureter.

These lesions of the ureter, especially ureteral calculi located high above the brim of the pelvis, are rarely ever confused with appendicitis. These conditions are rare, and it is only calculi of large size which usually present positive skiagraphic findings that occur in this part of the ureter. It is only those cases of retrocecal appendicitis in which the appendix curls back beneath the cecum along the course of the ureter which could produce misleading signs, such as hematuria or obstruction of the ureter from strictures or peri-ureteral contractures. The following are brief summaries of illustrative atypical clinical cases exhibiting either symptoms or signs of both lesions of the appendix and ureter.

CASE I.—Mr. B., aged twenty-eight years, travelling salesman. History of having four attacks of severe pain in right lower quadrant of the abdomen. Onset sudden, and attacks lasted from one to six days, accompanied by vomiting. After acute symptoms subsided, there remained more or less pain in region of the appendix. He was seen on the fifth day of a very severe attack, which had been diagnosticated by both his father and brother, who were physicians, as appendicitis. Urine showed erythrocytes and leukocytes. Skiagraph by Dr. Carman showed shadow in pelvic portion of the right ureter. Diagnosis, right ureter calculus. Combined operation. Appendix extended well over pelvic brim, adherent to parietal peritoneum over right ureter. The skiagraphic diagnosis of stone in right ureter was confirmed. Stone was located well down in the pelvic portion of ureter and was pushed into bladder. Stone was passed forty-eight hours after operation.

CASE II.—Miss D., aged twenty-six years, had suffered for two years with a recurrent pain in right side. The attacks at times were severe, and she was never free from pain. Examination revealed mild muscular rigidity over region of the appendix. Urine analysis showed erythrocytes and leukocytes. Skiagraphic examination was negative. A diagnosis of chronic appendicitis was made. Abdomen opened through gridiron incision. Appendix found well over pelvic brim adherent to parietal peritoneum over right ureter.

CASE III.—Mr. H., aged forty-eight years, broker. History of trouble dating back three years. Attacks came on suddenly with great violence, accompanied by vomiting and severe pain in region of the appendix. Pain radiating downward along the cord to testicle. Twelve years prior to last operation he had been operated on by a New York surgeon for a stone in the bladder, the crushing operation having been done. Urine examination negative. Skiagraphs (Figs. 5 and 6) showed shadow in the region of the right ureter. Three skiagraphs presented a shadow in a different location at each examination. The mobility of this shadow with normal urine was the basis for a diagnosis of chronic appendicitis with concretion in the appendix.

At operation an appendix eight inches in length with a concretion and constriction at the lower third was found. This case was especially interesting, as calculus in the ureter was excluded by the changing position of the skiagraphic shadow. The symptoms were undoubtedly due to appendicular colic, the appendix being long and unable to properly empty its contents.

CASE IV.—Mr. McC., aged forty-six years, blacksmith. This patient entered the hospital with the history of having been treated through several attacks of what had been diagnosticated appendicitis. He was just getting over a rather severe attack similar in nature to those from which he had previously suffered.

He complained of considerable pain in both right and left lower quadrants. There was some muscular rigidity on the right side and pain on deep palpation. Examination of urine showed erythrocytes and leukocytes. Skiagraphs showed a shadow in the pelvic portion of both right and left ureteral regions. Cystoscopic examination and ureteral catheterization showed right ureter free. Obstruction about two inches above entrance of left ureter into the bladder.

These plates here presented show the catheter in right ureter, and on the left side the catheter is shown curled up in the bladder due to obstruction met on left side. Combined operation, appendix over brim, non-adherent, but constricted and diseased. Stone removed from left ureter.

CASE V.—Dr. E., aged thirty-two years, had had several attacks of appendicitis. Skiagraph showed shadow in region of right ureter. Erythrocytes and leukocytes in urine. At operation the appendix was found adherent to ureter on right side and well over pelvic brim.

CASE VI.—Mr. N., aged thirty-nine years, wholesale lumberman, was referred from Arkansas by his family physician, who had observed him through a number of attacks of supposed appendicitis. The attacks were classical with regard to the ordinary symptoms and signs. The only positive finding upon examination was tenderness over McBurney's point. The skiagraph by Dr. Carman showed a characteristic shadow low down in the right ureteral region. Diagnosis of ureteral calculi was made. This patient later had same removed by Dr. Wm. Mayo.

CASE VII.—Mr. P., aged thirty-three years, farmer, was sent to St. John's Hospital from Illinois with diagnosis of intestinal obstruction. Two days previous to his entrance in the hospital he was taken with a violent attack of pain in the lower part of the abdomen, more marked on the left than on the right side. It was soon followed by abdominal distention and vomiting, which had frequently increased. Doses of catharsis which were given, failed to produce the desired evacuation. Upon examination he was found in this condition of marked abdominal distention, frequent vomiting, and more or less delirious, so that it was impossible to depend upon statements. Urine analysis showed marked hematuria. Skiagraph located shadow low down in the left ureteral region. Catheterization of the ureters, which was attempted with this examination, was unsuccessful. At operation a calculus was found in this location and removed. Combined operation, appendix normal.

CASE VIII.—Dr. E., aged thirty-two years, had had five attacks of abdominal pain followed by tenderness located in the right lower quadrant of the abdomen. The first three attacks were of short duration, not accompanied by fever, leukocytosis, or peritoneal irritation (duration two to six hours). Following the second attack, erythrocytes appeared in the urine with each subsequent one. A skiagraph showed a shadow located down in the region of the right ureter, after which the patient himself concluded he had ureteral calculi. The fifth attack was of longer duration and accompanied by two chills, fever, and slight leukocytosis. Erythrocytes and leukocytes continued to be present in the urine. After this attack another skiagraph was taken with stylets in the ureters, which demonstrated that the skiagraphic shadow was a considerable distance from the ureter. Diagnosis was then made—combined lesions of the appendix and ureter. At operation the appendix was found inflamed at its base and retrocecal. Since the operation of appendectomy, seven months ago, there has been no return of symptoms or abnormal findings in the urine.

DIAGNOSIS. In the diagnosis of those lesions which give symptoms referable to this quadrant of the abdomen, makes it necessary (1) to exclude those diseases which have no relation to the appendix or ureter, and (2) by special examination to differentiate between ureteral and appendiceal diseases. Among the general conditions which should always be considered as a possible source of error are tabes and the psychoneuroses. The *intestinal crises of tabes* can usually be recognized by numerous other signs of tabes. The *peculiar paroxysms of pain in neurotic individuals* associated with the menses are excluded by the stigmata of neuroses with negative local signs. Neurotic conditions, however, should not be held accountable for local symptoms when definite local lesions can be demonstrated, as they in themselves may be the cause for the general neurosis.

Among local conditions independent of the appendix and ureter those diseases, in the female, of *the uterus and adnexa* (salpingitis, tubal pregnancy, ovarian cyst, subserous fibroid, etc.) can usually be differentiated by bimanual examination, as definite tumefaction in the pelvis. It is unusual for appendiceal or ureteral diseases to produce tumefaction that can be palpated by this method. *Localized tenderness along the ureter can sometimes be elicited by rectal examination in calculi low down in the ureter. It is questionable, however, whether it is ever possible to palpate small calculi, even when within reach of the palpating finger in the rectum.* It was not possible in the clinical cases observed by the writers, and in the cadaver it was impossible to feel the stylet or small shot in the ureter although the skiagraph (Figs. 7 and 8) demonstrates them within reach of the finger in the rectum. Tenderness and occasionally bulging in the right fornix or pelvis is also present in lesions of a long pelvic appendix or pelvic abscess from this organ, but it is very exceptional that the appendix itself can be palpated. Skiagraph, Fig. 7, shows that the finger is barely able to reach to the top of an average size appendix through the rectum. *Pyelitis in pregnancy* gives a clinical picture which simulates appendicitis. It occurs more frequently in primipara, usually about the third month. Pyuria or local findings which soon occur about the kidney will clear up the diagnosis. As this disease is non-operable, it should receive the first consideration in the suspected appendicitis in early pregnancy. *Gall-bladder disease*, especially in those cases of ptosis of the liver or dependent gallbladder, are usually differentiated by the physical findings. *Ulcers and other lesions of the cecum* with an extension to the peritoneum, resulting in a localized peritonitis, should be suspected when the history of their causal disease is present elsewhere in the body, or the local findings have been preceded by large intestinal symptoms. *Mucous colitis*, which has been a very common cause for unnecessary operation upon the accessory organs of the intestinal tract, should always be considered as a possibility. The characteristic evacuation of large amounts of mucus following paroxysms of abdominal pain is sufficient upon which to base a diagnosis. *Tuberculous peritonitis* causing localized peritonitis should especially be suspected in children. A history of exposure and tuberculous lesions elsewhere in the body, Diazo reaction in the urine, etc., are usually sufficient upon which to base a positive diagnosis. *Chronic seminal vesiculitis and calculi in the seminal vesicle* may mimic both ureteral and appendiceal diseases. Periodic occurrence of pyuria which can be demonstrated by ureteral catheterization and cystoscopy as not due to the kidneys or the bladder itself, combined with pus massaged from the seminal vesicles, and skiagraphic findings will support such a diagnosis.

After these conditions have been given due consideration and positively excluded, many of these cases have symptoms and signs common to both ureteral and appendiceal lesion. It has been demonstrated by the illustrative cases given above that evidence derived from the subjective, physical, and urinary findings are not sufficient in some cases upon which to base a positive diagnosis. It is, therefore,

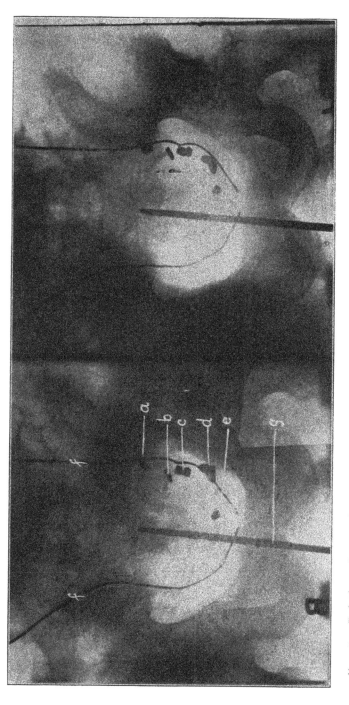

Fig. 1.—Relation of appendix to ureter: (*a*) base of appendix injected with mercury; (*b*) lead wire in distal end of appendix; (*c*) lead ball attached to and in the same plane with ureter; (*d*) lead balls about two inches anterior to ureter; (*e*) lead ball about two inches posterior to ureter; (*f*) lead wire in ureter; (*g*) sound in rectum (showing slight displacement of the sound to the left, throwing it slightly posterior to the ureters at their lower portion). (For examination with parlor stereoscope.)

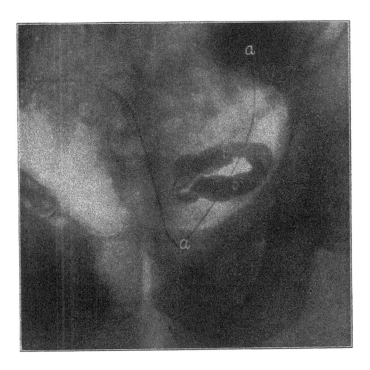

FIG. 2.—Relation of appendix to ureters: (a) stylet in ureter;
(b) appendix injected with bismuth paste.

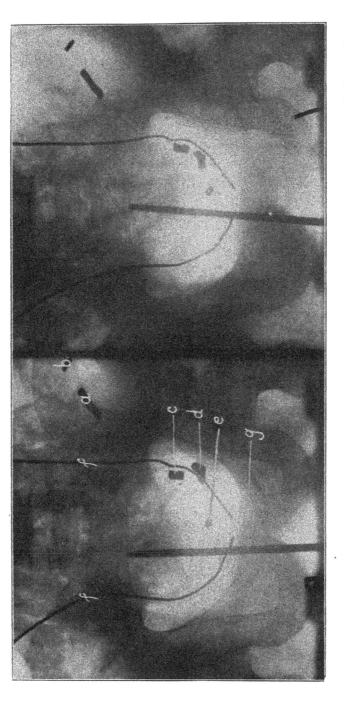

FIG. 3.—Relation of appendix to ureters: (*a*) base with the appendix injected with mercury; (*b*) lead wire in distal end of appendix; (*c*) lead ball attached to and in the same plane with ureter; (*d*) lead balls about two inches anterior to ureter; (*e*) lead ball about two inches posterior to ureter; (*f*) lead wire in ureter; (*g*) sound in rectum (showing slight displacement of the sound to the left, throwing it slightly posterior to the ureters at their lower portion). (For examination with parlor stereoscope.)

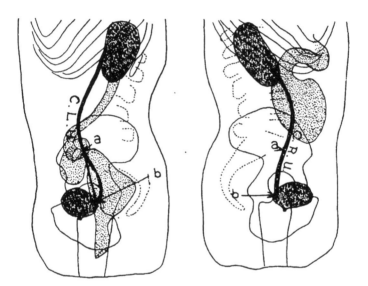

FIG. 4.—Diagrams showing, left (C. L. U.) course of left ureter; right (*C*. R. U.) course of right ureter: (*a*) synchondrosis; (*b*) prostate line from *a* to *b* represents plane in which sound lies when introduced into the rectum in position described.

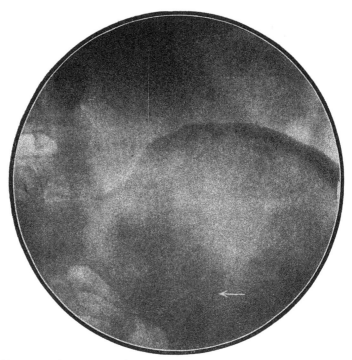

FIG. 5.—The arrow indicates shadow of concretion in appendix, external to the sacro-iliac synchondrosis over ilium.

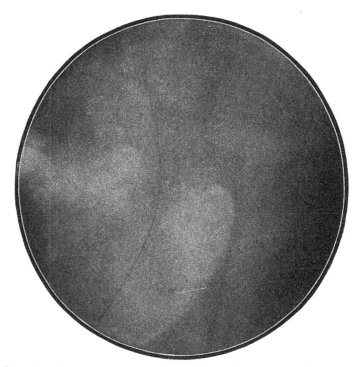

FIG. 6.—Skiagraph taken with stylets in the ureters. The shadow (indicated by the arrow) not in contact with the stylet in the right internal to synchondrosis ureter.

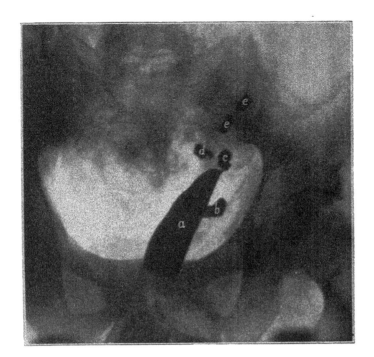

FIG. 7.—Skiagraph showing: (a) finger in rectum; (b) three lead balls about two inches anterior to ureter; (c) two lead balls attached to and on the same plane with the ureter; (d) lead wire in the tip of the appendix; (e) mercury in the proximal portion of the appendix.

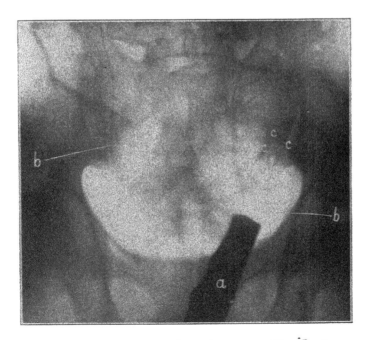

FIG. 8.—Skiagraph showing: (a) finger in rectum; (b) stylet in ureter; (c) appendix injected with bismuth paste.

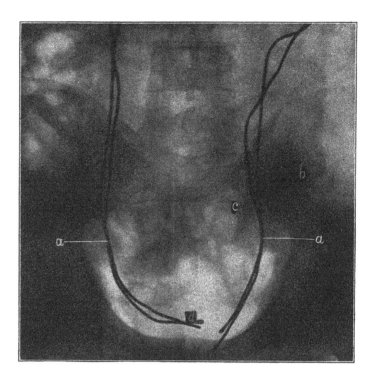

Fig. 9.—Skiagraph of double ureters: (a) stylets in bilateral double ureters; (b) mercury in the base of the appendix; (c) lead wire in the tip of the appendix; (d) lead ball posterior to the ureter.

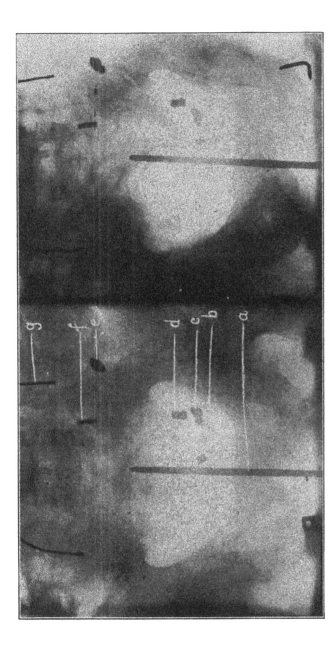

FIG. 10.—Skiagraph showing: (a) sound in the rectum in the proper position in the same transverse plane with the ureters; (b) lead ball about two inches posterior to sound in ureter; (c) three lead balls about two inches anterior to the sound and ureter; (d) two lead balls attached to ureter and in the same transverse plane with the sound; (e) base of the appendix injected with mercury; (f) lead wire in the tip of the appendix; (g) lead wire in the ureters withdrawn from the pelvic ureter. (For examination with parlor stereoscope.)

necessary to add to this evidence that procured by ski-
agraphy, cystoscopy, and ureteral catheterization. The
mere demonstration of a shadow along the course of the
ureter, with the positive findings in the urine and other
clinical evidences, is usually not sufficient for a positive
diagnosis. A skiagraph taken with stylets in the ureter
used as negative evidence is also not without some degree
of error. For example, stylets in the ureter not meeting
obstruction or in contact with a skiagraphic shadow is
not absolutely sufficient to exclude a stone in the ureters.
There are three conditions in which a stone might be
present in the ureter and the findings of a styletted skiagraph misleading. One is a calculus in a ureteral pocket
allowing the stylet to pass up the ureter and not producing
a skiagraphic shadow in contact with the stylet. Another
is the anomaly of a double ureter, as shown in Fig. 9. A
calculus might be present in one ureter and yet a stylet passed
up the other one would not be in contact with the shadow.
Ricketts has collected many cases of double ureter. The
third is a shadow appearing in contact with a stylet in the
ureter in a single skiagraph which can be demonstrated
to be either anterior or posterior to the stylet by stereoscopic skiagraph.

Original Method as an Aid to the Location of Skiagraphic
Shadows in the Pelvis.

It has been our misfortune to have so many reactions
from cystoscopy and catheterization of the ureters, either
from trauma or injection, that we have attempted other
methods of localization of the skiagraphic shadows in the
pelvis which occur in a considerable number of these cases.
While we do not wish to discredit the value of the skiagraph
of the styletted ureters as probably the most satisfactory
and positive way of localizing these shadows, we have become

convinced that if a more simple and practical method could be evolved, which would avoid these reactions, it would be of greater advantage, for the reason that it would be more frequently attempted. From personal experience we have found that the majority of skiagraphic shadows found in the pelvis are not in the ureters, as has also been shown by Parks and others. They are usually phleboliths in the papiniform, vaginal, and hemorrhoidal plexus of veins. The other common condition producing these shadows in the pelvis are calcified glands and enteroliths. Many of these shadows of extra-ureteral opacities are not on the same transverse plane with the ureter.

The male pelvis seems to be especially adapted to other methods of localization of ureteral calculi found within its bounds. This lies in the fact that the rectum running from the anus backward to the coccix, and then upward to the first sacral vertebra, will allow the introduction of a sound along the median line of the pelvis which will be on the same transverse plane of the ureters. As has been shown (Fig. 4), under the anatomical description, the ureters traverse the pelvis in a transverse plane extending from the base of the sacro-iliac synchondrosis to the posterior portion of the prostate gland. In taking advantage of these anatomical relations we have endeavored to demonstrate that when a sound in the rectum is brought beneath the crotch of the symphysis, and then passed directly upward for a distance of six inches, its tip will strike the first sacral vertebra just below the promontory of the sacrum, on the level and in the same plane with the ureters as they leave and pass forward from the posterior pelvic wall. The base of the sound in this position is against the prostate gland, and, therefore, on the same level with the ureters as they enter the bladder. The sound in this position then traverses the median line of the pelvis in practically the same transverse plane with the ureters, as shown in Figs. 1 and 3, provided their course is as constant as we have found it upon three subjects. Having thus determined the normal plane of the ureters by taking stereoscopic skiagraphs with the sound in the rectum in this plane, it can be determined whether a given skiagraphic shadow is in the same plane with the sound. If the course of the ureters is constant, then one would be justified in concluding that a skiagraphic shadow which was any considerable distance from this plane (anterior or posterior to the sound) would probably not be in the ureters. At the present time no definite claim can be made for this method, because it depends upon the constancy of the ureters, *i. e.*, whether they traverse practically the same plane in different individuals. This must be determined by extended anatomical and clinical investigations, which should be stimulated by this preliminary report. It is true that the lateral course of the ureter has already been demonstrated to vary considerably by skiagraphs taken upon clinical cases. This seems to be more pronounced in the female than in the male, probably due to the other conditions which are present causing the dislocation of the other organs. In the three bodies studied and the clinical cases observed by this method, so far the course of the ureters in the male seem to be remarkably constant in this plane. Therefore the liberty was taken to insert the method into this article as one that would be worthy of consideration in the diagnosis of these conditions. Providing it is of value, its simplicity and freedom from danger and reaction highly commend its trial.

TECHNIQUE. No preliminary catharsis is necessary. (If suspicious shadows are found, a second skiagraph should be made within two or three days, to exclude enteroliths.) An ordinary straight No. 26 French ureteral sound, graduated in inches, is introduced for the distance of six inches into the rectum, with the patient in the dorsal position. It is pulled up anteriorly until it impinges upon the subpubic ligament, directly in the median line. If the introduction of the sound is painful to the patient, caused by meeting obstruction in the folds of the rectum, the rectum can be inflated, which usually overcomes this difficulty. With the sound in this position, stereoscopic skiagraphs are taken in the usual manner.

TREATMENT.

The treatment of these lesions necessarily depends upon an accurate diagnosis, which will not only place positive indications for treatment, but will also indicate the absolute methods of the procedure to be undertaken, such as the location of the incision and the route of the operation. The treatment of definite lesions of the appendix is well established. Treatment of ureteral calculi is one that is not entirely established, and will depend to a considerable extent upon the findings in the individual cases. If the calculus is small enough to pass through the ureter, and there is no evidence of complications, such as pyelitis, hydronephrosis, etc., and repeated skiagraphic examination demonstrated the progression of the calculi toward the bladder, there is no imperative indications for surgical interference. On the other hand, if the calculus is complicated by secondary conditions of the kidney, or does not progress satisfactorily after a number of attacks of ureteral colic, indications are definitely fixed for radical removal.

The operations adapted for the removal of ureteral calculi are (1) the extraperitoneal operation; (2) the intraperitoneal operation; and (3) the combined extra- and intraperitoneal operation. In unquestionable cases of ureteral calculi a simple extraperitoneal operation should be attempted. Incision is made, according to the location of the calculi, along the external border of the rectus to the peritoneum. The peritoneum is separated (in pelvic calculi) down to the posterior surface of the bladder and prostate gland. The ureter is palpated with the *bare fingers*, beginning at the bladder and going upward.   If the stone is felt, a longitudinal nick is made in the ureter between the two fingers grasping the stone, through which the calculus is squeezed and removed. A cigarette drain is placed down to the opening in the ureter and the wound closed in the usual manner. If the calculus is not discovered by this extraperitoneal method, an opening should be made in the peritoneum at the site of the incision and bidigital palpation of the ureter, made with the finger in the abdominal cavity, and the thumb along the course of the ureter, extraperitoneally. If the stone is found, it is removed in the same way as extraperitoneal operation. If no calculus is found, the appendix and complete exploration of the abdomen should be made. In doing these operations it is necessary to remember that they should be done as soon after definite location is made of them, in order to be positive that they have not changed their position. It is not infrequent that after a catheterization of the ureters, ureteral colic, which is stimulated by the instrumentation, causes the stone to pass into the bladder. Many cases in which calculi have not been found during operation, which have been previously definitely located with a skiagraph of the styletted ureters, can be accounted for on this cause of change of position. In other cases the stone has been milked into the bladder without the knowledge of the operator.

DISCUSSION.

DR. HOWARD A. KELLY, of Baltimore.—I do not think so admirable a paper as this ought to be allowed to pass without discussion. I have looked through a thousand or more stereograms in the past two years, and while this method is full of promise I had not thought of applying it to this field, so I rejoice that a new and valuable diagnostic measure has been advanced.

Dr. Brown has done a great service in pointing out the liability of confusing a variety of affections on the right side, while the facility with which we do surgery in these days tempts us when there are two or three signs present suggestive of a particular condition to make a positive diagnosis, when of course, the appendix is usually the organ to suffer. Every one of us has seen patients who have come from other surgeons, and our patients have gone to other doctors, who have taken out their appendices when something else has turned out to be the matter. On the right side there are five or more pathological conditions which may be confounded with one another unless great care is exercised in making a diagnosis. We may have a localized inflammation high up in the corner of the bladder at the fixed point in the bladder which I call the cornu which causes trouble. Again, we have the tube and ovary on the right side, which may be readily confused with a trouble referable to an appendix deep in the pelvis; then we have the appendix itself and its diseases. We also have the ureter at the pelvic brim with a stone in it. I would insist above all things that we bear in mind sacro-iliac disease accompanied with pronounced pain at the pelvic brim. I recall several cases of sacro-iliac disease, and I must say that it is much more common than is accepted by any physicians today. When we review our cases and study them closely it is surprising how many complain of a loose sacro-iliac joint on the right or left side. Again, we may have a distended cecum. Most important of all, we have the kidney to take into consideration here also in making a differential diagnosis. We have also on this same side gallstones as well as diseases of the pylorus and duodenum. Diseases of the kidney and appendix, as well as ureteral and pelvic inflammatory diseases, are quite common in women. With the aid of the ureteral catheter alone are we enabled to differentiate certain of these pathological conditions. I recall one case in which a calculus caused the adherence of the appendix to the ureter, but I do not believe the appendix is ever the cause of a ureteral calculus.

DR. CHAS. H. MAYO, of Rochester, Minnesota.—Dr. Brown has certainly brought before us a most interesting subject; and Dr. Kelly has brought out the fact that sometimes people have two diseases at the same time. A patient may have a stone in the right ureter, which is overlooked, or he may have some pathological condition referable to the right side, and, of course, when that is the case the appendix is usually the first thing thought of. There is no question but what many people have been operated on for appendicitis who have had stones in their kidneys or ureters, but the fact remains that for a long time such patients may also have had trouble with their appendices, so that a thorough examination of the abdomen, when it is opened, will often disclose gallstones, which were really unsuspected. It will disclose the cause of so-called stomach troubles, such as gas in the stomach, indigestion, etc., troubles which do not localize themselves, the cause of which may be obstruction from a stone in the cystic duct, or other pathological conditions. The same thing holds true with regard to various other structures or organs in the abdomen. Many of us recall cases described in papers where patients have had a stone in the ureter, and yet they were operated on for appendicitis and had their appendices taken out. After the appendix was removed they continued to suffer the same as before. Such cases remind us that there may be something wrong with the appendix even though we operate for some other pathological condition. There may be nothing to show in the urine that a stone is present in the ureter. Even one or two examinations may not disclose anything definite, and these patients may come to us with unmistakable symptoms of appendicitis, and examination of the urine discloses nothing, and they are operated on for this disease, the appendix is removed, and found to be diseased and apparently the cause of the trouble. In our experience, twice we have found stones in the ureter in trying to dislodge a diseased appendix that was bound down by adhesions alongside the ureter. We could feel that the ureter was distended and obstructed with a stone, and there was an acute condition present in the appendix, so that today, if we operate for appendicitis, and we are going to operate on most of them, we must remember about the history, and if upon opening the abdomen we do not find an adequate cause we must look farther. I have not been satisfied when operating if I have not been able to relieve them of what they complained of. Adhesions do not amount to much in the minds of the laity, and yet they cause great distress, great suffering. When we open the abdomen, we should not hesitate, if we think it is necessary, to make our incision larger and search for stones in the ureter, because in this way we can locate them from the kidney down. One may search and search in some of these cases without being able to find ureteral stone. One of these patients the next day after operation passed pus from the bladder. The cystoscope was used, and it was found the stone had slipped out. In the other case, two weeks later, the stones slipped from the lowest position into the bladder.

I do not believe that the method which Dr. Brown has described is a very good one for those who do all kinds of work, but it is all right for those who are skilled in genito-urinary and ureteral work, as well as in the use of the cystoscope. It is difficult for a person to carry on many lines of work and become expert in all of them. Catheterization of the ureters is all right in the hands of the expert, and we depend upon it in the surgical work we do.

DR. WM. M. POLK, of New York City.—Referring to sacro-iliac disease, there is no doubt that we are beginning to realize that it is assuming proportions which we had not previously thought of, owing to the fact that we did not know much about it. As a matter of interest to those who may be interested in the orthopedic side of the question, there are many of us (gynecologists) who have had need for correct conceptions of sacroiliac disease on the right side, and I wish these gentlemen (orthopedists) would become sufficiently interested in it to develop something bearing upon differential diagnosis. I have been surprised to see how little interest, until within the last year or two, has been taken in this aspect of sacro-iliac disease—disease which may produce the kind of pain which so many report as being referable to the appendix; not that I think, gentlemen, we should refer the trouble to the appendix in such cases, because I happen to belong to a class who believe that it is possible to make a differential diagnosis between sacro-iliac disease and an inflamed appendix. But admitting that general surgery takes such a wide sweep we are apt to become confused in our efforts at differentiation, one would suppose that the orthopedists would take up the matter and lay down some absolute rules which would enable us to differentiate sacro-iliac disease from disease of the appendix. In view of the way in which this question is still held, I think this contribution of Dr. Brown is particularly valuable. In addition I would call attention to the fact that in this latter day, when we have so much to do with the rest cure, when many of such patients have sacro-iliac pains occurring upon the right side, or both sides, it would be a source of satisfaction for physicians to turn their attention to the possibility of this treatment, being responsible for some of these pains. By so doing, I think we would not only enlarge our horizon, but save ourselves occasionally from a certain degree of mortification on account of mistaken diagnoses. I have a case in mind.

DR. H. A. ROYSTER, of Raleigh, North Carolina.—To me the most important thing which I have heard at this meeting is the discussion relative to the question of diagnosis between appendiceal disease and right ureteral disease, as well as the satisfaction of knowing that a patient may have both in a given case.

We are all having cases of the type mentioned by Dr. Brown, in which the patient has had all the symptoms of stone in the kidney, and yet find an adherent appendix as the cause of the trouble. In one case of mine the appendix was adherent behind and directly to the kidney by means of the parietal peritoneum. In two other cases the appendix was found lying directly over the ureter, and in one case had ulcerated its way through, so that there was a communication between the appendix and ureter. If we could get some precise method of diagnosing these cases, we would solve one of the most difficult and important problems in the whole field of surgery.

Dr. Brown's paper covers the ground very thoroughly, and I believe he has developed certain definite facts.

DR. R. C. COFFEY, of Portland, Oregon.—I would like to put a question to Dr. Mayo and Dr. Royster, with reference to treatment. I have sent some of these cases to an orthopedist and have been surprised at the results obtained by bandaging. These patients who have been sent to an orthopedist have come back entirely satisfied, but whether or not the effect was psychological, or whether it was the bandaging or strapping that benefited them, I do not know. The orthopedist claims that bandaging does benefit these patients greatly, and the patients claim so, for the reason that the pain has returned after the bandage has been taken off.

DR. WM. P. MATTHEWS, of Richmond, Virginia.—There ought to be very little difficulty in making a diagnosis between sacro-iliac disease and appendicitis. Sacro-iliac disease is nearly always tubercular. Sometimes we will find that a loose sacro-iliac joint gives considerable trouble, but remembering that sacro-iliac disease, especially in children, is not common, and that you always find tenderness over the sacro-iliac joint, and the pain is referred down over the buttocks to the thigh, it makes the diagnosis rather easy. A simple little method we follow is a sharp blow upon the side of the pelvis, striking two bones together, which elicits pain always, which is never true in cases of appendicitis. We use a pelvic girdle in our orthopedic work and get splendid results, both from loose joint and from true sacro-iliac disease.

DR. CHAS. A. L. REED, of Cincinnati.—I rise simply to express my appreciation of the paper and to add one or two observations.

Recently I had occasion to observe an operator who made an effort to relieve a patient of a supposed ureteral calculus on the right side. No ureteral stone was found, although one had been definitely determined. The operator was consequently in a state of consternation. He had relieved the patient of ureteral symptoms by relieving peri-ureteral and perinephritic adhesions, and the results were satisfactory in a clinical way. After the operation, in making a control picture, he found that the disk, which, with the patient lying in the dorsal position, had registered along the line of the ureter, was found quite two inches in front of it when the patient was on the side. This emphasizes the importance of taking a control skiagraph with the patient lying on the side, as it leads to satisfactory conclusions.

My second observation reverts to the importance of studying diagnostic symptoms, as they are manifested, of the nervous system. We have paid too little attention to the question of pain as a symptom; we have given little attention to the definite localization of pain; we have given too little attention to the work of Langley in the elaboration of the autonomic nervous system. If we were to give more attention to this, we would be able to localize more definitely visceral conditions with which we may have to contend. For instance, in a case of kidney and ureteral complications, as compared with those in the appendix, we may rely upon the fact that a superficial algesia of the autonomic nervous system is related to kidney and ureter and corresponds to the distribution of nerves, not lower than the sixth dorsal nerve; whereas pain referable to the appendix corresponds to the distribution of the twelfth dorsal or the first lumbar spinal nerve. If we can remember these things and take them more definitely into consideration than we have done heretofore, we shall have, I think, a key for the interpretation of these symptoms more definitely than in the past. But I mention these things only in addition to the excellent work that has been presented by Dr. Brown. I think the observations and researches that have been presented by Dr. Brown this evening render the entire profession under obligations to him.

DR. BROWN (closing).—I quite agree with Dr. Mayo in his statement that the best way to clear up the obscure cases is by an exploratory incision, but I think it is much better and much more satisfactory to clear up some of them before making this incision. This paper was written for the purpose of stimulating more painstaking work in these atypical cases. There is no excuse for railroading the chronic cases to operation. It is bad enough to have to hurry the acute cases to operation. Where we have time, these cases should be gone over very carefully. We should make use of the laboratory and x-rays, the cystoscope and ureter catheter, so that an absolutely accurate diagnosis can be made before operation, if possible. If we are correct in our conclusions with regard to the relation of the appendix to the ureter, it will readily explain the urinary findings in many cases. It clears up a character of cases that heretofore have been rather puzzling. I wish to speak of the propriety of exploring these cases through a combined operation, that is, not only to do work on the ureter if there is a stone there, but make an incision sufficiently large to explore the appendix and gall-bladder and kidney, and to do such other intra-abdominal work as may be necessary.

In the rapid manner in which I went over this paper I did not have the opportunity to take up the differential diagnosis of these cases, as I have really done in the paper, and I hope this method I have described will prove of value to you.

THE DIAGNOSIS OF HYPERTHYROIDISM OR EXOPHTHALMIC GOITRE.

By *C. H. Mayo, M.D.,*
Rochester, Minnesota.

THE ancient history of hyperthyroidism or exophthalmic goitre amounts to a rather imperfect description of the disease by several observers of a few cases each. The condition was formerly considered as purely medical, and knowledge of existing conditions was derived solely from autopsies which necessarily presented many changes in structure throughout the body which were not present in the early stages of the disease. In fact, the condition of the thyroids did not seem to call for any unusual attention as compared with other organs, because microscopically they often resembled enlarged thyroids of the simple type.

For the last fifty years clinicians who have based their knowledge upon symptoms and upon terminal changes as found at autopsies have endeavored to classify certain cases of goitre within the narrow limits of the description of the few cases reported by those remarkable men, Parry, Graves, Basedow, and others nearly a century ago.

Today, even with the great progress in medical science we are lacking very much in our knowledge of the subject. Formerly only such cases as presented all the symptoms in a severe form were accepted as Graves' disease. The belief that the disease represents a condition *sui generis*, and thereby differs from nearly all other diseases, still prevails among many members of the medical profession. They pronounce well-marked cases as *fruste* or *pseudo* until the eyes became prominent. Should that feature have been delayed, even if all other symptoms are present, it is not until this condition appears that they are properly labelled as a disease, after all representing but a syndrome of symptoms.

It is now definitely shown that the condition is not one which involves all the organs at the onset, but that it is like other diseases in presenting acute, chronic, mild, severe, and irregular or remittent types of the disease.

In the development of the surgery of simple goitre during the last thirty years, many patients have been operated upon who either had at the time of operation or previously, many if not all the symptoms of exophthalmic, goitre. If symptoms of hyperthyroidism were the main indications for operation, the cases were classified accordingly; otherwise they were considered as simple or encapsulated goitre with partial or temporary hyperthyroidism.

The result of the accumulated knowledge in the examination of all forms of thyroid disease the world over is that there is a definite increase in the parenchyma of the gland in some forms of exophthalmic goitre, with evidence of overactivity of cell secretion. This evidence may present itself in several forms—(a) increase of cells in the alveoli, (b) increase in the number of alveoli, (c) by papillomatous invagination into the vesicles of the gland. All of these changes may be throughout the gland or only in areas of it. Pathologists who are experienced in this class of laboratory work are usually able to give the symptoms and stage of the disease from a typical microscopic slide, and from the form of degeneration of the tissues in some cases can estimate the probable condition of the heart, liver, and essential organs.

It seems probable that a thyroid which presents this condition of hyperthyroidism and does not destroy the life of the individual or destroy itself must, at some period of its activity, revert back to simple goitre. Then colloid will be deposited with iodothyroglobin, and the gland will lose its apparent cell activity.

From the examination of a great many thyroids of this type it would appear that this change or reversion may occur at any period, and that certain exceptional individuals are able to withstand the disease until there is a degeneration of the parenchyma, and a positive loss of secretion or hypothyroidism, shown by varying degrees of myxedema as a terminal condition following a former hyperthyroidism. There may be wide variations in the quantity of thyroid secreted in simple and cystic goitres, within the limits of health. Theoretically, in the one case there should be hypothyroidism, in another, hyperthyroidism, yet neither of these conditions can be constantly recognized. The break in the equilibrium of the associated ductless glands to produce hyperthyroidism under such conditions is seemingly brought about in the majority of cases by some infectious disease or severe illness, although a considerable number of cases exhibit the first symptoms through a change in the nervous system following a severe mental shock.

In fact, there has been but little added recently to our knowledge of the etiology of simple goitre, and concerning that of exophthalmic goitre much has been written and little is known. Heredity appears to be an important factor in some cases. We still lack the knowledge as to whether the stimulus is from without or within, as a chemical irritant or hormone messenger. The gland elaborates iodine, of which there is less in the gland of hyperthyroidism than in the normal gland, but Ried Hunt has shown that in such cases there is more iodine in the blood, it being produced, delivered, and slowly excreted from the system contrary to its usual rapid elimination. It is also shown by Marine and others that colloid goitre contains more iodine in the whole gland than in the normal thyroid, but bulk for bulk the colloid goitre contains less iodine. It is possible that colloid is capable of holding the secretion of the gland without suffering destruction, and in the retention of the secretion with colloid the size of the thyroid is necessarily increased. Marine believes that hyperthyroidism is induced by a lack of some essential secretion of the thyroid considered as a complex substance, and in the effort to restore this, an excess of some component part of the secretion is produced to a toxic degree.

Reviewing briefly the most important manifestations of hyperthyroidism we have tachycardia as the most usual heart condition. In advanced cases the heart may be irregular in rhythm, and the pulse of low tension. Dilatation of the heart must be differentiated from dilatation with hypertrophy and compensation, and from pure myocardial disease as well.

The eye symptoms are numerous and may appear early or late, and one or all of them may be present. These symptoms consist of prominence, a widening of the palpebral fissure (Dalrymple), staring without winking (Stellwag), lagging of the lids with eye movements (Graffe), or insufficiency of accommodation at near point (Mobius). Rarely there is dislocation of the globe. Ulcer of the cornea is not uncommon in marked cases.

Myocardial changes and Bright's disease may also produce some of these symptoms.

Tremor is nearly always present, eight or nine to the second, and may be associated with chorea-like movements in extreme cases, with, as a rule, great muscular weakness.

As to goitre, the thyroid may be but little enlarged in the early cases, or enlargement may be the first symptom. If it is present a long time previous to the onset of Graves' disease the microscopic changes will be parenchymatous increase of cells projecting into the colloid retention in the vesicles. From these cells the secretion is derived. Operative deductions from certain cases would indicate that a wonderful cell increase may occur with but little enlargement of the thyroid as a whole, and it is apparent that the secretion is delivered and not retained.

The general symptoms are sweating, anemia, emaciation, and loss of strength in the majority of cases. Vomiting and diarrhea without apparent cause are common and transient symptoms. Pigmentation of the skin is often seen, and a bronzing is not unusual.

Urine is small in amount. Albumin is found occasionally in many cases. Patients in advanced conditions may have it in considerable amounts, as well as hyaline and granular casts. Transient glycosuria is often noted, and occasionally a true diabetes. Irregular fluctuations of temperature, tending to normal, yet often up one or two degrees, are common.

Nervous Symptoms. There is often excitable or nervous irritability, and sometimes altered disposition with mental depression or signs of mania.

It must be remembered that malignant goitre may at times present the most aggravated picture of hyperthyroidism.

In the diagnosis of the condition Professor Kocher regards leukemia of the neutrophilic polymorphonuclears as an important early symptom, also a percentage and absolute increase in the lymphocytes. In over two hundred tests made from patients with goitre, mostly with hyperthyroidism, we have at times found such changes most marked, although some of the advanced cases varied greatly, sufficiently so to classify the condition in the same category with other laboratory tests which are employed for other conditions as a means of diagnosis in association with other signs and symptoms.

Notwithstanding the fact that many patients with the disease are cured spontaneously, and many are improved or cured by some type of medical, semimedical, or a form of serum treatment by cytolysis, the condition known as hyperthyroidism has stepped boldly into the field of surgery.

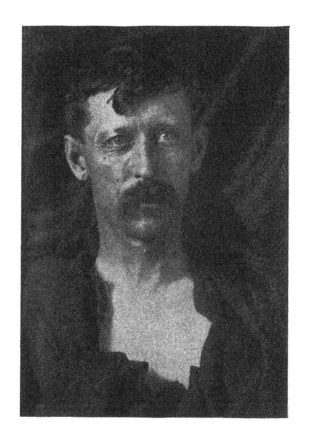

FIG. 1.—Hyperthyroidism with little glandular
enlargement and no exophthalmos.

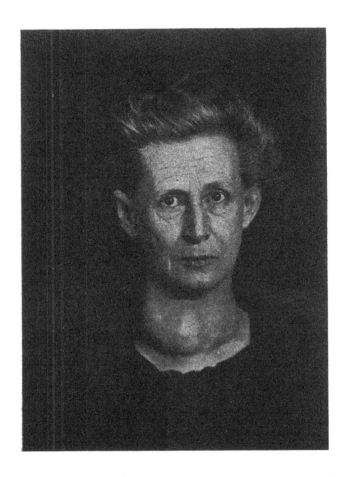

FIG. 2.—Hyperthyroidism with thyroid enlargement but
no exophthalmos.

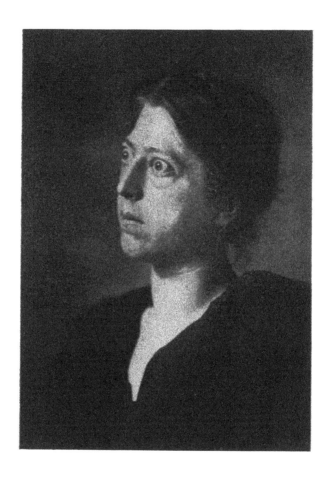

FIG. 3.—Hyperthyroidism with little glandular enlargement but marked exophthalmos.

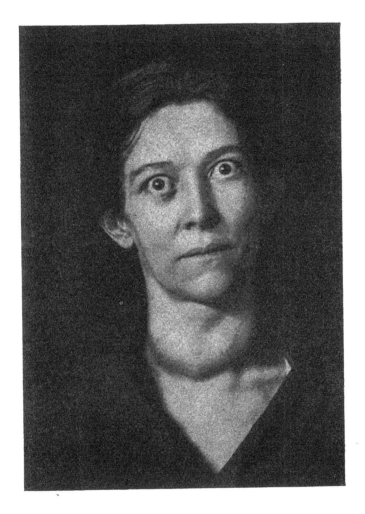

FIG. 4.—Hyperthyroidism with both thyroid enlargement
and exophthalmos marked.

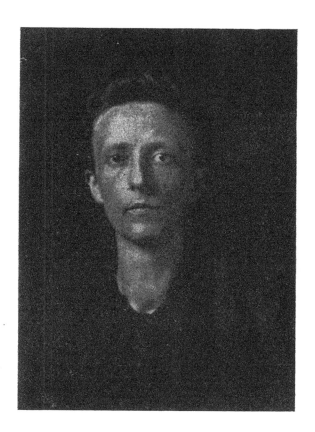

Fig. 5.—Hyperthyroidism, terminal results; chronic toxemia now abated, but leaving myocardial and general degenerative changes.

It must be conceded that the operation is a serious one, and that operating on those suffering from hypothyroidism, because they still have some signs of Basedow's disease, will not benefit the patient, the surgeon, or surgery. Operations upon advanced cases of hyperthyroidism will not cure fatty degeneration of the heart muscle, nor fatty degeneration of the liver, or advanced changes in other organs, although the disease may be checked by reducing the toxemia. Altogether too much is expected, especially by those personally interested, from operations made under such conditions. The responsibility of the operator being great, the diagnosis of the condition, the accurate estimate of the stages of the disease, and the approximate condition of the gland and essential organs must now be weighed with much more care than when the condition was considered purely medical and a death from it the "will of God."

The physician's judgment in his estimate of the patient's condition may lead him to first advise some form of non-surgical treatment, e. g., therapeutic, hygienic, etc. If improvement does not soon follow these measures, a surgeon should be called in consultation, who may, from his standpoint, advise immediate operation or a continuation of or additional treatment as a part of the preparation of the patient in case some form of operation is indicated either upon the blood supply of the gland or upon the gland itself, at a later period.

DISCUSSION.

DR. GEORGE W. CRILE, of Cleveland.—Whenever Dr. Mayo speaks we always hear a great deal of valuable and authoritative information on any subject he may elect, and particularly the subject of hyperthyroidism or Graves' disease. There is very little I can add in the way of discussion, because Dr. Mayo has covered the entire field so well.

In the few minutes allotted to me I shall discuss one or two features which were presented by the pictures on the screen, and particularly the question of malignancy. Dr. Mayo referred to the fact that in one case of his malignant disease had been cured. I would like to ask him whether it was possible for him to have diagnosticated the case as malignant before operation. I have heretofore made the statement, based upon my own experience and particularly on the literature, that when malignancy of the thyroid gland is accurately diagnosticated it is usually incurable. I, myself, have a record of a case that was cured for four years of cancer, then dying of another disease. Cancer was discussed, but a diagnosis of cancer was not made.

The psychic cause of hyperthyroidism, it seems to me, is a factor of the greatest importance. As Dr. Mayo has said, something happens in the patient from various causes, which may break the apparent normal relations, that is, breaking the physiological relations in some ductless gland, perhaps through its hormone relation. From my own studies it seems to me that one of the most prominent factors of this break is the psychic. Many times we see cases, as Dr. Mayo has pointed out, in which the disease is produced spontaneously by some event of great psychic importance, and no one has yet been able to show the method of operation of such causes. However, we may draw from the psychic factor in the cause of the disease a very important indication in the management of these cases, namely, that the psychic relations afterward, and especially during treatment, are of equally great importance.

In conclusion I want to express my personal indebtedness to Dr. Mayo for his contribution.

Dr. JOSEPH C. BLOODGOOD, of Baltimore.—There are one or two points to which I would like to call attention. I have been disappointed now and then by the failure of lobectomy combined with the best medical treatment to arrest the disease, even in very early cases. You cannot always tell, either from the clinical picture or the pathological examination of the gland removed as to what the result will be, and I think the family of the patient and the physician should be cautioned as to the possible necessity of a second operation, so that the patient will get the benefit of this before there is too much delay. It seems to me it is just as important to perform the second operation, if indicated, quickly as to operate in the early stage primarily. The second operation in some instances may consist of ligation of the vessels only, but there are cases in which it is wiser to remove at the same time some of the remaining lobe. Of course, in very desperately ill patients one should, at the first operation, ligate the vessels only. But in the majority of instances there is no necessity to delay until the patients are in a desperate condition.

As to the technique of the second operation, I have found it convenient to separate the remaining lobe so that it is held by its vascular supply only; then, with the cautery, I remove a portion of the thyroid toward the median line, leaving the poles and outer portions of the body in the shape of a half-moon; in some instances I do not even ligate the vessels. This method has impressed me as one which reduces the risk of any injury to the parathyroids to a minimum. Then this crescent piece of thyroid gland is approximated with catgut, so that it becomes a spherical mass, which is fixed in the middle line over the trachea with catgut. Such a maneuver reduces the deformity in the neck.

DR. MAYO (closing).—As to the point brought out by Dr. Crile of the possibility of a cure if we should diagnosticate cancer of the thyroid, I agree with him that it is impossible to cure cancer of the thyroid when it has reached such a stage that we are quite positive it is cancer. It is the occasional case where you think from the allied symptoms and from the difference in tension on the glands there is a possibility of carcinoma. I will speak of the case of a little girl, aged two years, with goitre, on whom I operated and removed two small round adenomata from the thyroid. This child came to me at the age of twelve with a large follicular goitre. I took out the right lobe, which was larger than the left, and in the upper pole of that I found carcinomatous tissue, as reported by Dr. Wilson, who made the microscopic examination.

In the cases Dr. Bloodgood speaks of, where there is occasionally a relapse of the goitre, especially in the early cases, we cannot get our judgment just right as to the type when we are operating, and the type of case we are dealing with can only be cleared up by careful microscopic examination. There are certain conditions over which we have not full control. We remove the right lobe and isthmus, and in the occasional case there will be relapse at the end of a year. In one case there was a relapse after fifteen years, and in several cases relapses have occurred in two years, four years, and five years. If it is an old case there is usually considerable colloid in the gland, and one can resect the gland in that type of case in simple tumors, but in the more acute conditions I prefer to ligate the upper pole of the remaining lobe, and if sufficient benefit or improvement does not take place after, say, five months, one should resect that and find considerably more colloid present than would have been found had the operation of resection been made before ligation, and a safer operation.

Dr. Crile.—Will you explain why the right lobe is more frequently enlarged than the left?

Dr. Mayo.—In all descriptions of the thyroid the right lobe is said to be about three-fifths and the left two-fifths of the gland, and why it is that the right lobe is larger than the left I would like to have Dr. Crile explain, because I think he has something up his sleeve.

HYPERNEPHROMATA.

By Louis B. Wilson, *M.D.*,
Rochester, Minnesota.

During the eight years ending December 31, 1909, 36 tumors of the kidney have been removed entire, and specimens for microscopic examination from 3 others, making 39 in all, in the clinic at St. Mary's Hospital, Rochester. One of these was a mixed embryoma, 3 were papillo-adenocarcinomata, 2 were flat-celled carcinomata secondary to stone, 2 were sarcomata, and 31 were hypernephromata. It is the latter group which I wish to report, at present drawing attention only to those pathological conditions on which rest the diagnostic clinical data.

Of the 31 cases of hypernephromata, 15 were males and 16 females. All the cases occurred in patients between thirty and sixty-four years of age, there being 7 between thirty and forty, 9 between forty and fifty, 12 between fifty and sixty, and 3 between sixty and seventy years. The left kidney was involved in 13 cases, and the right in 18 cases. There was a definite history of precedent injury over the affected kidney in 4 cases. There was history of pain in the kidney region in 28 cases, arising in 20 of the cases in what was probably a somewhat early stage of the development of the tumor. Twenty-seven cases passed perceptibly bloody urine. In 19 cases a tumor had been noticed by the patient, and in 30 cases it was palpable on physical examination. One of the cases is still in the hospital. Of the remaining 30, 2 have not been heard from since they left the hospital, 9 are known to be dead, 3 dying before leaving the hospital, 2 two months after operation, 1 five months, 1 eight months, and 2 two years after operation. The latter 6 all died from metastatic recurrence. Of the 20 cases still alive, 12 have been operated on less than a year, 3 between one and two years, 2 between two and three years, 1 three years, 1 four years, and 1 five years.

Pathologically, the tumors were all apparently primary in the kidney cortex, though in some cases the disease was so far advanced as to prevent an accurate determination of this point.

In the following presentation of protocols I have grouped the cases somewhat with reference to their pathological anatomy at the time of operation, since in this manner we may be able to compare the findings with the clinical histories of the cases. In the first group (15 cases) will be found those cases in which the tumor has arisen at one or the other pole of the kidney, and has deformed to a greater or less extent the pelvis of the kidney from its point of origin as it has advanced in growth. In the second group (6 cases) will be found those cases in which the tumor has developed near the middle of the kidney and has advanced into the renal pelvis from the side. In the third group (2 cases) are those cases in which the tumor, more or less pedunculated, has developed almost wholly outside the kidney substance. In the fourth group (8 cases) are those cases in which the tumor was so far advanced at the time of operation that its initial site was undeterminable.

PROTOCOLS. GROUP I (TUMORS ARISING FROM POLE).

CASE I (18,549).—Mr. N. S., farmer, aged forty-six years. About two years ago was kicked by a horse in lower right chest. One and one-half years ago began to pass some blood in urine, then not again until six weeks ago, when hematuria returned, accompanied by pain in back and groin. Has had some irritability of bladder twice, for a week at a time, during the last six weeks. Is now tender in right side of groin and back. There is a palpable tumor mass in the right side. The urine shows much blood. (Fig. 1, Plate I) shows the tumor to be a very small one in the upper pole of the kidney, producing practically no deformity of the pelvis. There is no extension into the renal vein. The tumor is surrounded by a dense capsule of compressed kidney tissue. Histologically, the tumor is typical hypernephroma. The patient was operated on May 21, 1906, was alive and well without recurrence October 23, 1909.

CASE II (14,238).—Mrs. J. H., housewife, aged fifty-two years. Well until six weeks ago, when developed sharp pain in right side and back, and two weeks later noticed blood in urine. On examination a palpable tumor mass is found in the kidney region of the right side. The urine shows much blood. The kidney on removal (Fig. 2, Plate I) shows a tumor of the upper pole, which extends through the kidney substance rather diffusely, having evidently broken past the condensation band of tissue usually surrounding these tumors, and advanced well into the renal pelvis. Section showed rapidly growing hypernephroma with distinct alveolar arrangement. Though the encapsulation of the tumor is perfect at some points, in others the newgrowth has passed well beyond any barrier. This patient died two years after operation from metastatic recurrence.

CASE III (32,106).—Mr. B. S., implement dealer, aged fifty-seven years. Was operated nine years ago for appendicitis. Nine months ago began passing nearly pure blood in urine; three days after first bleeding, another attack, and a third three weeks later. Two months later was examined by physician and no trouble found. For last two months has had almost constant pain in right kidney region. Last week noticed a tumor mass in right side. Has lost thirty-pounds in weight within the last six months. There has been no blood in the urine during the last two months, until within the last twenty-four hours; now urine shows much blood. On removal, the tumor (Fig. 3, Plate I) is found to involve the upper pole of the kidney. It has broken through the kidney capsule and the perirenal fat is involved. The renal pelvis is much deformed. The renal vein contains some of the newgrowth. Histologically, the tumor is a typical hypernephroma. This patient was operated upon September 23, 1909; December 23, 1909, reports that he has been in bed all the time since the operation, and has considerable pain in his back.

CASE IV (29,730).—Mr. G. M., real estate agent, aged fifty-one years. Fifteen months ago after severe exertion noticed blood in urine. Eight hours later sudden, severe left lumbar pains. Vomited all night, requiring morphine for relief of pain. Was in bed one week after this attack. Partially recovered, but did not feel well again. Had second severe spell of pain accompanied by increase of blood in urine six months ago. At present occasionally has to use catheter to draw urine; at other times urination is frequent. Pain extends through bladder to kidney. Has lost thirty pounds in weight. Has noticed no tumor mass. On examination a large tumor mass is found in right side. The urine shows much blood. The tumor in this case (Fig. 4, Plate II) involves the whole upper pole of the kidney, obliterating the upper renal pelvis, which has been correspondingly distended posteriorly. The renal vein at its exit from the kidney is filled with a tumor mass. Sections show typical hypernephroma with loose structure containing many blood spaces, particularly along the outer border. This patient was operated on April 5, 1909, and was still alive when last heard from.

CASE V (32,300).—Mrs. B. F. L., housewife, aged fifty-eight years. Has two children alive and six dead. Passed menopause twelve years ago. Nine years ago says she noticed a lump in left kidney, which did not appear to grow any until two years ago, then began rapid growth. Has had a dragging sensation in left side, but no real pain. Has had constipation, apparently from obstruction in the sigmoid. Has had some blood in the urine during the past four months, when hemorrhage has been sufficiently free to produce considerable weakness. General health has been bad only at times of bleeding. On examination a large tumor is found in the lower left kidney region. The urine shows much blood. On removal (Fig. 5, Plate II) the tumor was found to be very large, and growing from the middle of the lower pole of the kidney. It has encroached upon the renal pelvis from below, and has invaded, to some extent, the renal vein. Section shows alveolar hypernephroma with very large blood spaces. Some areas have an arrangement of cells suggesting carcinoma. This patient was operated on October 5, 1909, and is still alive.

CASE VI (28,980).—Mr. N. A. F., farmer, aged forty-three years. For the past three years has had some pain in right kidney region, and at intervals has noticed some blood in urine. Recently urine has occasionally appeared to be almost pure blood, clear or in clots. For the last four months has had spells of acute pain, commencing over right kidney and passing downward to penis. After bleeding spells attacks of colicky pain, lasting one hour or so, have been common. During last two months has lost much strength and twenty-five pounds in weight. On examination a large palpable tumor is found. The urine shows little blood. The tumor in this case (Fig. 6, Plate II) has arisen near the superior pole of the kidney and advanced laterally and toward the inferior pole. The pelvis has been much elongated, and though somewhat encroached upon from the side, it is well marked, as though it had been distended. There is no involvement of the renal vein. Section shows typical areas of hypernephroma tissue. Some cells show much fat with crowded nuclei. The thin-walled capillaries have ruptured in many places, giving large areas of extravasated blood. Six months after operation this patient is alive and much improved.

CASE VII (31,867).—Mrs. W. B., farmer's wife, aged fifty-seven years. Has four children alive, one dead, and has had two miscarriages. Passed menopause nine years ago. Seven years ago began to have pain in left side and back, with dull ache in the left kidney. Two months ago felt tumor mass in her left side herself. Says this has grown rapidly

PLATE I

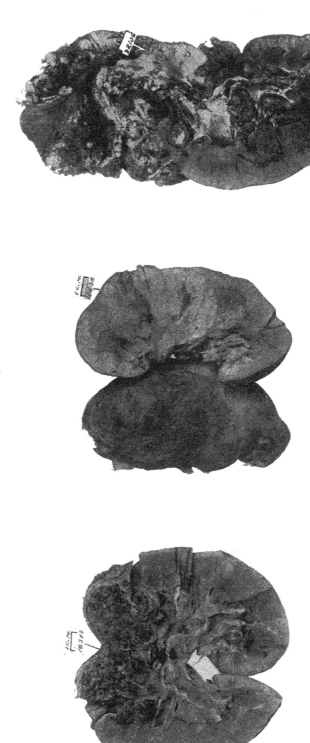

Fig. 1, Case 1. (18549)

Fig. 2, Case 2. (14238)

Fig. 3, Case 3. (32106)

PLATE II

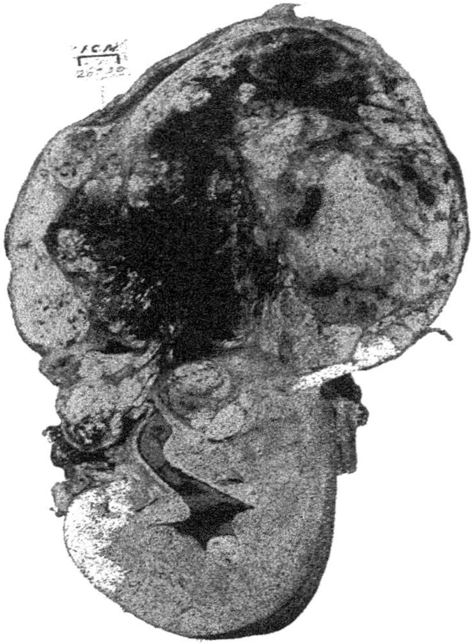

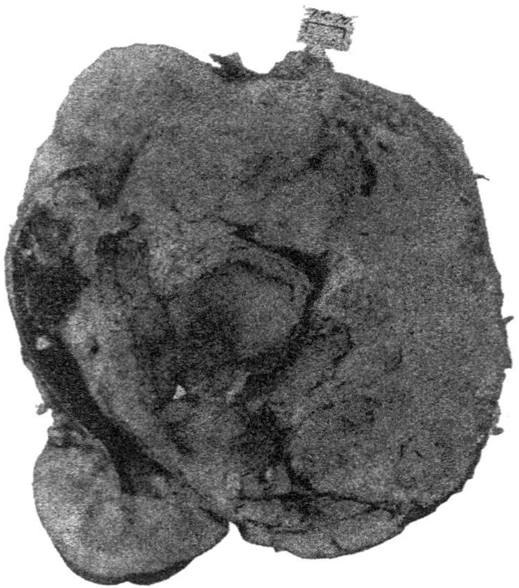

FIG. 6, CASE 6.   (28980)

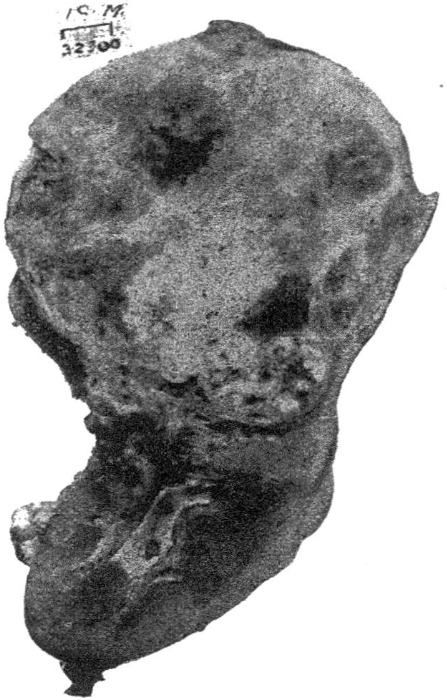

FIG. 5, CASE 5.   (32300)

FIG. 4, CASE 4.   (29730)

PLATE III

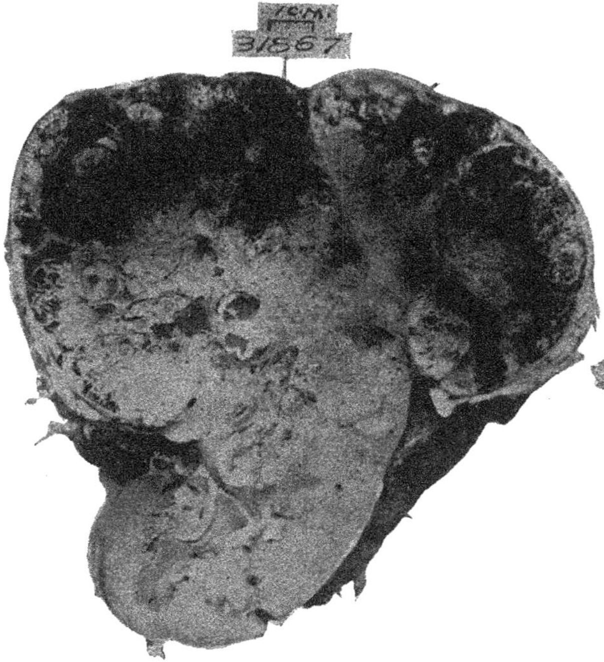

FIG. 7, CASE 7. (31867)

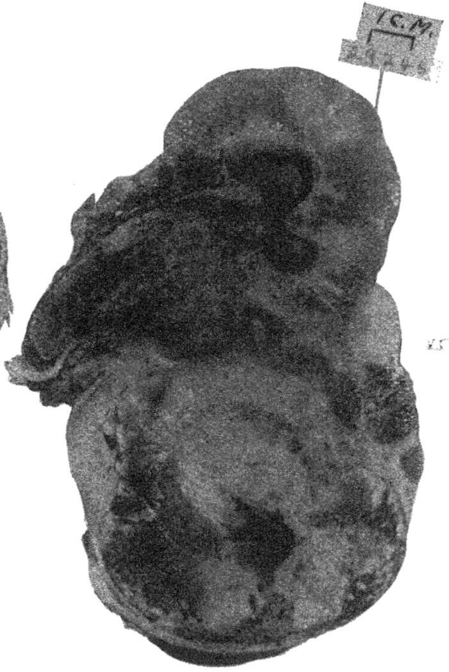

FIG. 8, CASE 8. (29245)

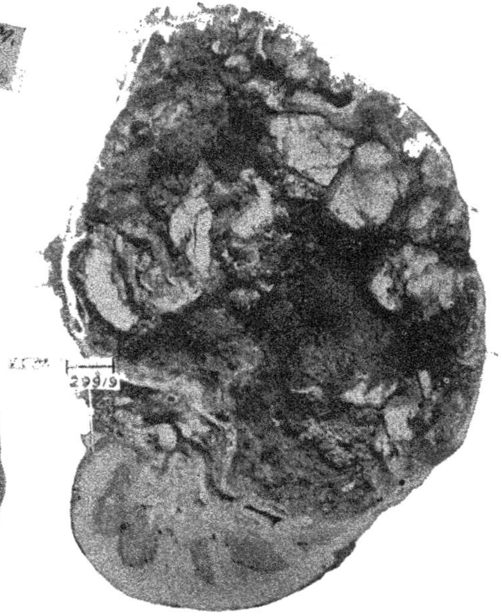

FIG. 9, CASE 9. (29919)

PLATE IV

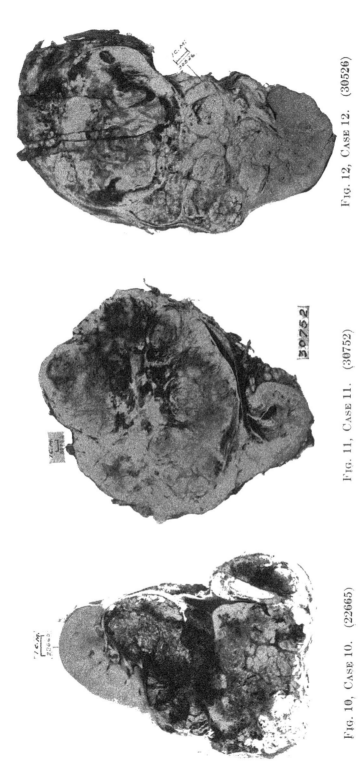

Fig. 10, Case 10.   (22665)

Fig. 11, Case 11.   (30752)

Fig. 12, Case 12.   (30526)

PLATE V

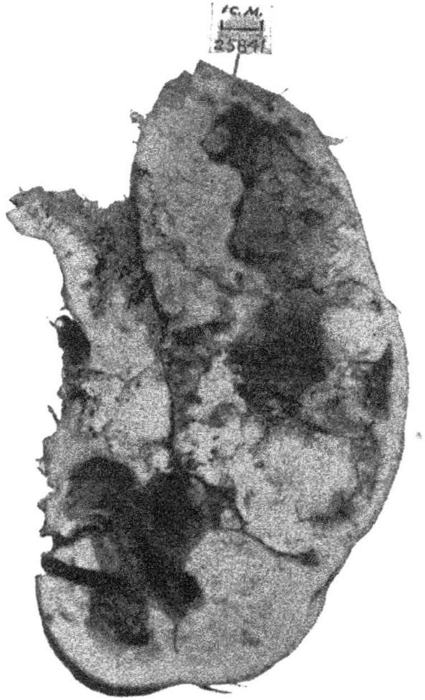

FIG. 13, CASE 13. (25841)

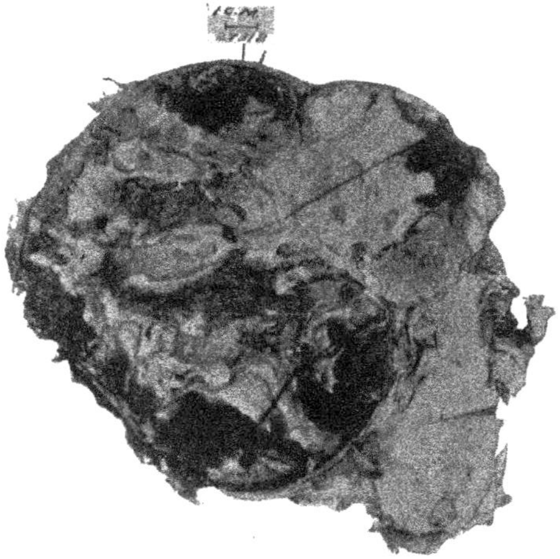

FIG. 14, CASE 14. (27312)

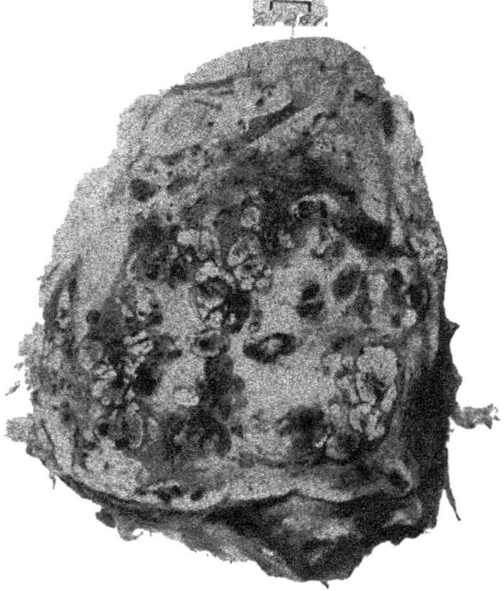

FIG. 15, CASE 15. (27267)

PLATE VI

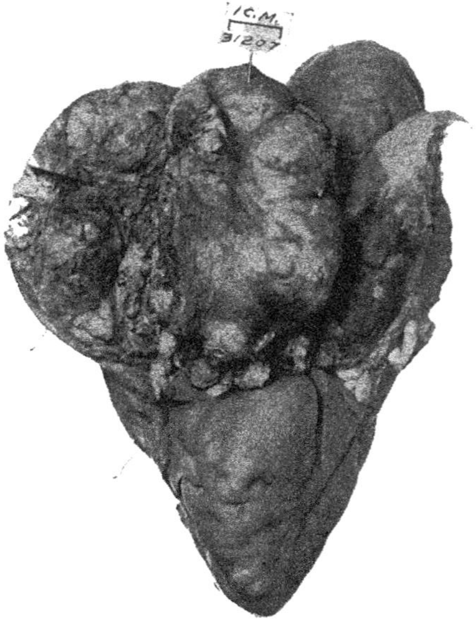

FIG. 16, CASE 17. (31207)

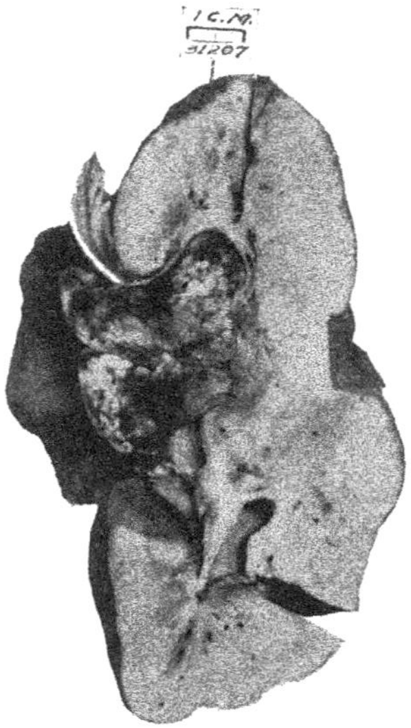

FIG. 17, CASE 17. (31207) SECTION

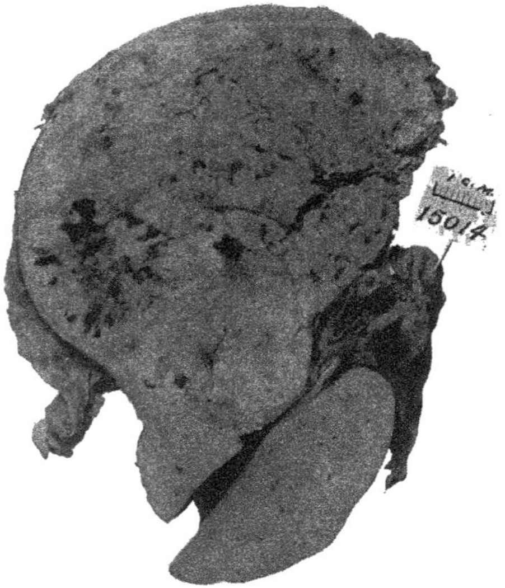

FIG. 18, CASE 18. (15014)

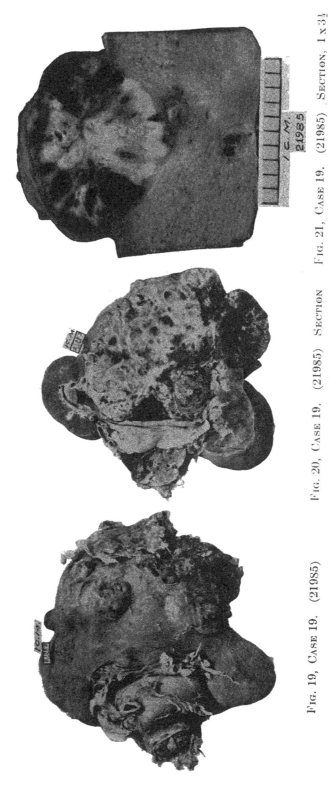

PLATE VII

FIG. 19, CASE 19.   (21985)

FIG. 20, CASE 19.   (21985)   SECTION

FIG. 21, CASE 19.   (21985)   SECTION, 1 x 3½

PLATE VIII

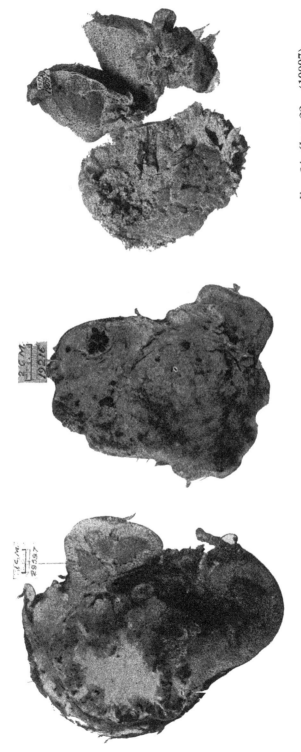

Fig. 22, Case 20.　(29597)

Fig. 23, Case 21.　(19216)

Fig. 24, Case 22.　(19097)

Fig. 27, Case 25. (17995)

Fig. 26, Case 24, (22074)

Fig. 25, Case 23. (8938)

PLATE X

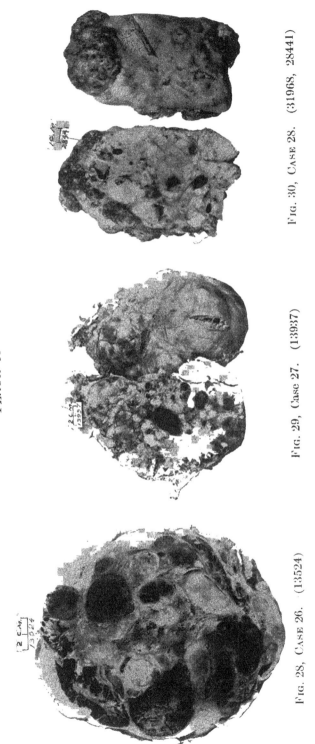

FIG. 28, CASE 26.   (13524)

FIG. 29, CASE 27.   (13937)

FIG. 30, CASE 28.   (31968, 28441)

PLATE XI

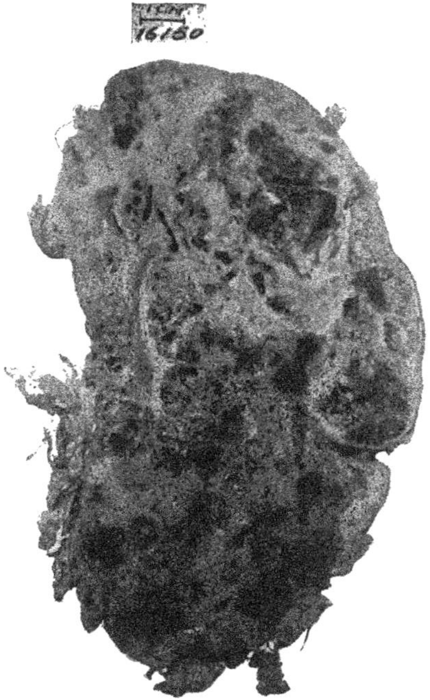

FIG. 31, CASE 29. (16150)

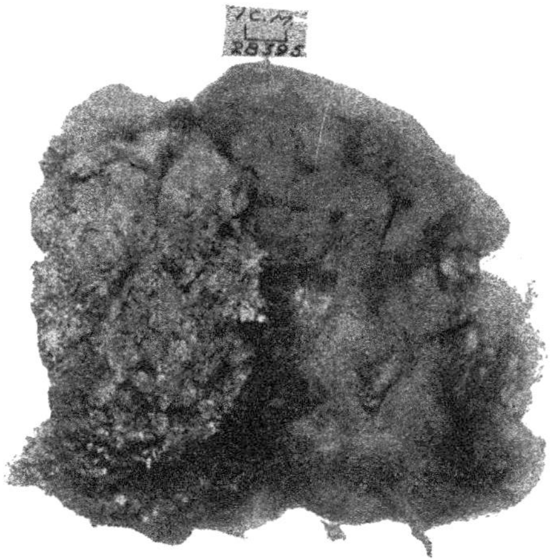

FIG. 32, CASE 30. (28395)

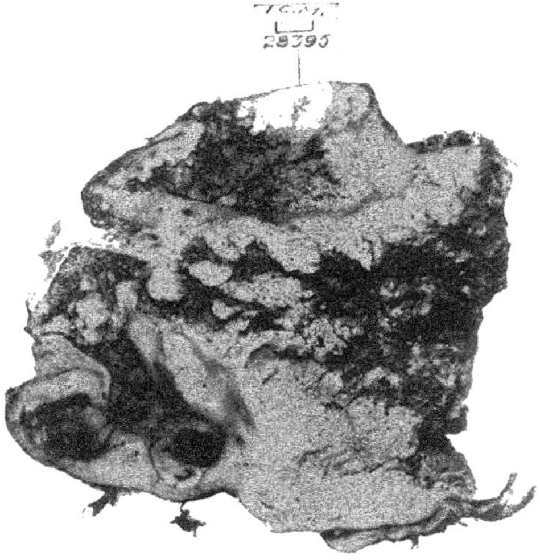

FIG. 33, CASE 30. (28395) SECTION

since. The urine varies in quantity and has contained blood at intervals for the last two months. *P*atient has lost about twenty-five pounds in weight. Examination shows a large palpable tumor in left kidney region. The urine shows much blood. The tumor (Fig. 7, Plate III) is a large one, involving the whole of the upper pole of the kidney. It has apparently developed first on the upper mesial aspect of the organ, then broken through its capsule laterally and formed a secondary extension of considerable size. Though the tumor is so large and has involved so much of the kidney substance, it has not deformed the renal pelvis as greatly as other tumors of smaller size. Microscopic sections show typical hypernephroma tissue. In many areas connective tissue stroma is in preponderance. To this has probably been due the slow development of the neoplasm. This patient was operated on September 3, 1909, and has been much improved in health since.

CASE *VIII* (29,245).—Mr. L. E., hotelkeeper. aged forty-three years. *F*ive months ago noticed a gradual physical decline, with loss of weight, loss of strength, and frequency of urination. Three months ago had a severe hemorrhage from the bladder, followed by pain in the right kidney region, passing downward to the right testicle. A similar severe attack one month later, lasting twenty-four hours. Night urination increased to every hour; day, every two hours. Has lost twenty-five pounds in weight. The tumor (Fig. 8, Plate III) involves the lower pole of the kidney and completely fills the renal pelvis. It extends out into the renal veins, which have been dissected off from the vena cavæ. Much of the tumor tissue has degenerated, so that mere outlines of the walls are visible. Other areas show characteristic hypernephroma structure still well preserved. This patient was operated on *F*ebruary 25, 1909, and died *D*ecember 5, 1909.

CASE IX (29,919).—Mrs. E. H., hardware merchant's wife, aged sixty-four years. *F*irst noticed a tumor in her right side three years ago. Had attack of la grippe six months later, and tumor apparently became smaller. Has had no pain at any time. *D*uring the last few weeks tumor has grown larger. Has a sense of discomfort in the right side. Has had no loss of appetite or weight and no urinary symptoms. On examination, large palpable tumor mass is found in right kidney region. No blood present in urine. On removal the tumor (Fig. 9, Plate *III*) is found to be a large one, involving all of the upper pole of the right kidney. It has obliterated the upper half of the renal pelvis. It has not grown into the renal pelvis nor into the renal vein. Its capsule is heavy, and apparently has not been passed at any point. Histologically, the tumor is a large degenerated hypernephroma, with the better preserved portions showing a marked papilliferous arrangement of single rows of cuboidal cells along thin-walled capillaries. This patient was operated on April 17, 1909, and when last heard from, August 4, 1909, was much improved in health.

CASE *X* (22,665).—Mrs. S. L., housewife, aged forty-nine years, has one child, aged seventeen years. Thirteen months ago had suffered renal colic, followed by passing blood in urine for a month or more. No further attacks of pain or hemorrhage until three weeks ago; then had very severe pain for one hour, followed by passage of blood in urine for three weeks. Five months ago discovered hard lump in right kidney region, which has not seemed to have increased in size. Examination shows palpable tumor and some blood in urine. The tumor (Fig. 10, Plate IV) is found to involve all except the upper pole of the kidney. The renal pelvis has been almost completely obliterated. The tumor extends into the renal vein. Many areas of the tumor tissue show typical hypernephroma arrangement, large blood sinuses, and many hemorrhages. Fatty degeneration is extensive. The tumor is well encapsulated. This patient was operated on July 7, 1907, but follow-up letters have brought no reply since that time.

CASE XI (30,752).—Mr. *C.* H. A., saw filer, aged fifty-three years. Five years ago patient fell from a horse, striking on left side. Three months later a swelling appeared in left side. This has become larger during the last twelve months. For last four years has had spells of intermittent fever, temperature rising to 103. These have been relieved by purgation. Two years ago noticed blood in urine for several days. Similar occurrence eighteen months ago. On examination, large palpable tumor in left side is found. Urine shows but little blood. The tumor (Fig. 11, Plate IV), almost as large as an adult human head, involves the superior pole of the left kidney. The mesentery of the sigmoid is adherent to the tumor. The upper portion of the renal pelvis is reduced to a long, narrow slit. The lower portion is fairly normal in shape. The renal vein is invaded. The tumor is quite dense in structure, and, though showing numerous hemorrhages, it is composed largely of well-staining hypernephroma tissue. The patient was operated on June 20, 1909, and died the next day after operation.

CASE XII (30,526).—Mrs. F. L. B., laborer's wife, aged thirty-three years. One year ago developed pain over right kidney, especially when working. Pain gradually grew worse. Has noticed some blood in urine at intervals during the last year. For past three weeks has lost weight, twenty-two pounds. Is weak and easily exhausted. First noticed tumor mass over right kidney one week ago. Examination shows palpable tumor. The urine contains no blood. Operation reveals large tumor (Fig. 12, Plate IV) of superior pole of right kidney. The pelvis of the kidney has been completely obliterated by pressure of the neoplasm, which also has invaded the renal vein, as is clearly shown in the cut. Several interrupted capsules (*i. e.*, remains of condensed kidney tissue) are present, showing how the tumor has broken through its boundaries at different intervals, involving from time to time more and more tissue. Microscopic sections show the bulk of this tumor to be of ordinary hypernephroma type, but some are as shown typical spindle-cell sarcoma (see Fig. 39, Plate XII). This patient was operated on June 17, 1909, and died August 29, 1909.

CASE XIII (25,841).—Mrs. J. W. B., farmer's wife, aged thirty-one years. Four years ago noticed blood in urine and painful urination occurring twice within a year. Has been troubled similarly at intervals of two to four months since. Bad attack eight months ago, at which time also noticed tumor in region of left kidney. Tumor has been getting larger ever since. Lost fifteen or twenty pounds in weight during the last year. Examination shows palpable tumor and much blood in urine. At operation large tumor (Fig. 13, *Plate* V) of left kidney is removed. This involves almost the entire organ. Its advance is marked off by remains of capsules. The interior is soft and necrotic. The cystic necrotic centre connects with the kidney pelvis. There is no growth of the tumor into the renal vein. The microscopic appearance of the recently developed portions of the tumor is shown in Fig. 36, *Plate* XII, consisting of epithelial masses within connective tissue stroma. From the walls of these cyst-like structures project numerous thin-walled capillaries, along the sides of which are arranged the large cuboidal cells, giving a papilliferous appearance to the structure. Some areas show dense columnar arrangement of the cuboidal cells and varying grades of compression of kidney tissue. This patient was operated on May 11, 1908, and when heard from, September 9, 1909, was "feeling fine."

CASE XIV (27,312).—Mr. W. B., owner of carriage shop, aged fifty-three years. Has had some pain in region of left kidney for a year. First noticed lump there about nine months ago. Urine has been cloudy at times and micturition somewhat frequent. Examination reveals a large palpable tumor in left kidney region. The urine shows no blood. Operation reveals a very large tumor of the left kidney, involving the upper pole and advancing toward the mesial side. The pelvis is almost completely obliterated. There is no growth of the neoplasm into the renal vein. The tumor (Fig. 14, *Plate* V), though very large, is well encapsulated, and distinctly separated from the remaining portion of the kidney. Histologically, the structure is much like that in Figs. 36 and 38, *Plate* 12, the stroma consisting principally of thin-walled capillaries lined with large cuboidal cells. Several large cysts mark areas of hemorrhage and degeneration. This patient was operated on December 12, 1908, and August 1, 1909, reports himself well.

CASE XV (27,267).—Mrs. A. H. P., housewife, aged fifty-four years, mother of five children, youngest aged twenty-three years. Menopause six years ago. Six years ago had rather free bleeding in urine and a good deal of pain on right side. Four years ago passed blood in urine again, but had no pain. Two years ago had rather severe pain and passed a good deal of blood. No hematuria since then. Has noticed mass in right side for several months. Has heavy feeling of distress in that area. Examination reveals large tumor. Urine shows some blood. Nephrectomy required extensive dissection. There were close attachments to the vena cavæ. The renal vessels were huge. The left kidney was explored and found apparently normal. The tumor (Fig. 15, *Plate* V) had its initial development in the lower pole. Though very large, it had not completely obliterated the renal pelvis. Much of the centre of the tumor shows hyaline degeneration. Histologically, the tumor shows alveolar arranged papilliferous groups. This patient was operated on September 7, 1908, and was reported well, except for some pain on the other side, December 1, 1909.

GROUP II (TUMORS OF MID-PORTION OF KIDNEY).

CASE XVI (33,295)—Mr. *D. M.* B., farmer, aged fifty-two years. Three and one-half years ago had typical gall-bladder attack with jaundice. Patient recalls seeing some blood in urine once or twice during last two years. Five weeks ago noticed tumor just below right costal arch. Has no pain nor tenderness, but feeling of weight or pulling. Micturition all right. Eats and sleeps well. Weight normal, gaining a little, if anything, during the past few months. Physical examination reveals hard, firm tumor lying under right ribs, and coming down to level of umbilicus on deep inspiration. Tumor is not through to back, and can be held down with fingers above it on deep inspiration. Urine shows no blood. Exploratory operation reveals large hypernephroma of right kidney. The tumor (Fig. 36, Plate XII) involves the ventral side of the kidney, somewhat nearer the lower than the upper pole. It has pressed upon and deformed the renal pelvis, though not breaking through the pelvic wall. The renal vein is filled with a conical plug of the neoplasm. The color and gross structure of the tumor is accurately shown in Fig. 36, and the histologic appearance of it in Fig. 35. This patient was operated on December 28, 1909, and has made an uneventful recovery, though recurrence is to be expected from the involvement of the renal vein.

CASE XVII (31,207).—Mrs. H. E. S., glove manufacturer's wife, aged thirty-three years. Large, strong, very athletic woman. Has four children, youngest two years. Three years ago had scarlet fever and nephritis. Three months ago began to feel some pain in left side of abdomen and around to left loin. Two months ago got worse for a couple of days, and noticed a little blood in urine. Pain disappeared in a couple of days, recurring again three weeks ago for a couple of days, but with no blood noticed in urine. One week ago another attack of pain, and passed a large amount of blood. Weight good; no fever, chills, sweats, or increased frequency of micturition. Patient under physicians' observation two and one-half months, during which time two x-ray examinations and two cystosopic examinations were made, both negative. Ten urinary examinations during time showed small amount of pus and a very few red blood cells. Exploratory operation reveals small hypernephroma in left kidney. The tumor (Figs. 16 and 17, Plate VI) involves the middle portion of the ventral side of the kidney. It has grown into and filled the upper half of the renal pelvis and extends into the renal vein. The lower portion of the renal pelvis is normal in size and contour. Histologically, the tumor is a typical hypernephroma. This patient was operated on July 19, 1909, and was reported in fairly good health six months later.

CASE XVIII (15,014).—Mrs. *C. H.*, housewife, aged thirty-four years. Patient has noticed some dull aching pain in right kidney region for about three months. Thinks she felt a lump in the region about the time pain commenced. Has noticed no blood in the urine. Physical examination reveals a small, freely movable tumor in right kidney region. The urine shows no blood. At operation there was found a tumor (Fig. 18, Plate VI) involving the middle of the right kidney. It has deformed, but not invaded the pelvis of the kidney, and has not extended into the renal vein. The tumor is thoroughly solid and is composed largely of hypernephroma tissue, similar to that in Fig. 37, Plate XII. This patient was operated on March 10, 1905, and reports herself in good health August 1, 1909.

CASE XIX (21,985).—Mr. J. S., railroad superintendent, aged forty-eight years. Four years ago had attack of sharp, stabbing pain over left kidney, which lasted for a few hours, followed by blood in the urine every two or three days. Was in bed one week. Two years later had a second attack similar to preceding one, then entire relief until seven months ago, when he had a third attack. Five months ago he had a fourth attack, followed by marked bleeding and extreme weakness. The fifth, and last, attack occurred one week ago, when he was in bed two days. Has lost no weight. His general health between attacks is good. Bladder fills with clots, which cause stoppage of urine after attacks of pain. Has noticed no tumor. Physical examination shows palpable tumor in the left kidney region. The urine contains numerous small clots of blood. At operation there is removed a tumor (Figs. 19 and 20, Plate VII) involving the middle portion of the kidney, having apparently arisen from the outer convexity of the organ. It has extended throughout the middle portion of the kidney, leaving only the two poles undisturbed. It fills the renal pelvis, but not the renal vein. This tumor is peculiar in that it contains a number of nodules apparently completely separated from each other and from the main mass of the neoplasm. Some of these are quite small. One is shown in Fig. 21, Plate VII, magnified 3 diameters. Histologically, much of the tissue shows dense, cellular, encapsulated areas. In others the alveolar groups contain looser tissue, with thin-walled capillaries, bordered by cuboidal cells. This patient was operated on May 15, 1907, and reports himself in good health August 1, 1909.

CASE XX (29,597).—Mrs. J. McN., machine agent's wife, aged fifty-five years. Seventeen years ago had a period of three months of urinary frequency with pain in kidney region. Recovered under medical treatment. No further trouble until seven weeks ago, when pain returned in left kidney region. Urine has been highly colored at times for years, but no red blood has been noticed until within the last seven weeks. Three weeks ago tumor was discovered by physician

in left hypochondrium. Patient has had failing appetite and has lost
twenty-five pounds during last six months. Physical examination
reveals large tumor in left kidney region. Urine shows much blood·
At operation a large tumor of the middle portion of the kidney is removed. The spleen appears to be twice its normal size. The tumor
(Fig. 22, Plate VIII), is round, with most of its circumference well walled
in with dense kidney tissue. At its lower border, toward the renal
pelvis, it has broken through, and now invades, as well as deforms, the
renal pelvis and extends into the renal vein. Its central portion shows
a large area of hyaline degeneration. This patient was operated on
March 23, 1909, and died three months later of metastatic recurrence.

CASE XXI (19,097).—Mr. J. O., hotelkeeper, aged fifty-five years.
Three years ago noticed reddish color of urine and some small blood
clots; attack lasted a day or so. After a month or two of freedom blood
returned in urine again for a day or two. One and one-half years ago
a sharp, shooting pain started on left side. Trouble lasted longer than
before, perhaps a week at a time. There is now some pain upon urination
when clots appear. Physical examination shows a palpable tumor and
much blood in the urine. At operation a very large tumor of the left
kidney is removed. The neoplasm (Fig. 24, Plate VIII) has apparently
started on the ventral side of the kidney, midway between its poles. It
has almost completely obliterated the normal kidney tissue, leaving only
small lines at either pole. It has involved the pelvis and the renal vein.
Most of the tumor is very soft and broken down. Histologically, the
typical alveolar arrangement of thin-walled capillaries supporting
cuboidal cells and contained within a more or less well-marked connective tissue capsule is present where the tumor has not completely broken
down. This patient was operated upon July 16, 1906. He recovered
from the operation, but died two months afterward from metastatic
recurrence.

GROUP III   (GREATER PORTION OF TUMOR OUTSIDE KIDNEY).

CASE XXII[1] (8938).—"Mrs. M. F., housewife, aged forty-five years.
Mother of twelve children, youngest two years old. Twelve years ago
patient was kicked in left side by a cow. Has had occasional attacks
of pain in kidney region ever since. Two years ago she noticed an
enlargement, and for the past four months has had steady pain in the
side. Now has difficulty in moving bowels and trouble with frequent
micturition. Physical examination shows palpable tumor in left kidney region. Urine from right kidney is normal in amount and quality;
that from left about quarter as much as from right, and contains pus
and blood. Springing from the upper pole of the kidney (Fig. 25,
Plate IX) and extending into the abdomen is a smooth growth of firm
consistency measuring 10 x 24 x 28 cm. It is included in the kidney

[1] This case has been previously reported. See Herb, Amer. Jour.
Med. Sci., 1905, cxxix, 1010.

capsule. The stroma is composed of a delicate network of capillaries, in the meshes of which are round or polygonal cells, with a distinct cell wall and a large amount of protoplasm. There are large venous sinuses with well-developed walls. This patient was operated upon December 2, 1901. Two and one-half years later there were no signs of recurrence or dissemination."

CASE XXIII (22,074).—Mrs. T. McM., grain buyer's wife, aged thirty-five years. For the past two years has had attacks of dull pain in right upper hypochondrium with soreness. Sometimes has had sharp pain in abdomen, lower down in appendix region, referred down leg. Five months ago had severe attack of sharp pain in right kidney region, with severe headache and frequency of urination. This attack lasted three days. Since then has had dull pain and soreness in upper right side, with a dragging sensation. Discovered a tumor mass in right kidney region five months ago. Operation reveals tumor attached to upper pole of right kidney. It simply indents (Fig. 56, Plate IX) the kidney without being attached, except by fibrous connective tissue, to the organ. The gross structure of this tumor resembles the more dense portions of the hypernephromata previously reported. Histologically (Fig. 57, Plate XII), it consists of bands and columns of cuboidal cells arranged about thin-walled capillaries. The tumor held the position of the suprarenal, but it is difficult to determine from examination of the specimen whether it is a tumor of the suprarenal or of the kidney proper. Aside from the absence of degenerated areas, it is a counterpart of the other tumors herewith reported. This patient was operated on May 24, 1907, and July 28, 1909, reports herself in good health, having passed successfully through pregnancy, beginning six months after her operation.

GROUP IV (INITIAL SITE OF TUMOR NOT DETERMINABLE).

CASE XXIV (17,995).—Mrs. H. W., railroad employee's wife, aged thirty-four years. One year ago developed sharp, lancinating pain over left kidney region. Some pain at all times since, with frequent exacerbations. Noticed some blood in urine four months ago. Physical examination shows large tumor in region of left kidney. Urine shows no blood. Operation reveals large tumor (Fig. 27, Plate IX) involving whole of kidney to such an extent that its point of origin cannot be determined. The renal pelvis is involved, but the renal vessels slightly if at all. Some areas show microscopically alveolar groups of typical hypernephroma cells, but much of the tumor is in an advanced stage of fatty and hyaline degeneration. This patient was operated on March 19, 1906, and died August 5, 1908, of metastatic recurrence.

CASE XXV[1] (13,524).—"Mrs. S. McD., housewife, aged sixty-four years. Mother of five children. A year and a half ago began to pass

[1] This case was previously reported. Herb, Amer. Jour. Med. Sci., 1905, cxxix, 1010.

bloody urine. First attack lasted four days, two others not so long. Pain at this time referred to bladder region. Recovered and felt fairly well for one year. During last six months has had more or less pain in bladder. Two months ago noticed tumor in right side, which has rapidly increased in size, but is not especially sensitive. On physical examination large tumor mass in right side was palpated. The urine from the left kidney was normal, and none was being excreted on the right side. Operation reveals large tumor involving the entire kidney. Section (Fig. 28, Plate X) shows group of lobules more or less separated from each other by bands of connective tissue. Many of these show the hypernephroma tissue in advanced stages of fatty or hyaline degeneration. A few contain well-preserved tissue in which the alveolar arrangement of cells is well marked. Patient was operated July 6, 1909, and died seven days after the operation."

CASE XXVI[1] (13,937).—"Mrs. H. P. R., housewife, aged sixty-one years. Has passed bloody urine for ten years. Noticed an abdominal tumor four years ago, which she thinks has increased fully one-half in size in the last six months. Complains of dull pain for last four years, starting in right side and extending to suprapubic region. Physical examination reveals a large palpable tumor in right kidney region. A mixed specimen of urine contains pus and blood. That from the left kidney is normal. Some pus and blood with no urine obtained from right kidney. At operation a very large tumor involving the entire kidney is removed. On Section (Fig. 29, Plate X) this tumor shows a similar gross structure to that in Case XXV. Degeneration, both fatty and hyaline, is well marked. Histologically, except in degenerated areas, there is typical alveolar arrangement of hypernephroma cells resting on thin-walled capillaries."

CASE XXVII (31,968).—Mr. A. J. B. Fell from a bicycle five years ago. Noticed blood in urine shortly afterward, which lasted a few days. Then well until one and one-half years ago, when again noticed blood in urine and had pain in right kidney region. Has had more or less pain constantly ever since, with two or three periods of blood in the urine. Has noticed no tumor. Has become weak and lost weight, about twenty-five pounds. Physical examination shows no tumor. The urine contains blood. Operation shows large tumor of right kidney involving entire organ. Section of the tumor (Fig. 30, Plate X) shows a large degenerated tumor. Some areas still show fairly typical hypernephroma arrangement. The patient was operated on September 10, 1909, and November 20 patient reports himself in good health, having gained twenty pounds in weight.

CASE XXVIII (16,150).—Mr. J. S., farmer, aged sixty-four years. Two years ago began to pass some blood in urine. This stopped after a short time. Nine months ago began to have pain in left side. This

---

[1] This case has been previously reported by Dr. Herb, Amer. Jour. Med. Sci., 1905, cxxix, 1011.

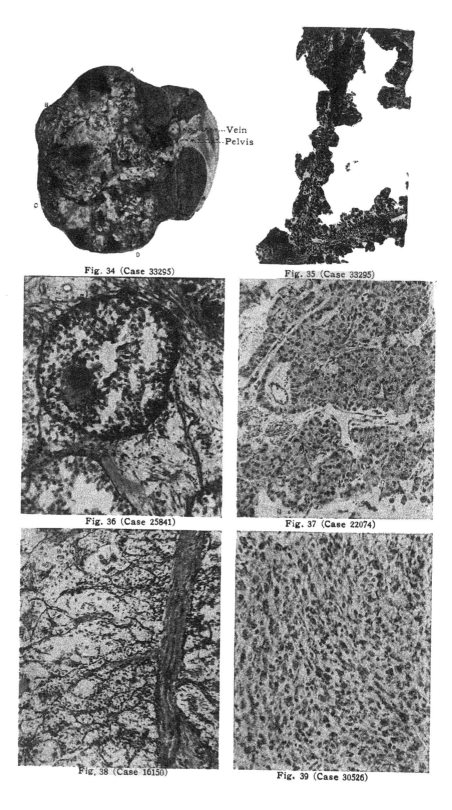

Fig. 34 (Case 33295)

Fig. 35 (Case 33295)

Fig. 36 (Case 25841)

Fig. 37 (Case 22074)

Fig. 38 (Case 16150)

Fig. 39 (Case 30526)

was worse at night. Has never noticed any tumor. On physical examination a very large tumor in the left kidney region is made out. The urine shows much blood. On account of weak condition the patient is advised not to submit to operation, but insists that he be given the possible chance. Operation reveals very large tumor involving the entire left kidney, extending into the renal vessels and involving their walls to such an extent that it is almost impossible to form a stump. The tumor is adherent to the surrounding tissues and the capsule is highly vascular. Section of the tumor (Fig. 31, *Plate* XI) shows its structure to be much degenerated. Histologically, aside from degeneration, there are some areas which show alveolar arrangement with numerous bloodvessels. The wall and a portion of one of these is shown in Fig. 38, *Plate* XII. Thin-walled capillaries, on which rest cuboidal cells forming papilliferous projections out into the cyst-like structure, are clearly shown. This patient was operated on August 4, 1905, and died eight hours after the operation. Autopsy showed death to have occurred from hemorrhage from the meshwork of much distended vessels, which had been connected with the capsule of the tumor. There were numerous small metastases in the liver and in abdominal lymph glands.

CASE XXIX (28,395).—Mr. O. G., lumberman, aged thirty-one years. Eight months ago began to pass blood in urine. This was accompanied at times by colicky pains. Had four or five such attacks, with short duration, but gradually dull pain became prevalent all the time. Blood in urine three months ago. Has been in Lumbermen's Hospital last thirteen months for treatment. Has lost twelve or fifteen pounds in weight. Is weak and run down. There is a large palpable tumor in the region of the right kidney, and the urine shows some blood. Operation reveals a tumor which involves the entire kidney and has broken through the capsule of that organ, projecting in a fungous mass into the abdomen. Section of the tumor (Fig. 33, *Plate* XI) shows it to be of a papilliferous character in some areas and in others dense and solid, though much degenerated in structure. The renal pelvis is much encroached on; the vessels appear to be free. Histologically, there are many areas showing typical hypernephroma tissue. Other areas are indistinguishable from ordinary spindle-cell sarcoma, and similar to that shown in Fig. 39, *Plate* XII. This patient was operated on December 15, 1908, and was alive and in fairly good health August 15, 1909.

CASE XXX (18,748).—Mr. H. C. S., farmer, aged forty-six years. Six years ago began to have pain in back and right side. Blood appeared in urine, which frequently contained clots. The pain at times was very severe, causing nausea and vomiting. At times voids large quantities of urine, after having passed small clots for a day or two. Has never noticed any tumor. On physical examination a very large tumor is palpable in the region of the right kidney. The urine contains much blood. Exploratory operation only reveals large tumor of right kidney so adherent to adjacent structures as to be inoperable. Small piece of tissue removed for examination shows typical hypernephroma tissue and one area resembling round-cell sarcoma. Though the entire tumor is not removed, a diagnosis of hypernephroma is warranted from the gross appearance of the tumor, and from the test specimen removed. This patient was operated on June 9, 1906, and died two months after return home.

CASE XXXI (30,897).—Mrs. *D. J.* McM., cigarmaker's wife, aged forty-three years. *Patient has had stomach trouble (i.e.,* distress after eating, bloating, sour eructations, vomiting of food, etc.) *for the last eight years. Sometimes great pain two or three hours after meals. Has had pain over right kidney during past year.* First noticed a lump in the right side eight months ago. *Physical examination reveals large tumor in right hypochondrium. The urine shows no blood.* Operation reveals very large tumor of the kidney, extending well up behind liver, which organ is elevated. Tumor has gross appearance of hypernephroma. Piece removed for microscopic examination shows hypernephroma. *Patient was operated on June 29, 1909, and is reported alive and somewhat improved in health October 18, 1909.*

An examination of the preceding protocols and the accompanying illustrations will serve to make plain the pathologic reasons for certain points important to the diagnostician and surgeon.

1. The small solid tumor well away from the renal pelvis is likely to cause no hematuria and no pain. From such there should also be no venous metastases. Since they are apt to be symptomless, their surgical discovery is an accident. But granting that all hypernephromata probably pass through such a stage, the nearer we can come to recognizing it the better it will be for the patients.

Small amounts of blood in the urine usually come from the kidney side of the condensation "capsule" of the tumor. Large renal hemorrhages are from the thin-walled capillaries of the tumor where it has broken through the capsule into the kidney tissue, or into the renal pelvis.

3. The compression by the tumor of the remainder of the kidney, of the renal pelvis, or of adjacent nerves, as well as the presence of clots in the ureter, explains the various types of pain.

4. Tumors of the superior pole are apt to cause the more early distortion of the renal pelvis and apparently also earlier and more pronounced pain, owing to the relationships of liver and diaphragm.

5. Tumors of the mid-ventral side of the kidney are apt to develop slowly and cause only small amounts of hematuria and pain.

6. Tumors of the lower pole may be large enough, before the kidney tissue is all destroyed, to block the ureter and cause varying degrees of hydronephrosis.

7. The renal pelvis may be encroached upon from above (Group I), from below (Group I), or from the side (Group II). In either event there is more or less of a compensatory enlargement in other directions, even where no ureteral obstruction is demonstrable. On the other hand, there may be no deformity of the renal pelvis (Case I and Group III), or it may be entirely obliterated (Group IV). These points are of importance in interpreting the Röntgen pictures of the renal pelvis made after collargol injections, a method of diagnosis so satisfactorily developed by my colleague, Dr. Braash.[1]

8. Early extension of the tumor into the renal vein may temporarily lessen the pressure in the renal pelvis. The capsule of the portion of the tumor projecting into the vein is apt to be very thin. Extensive renal vein involvement at the time of operation usually means the early death of the patient from metastatic recurrence.

A further study of the morbid histology and the comparative embryology of these tumors will be presented in a subsequent paper.

I desire to thank Dr. W. F. Braash for the use of clinical data, and Dr. B. C. Willis, assistant pathologist, and Mr. H. C. Andrews, photographer, for their efficient help in preparing the material and illustrations for the foregoing paper.

[1] Annals of Surgery, March, 1910.

DISCUSSION.

DR. THOMAS S. CULLEN, of Baltimore.—We are greatly indebted to Dr. Wilson for this careful and exhaustive presentation of the subject. His photographs and histological pictures are remarkably clear, and I have never seen color photography come out more perfectly.

I would like to ask Dr. Wilson how the clinical diagnosis was made in early cases of hypernephroma. I would also like to ask what incision is made when these very large renal tumors exist.

Dr. Kelly will refer to hypernephromata of large size. Personally I have only had one case of adenocarcinoma of the kidney. The growth was a very large one, situated in the left side, and it was necessary to make an incision almost from the vertebral column to the median line in front. We knew we had not gotten the entire growth out. A little more than half a year later there was a lump in the right hypochondrium which proved to be a growth in the liver. We took it out.[1] A year or two later there was a large growth in the left side. This persisted for several years and filled the entire left half of the abdomen. At autopsy—three years after the liver operation—we found two small metastases in the liver. These were of recent date, showing that the original metastasis in the liver had been a single one and that there had not been a continuous growth of the original renal tumor, so that, so far as any liver complications were concerned, she would have remained perfectly well.

DR. JOHN C. MUNRO, of Boston.—I would like to ask whether the risk of metastases in these hypernephromata cannot be minimized by ligating the pedicle as a preliminary step, thus shutting off the blood supply before any handling of the tumor takes place?

DR. WILSON (closing).—With reference to the question which was asked by Dr. Cullen, I will say that cases one and two are extremely early ones.

The growths in the liver are a most interesting study by themselves. We have had one case of primary hypernephroma of the liver, which I have not included in this kidney series.

---

[1] Large Carcinomatous Tumor of the Liver, Jour. Amer. Med. Assoc., April 22, 1905.

This was in a child nine years of age. The child is well two years and a half after operation.

As to Dr. Munro's question of the possibility of preventing metastases by early ligation of the pedicle before bringing the tumor up into the wound, that would seem to be important and feasible with tumors in early stages, but with tumors in the stage of some of those here presented it would be impossible to make the ligation before manipulating the organ. With certain tumors there is liability of rupturing the capsule into the renal vein during manipulation.

INCISIONS IN THE ABDOMINAL WALL TO EXPOSE THE KIDNEY: INCISIONS IN THE KIDNEY TO EXPLORE ITS PELVIS.

By Howard A. Kelly, M.D.,
Baltimore, Maryland.

I THINK the crux of our kidney work for the present lies in two directions, indicated by the title of my paper. First, it will be of great value in furthering the progress of renal surgery if we can generally agree upon certain types of incisions to expose the kidney for exploration or for removal. Secondly, the most serious difficulties in exploring the kidney itself are the immediate hemorrhage and the subsequent infarct destroying the tissues; obviated when some satisfactory method has been discovered by which an exploration of the kidney, its calices, and its pelvis can be effected simply and safely. I confine myself to these important subjects today.

INCISIONS TO EXPOSE THE KIDNEY. Anyone looking through the literature of this subject will at once be struck by the great variety, the apparent want of uniformity, in the methods adopted in exposure of the kidney. Renal work having followed other abdominal work in the order of time, the first natural impulse was to approach the kidney trans-peritoneally by an anterior incision. This method has been almost universally abandoned, and I think rightly, because of the two wounds made in the peritoneum, and the awkwardness of getting at the vessels high up in the lumbar region, added to which was the serious danger of peritonitis in infected cases, which constituted so large a part of renal surgery. I believe today that any opening in the peritoneum should only be made as a temporary expedient for the purpose of exploring the upper part of the kidney, of examining the vessels at its hilum, to detect any neoplastic infiltration, and also to note the condition of the opposite kidney, and of the other abdominal organs. Such a wound should be carefully closed at once, as soon as it has served its purpose, and the remainder of the operation conducted wholly extraperitoneally. It is sometimes advisable, also, to open the peritoneum for the purpose of drawing the cecum down into the wound to remove a diseased vermiform appendix, as so often done by Edebohls, who attributed considerable importance to causal relationship between displaced kidney and appendicitis.

What we desire most in our surgical work on the kidney is an incision so placed and large enough to give good exposure of the retroperitoneal space and to afford the easiest possible access to the kidney, and, most important of all, to the vessels at its hilum. Where the kidney has its normal mobility the incision should be located somewhere well posteriorly in the soft tissues in the interval between the margin of the ribs and the crest of the ilium. The kidney can be safely drawn out of such a wound, pulling and stretching its vessels to complete the luxation without risk of rupturing them. Where it is high up and more or less fixed by inflammation about its upper pole or by an infiltrating neoplasm, then it is necessary for the operator to devise some form of incision which will fall more directly over the affected organ. Such an opening, for example, as is secured by cutting through the last ribs or by carrying the incision upward, skirting the margins of the ribs, or by extending it straight out to the semilunar line and then up to the ribs.

The choice of the best incision is, therefore, a question of election for the individual case with which a surgeon has to deal. I think that thr e or four types of incision can be described, out of which one can always be selected as the best for any given case.

I here offer as the unit or basis from which to calculate all operations for the exploration or removal of the kidney a well-defined anatomical landmark, the superior lumbar triangle, which I have used in all this kind of work for about fifteen years past. I call this the unit of calculation, as it is the best basis or starting point for all incisions whether large or small. From this point the opening may radiate outward, either downward and forward, parallel to the crest of the ilium, or straight out to the semilunar line and upward, or back along the last rib.

The superior lumbar triangle is made up of the tendinous aponeurosis of the oblique and transverse muscles to the point where they meet the quadratus lumborum and the last rib. It is a narrow triangle with the base upward at the rib. It is in a sense complementary to, but not to be mistaken for, Petit's triangle, which rests with its base upon the crest of the ilium. The superior lumbar triangle is covered in by the latissimus dorsi muscle, which has to be lifted in order to expose it. The last dorsal which divides into the ilio-inguinal and the iliohypogastric nerves is the most important anatomical structure in the region, lying as it does just under the margin of the quadratus muscle, where it is accompanied by an artery and a vein.

The method of exposing the superior lumbar triangle is as follows: The patient lies on the inflated rubber cushion (Edebohls), inclined a little to the opposite side, with the body gently sloping downward in both directions from the lumbar region, which is prominent. I then palpate the tissues of the side to be opened to locate the grosser landmarks, the spinal column with the transverse processes, the erector spinæ and the quadratus forming a strong resisting vertical column, the eleventh and twelfth ribs, the crest of the ilium, and out toward the navel the yielding oblique muscles. I then feel with my fingers for the little, soft, yielding spot up in the angle between the last rib and the quadratus lumborum. This lies just external to the margin of the erector spinæ and quad-

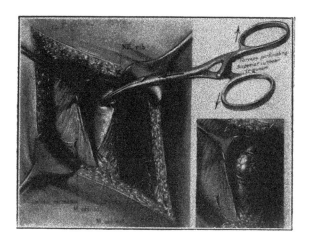

FIG. 1.—Showing incision of simplest type to
superior lumbar triangle.

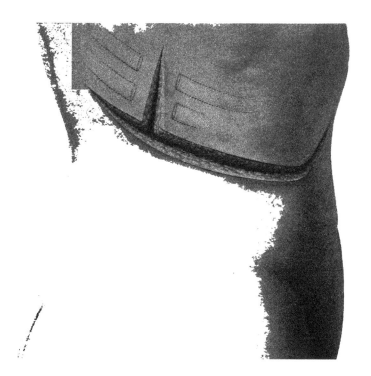

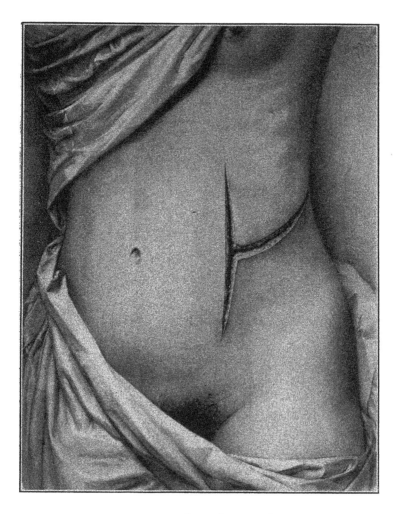

FIG. 3.—Incision for large hypernephromata.

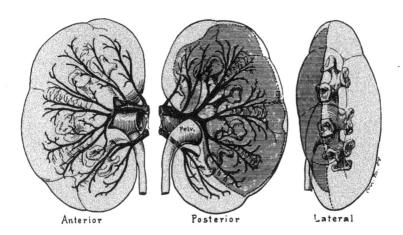

Anterior   Posterior   Lateral

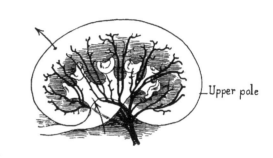

Upper pole

FIG. 5.—Showing use of silver wire in nephrotomy.

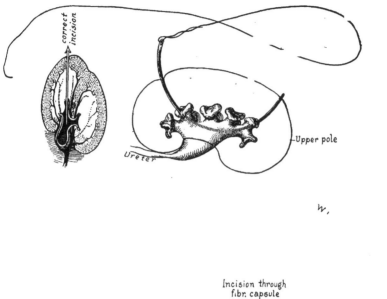

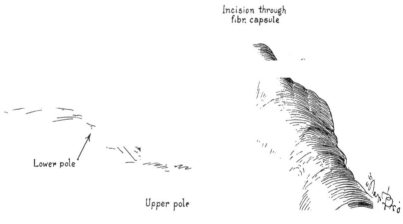

FIG. 6.—Second cut with wire, opening entire kidney.

ratus lumborum muscles, and yet not far enough away from the firmer edge of these muscles to fall wholly within the region of the softer muscular oblique muscles. Having fixed this point, I make a somewhat curvilinear incision from 7 to 10 cm. in length, beginning just above the triangle and extending downward and outward in the line of the fibers of the external oblique. As soon as the skin and fat are cut through, the lamella of the thin latissimus dorsi appears. This is recognized by the more up and down direction of its fibers, the whitish edge of the fascia distinguishing it from the external oblique which lies on a plane just beneath it. Not infrequently one or two vessels rise through the fascia from beneath the muscle, becoming superficial and spreading out on it. The next step is to deal with the latissimus in one of three ways (Fig. 1). In a suspension of the kidney I prefer to lift its margin, dissecting it free from the underlying tissues, simply lifting it up like a lid and retracting it until the tendinous yellowish-white superior lumbar triangle comes into view. Another method is to split the fibers and pull them apart by a blunt dissection, so exposing the triangle immediately beneath. In more serious operations I often cut straight through the muscle, dividing it for from 3 to 5 cm. When the triangle is laid bare, I take a pair of sharp-pointed forceps and plunge them through the fibrous tissues at its outer edge, avoiding the quadratus, which may overlap the inner part. Then opening the forceps, a little round hole is left, through which the golden-yellow retroperitoneal fat pops out—quite a characteristic sign. The index finger is thrust in, then two fingers are inserted, and the wound pulled open and made larger by strong traction in opposite directions with the fingers; to make the wound of considerable size, perhaps large enough to introduce the whole hand, the assistant standing opposite to the operator inserts three fingers, while the operator also inserts three opposed, when considerable steady force is used until the wound is large enough to introduce the entire hand. In the separation the opening is not made close along the border of the quadratus muscle, but extends downward and outward. The finger is then carried in and the elastic web of Gerota's fascia recognized, caught on the end of the finger, and broken through. The lemon-colored fat surrounding the kidney then appears in marked contrast to the golden yellow retroperitoneal fat. I have called attention to this little anatomical fact for many years, and can confirm the observation of Dr. W. W. Keen.

Any ordinary operation upon the kidney can be done through opening made in this way.

If the kidney is a large pus one, after evacuating the abscess the organ can be collapsed and brought out of this wound. A big hydronephrotic kidney can also be treated in the same way.

The opening thus made can be readily closed with one or two figure-of-eight sutures uniting the rounded edges of the oblique muscle on the outer side of the incision to the quadratus and spinous muscles on the inner side, always avoiding the nerve under the edge of the quadratus.

When the kidney is large and solid or fixed, then this superior lumbar triangle opening is either not big enough or not sufficiently under the kidney to enable the surgeon to handle it safely in dealing with any serious adhesions, or above all to afford perfect control of the vessels. In a stone or pus kidney, therefore, which cannot be collapsed and pulled down and out of the smaller incision, I enlarge my incision in a direction downward and outward by parting the fibers of the external oblique muscles and by cutting through the internal oblique and the transversalis. The transversalis is often so thin here as not to demand separate consideration. An important enlargement of this incision in the opposite upward direction is effected by dividing the quadratus from the last rib to the extent of 2 or 3 cm. This detachment enables the operator occasionally to avoid re-secting the rib. When this does not suffice, and the vessels are still inaccessible, I then separate the periosteum of the twelfth and eleventh ribs, if necessary, and cut through these ribs without injuring the pleura, thereby securing an exposure of the renal vessels.

Where the kidney is large and fixed, as in carcinoma and hypernephroma, while the longest incision I have just decribed will, as a rule, suffice for its exposure and safe removal, I think it better to adopt the rule of attempting to treat these organs more *in situ*, to secure better control of both the hilum and the numerous small vessels which have often been exaggerated to an enormous size by congestion. For such cases I have two incisions to propose, still using the superior lumbar triangle as the unit from which to carry the incision in one direction or another.

1. Having opened the retroperitoneal cavity at the point of the superior lumbar triangle, I carry the incision around in the direction of the umbilicus about half way between the ribs and the crest of the ilium until it meets the semilunar line. The incision is then carried up along this line close to the margin of the ribs. Pushing away the peritoneum so as to expose the kidney and retract the abdominal wall, the opening made in this way affords an excellent exposure of large, high-seated kidneys.

2. Where this incision is insufficient, I have adopted the plan shown in the figures of cutting through the last of three ribs directly upward from the superior lumbar triangle opening (Fig. 2). Such an incision, associated with the incision running out to and up the semilunar line, enables one to reflect the entire margin of the ribs, with the diaphragm as a sort of large bony flap, giving wonderful exposure of the entire retroperitoneal area under consideration.

Again, in a case of an enormous and exceedingly vascular hypernephroma, where engorged giant capillaries coursed under the capsule and threatened the death of the patient from hemorrhage in case of injury, I made the incision outward and around to the semilunar line in the manner described, and then cut up and down in this line, making a large ⊣-shaped wound—what we called when I was a cowboy in Colorado a lazy T. In this way securing splendid exposure and a corresponding control over the untoward conditions, I got the patient safely through a most threatening and forbidding operation.

The closure of these large incisions offers no particular difficulties. If the patient's condition permit, the wound can be closed in layers with careful apposition of homologous structures with catgut; if the condition is bad, it can be approximated with silkworm-gut sutures passed at intervals of 2 or 3 cm., embracing all the tissues.

EXPLORING THE KIDNEY ITSELF. The one serious operation performed upon the kidney itself, which may be described as typical and fairly common, is the exploration of renal tissues, the calices and the pelvis. This may be called for when one of the poles of the kidney contains abscesses and it is uncertain how far the disease may extend down through the rest of the renal tissues, which it is desirable to conserve. It may be necessary to determine the extent of a tuberculosis in the kidney tissue, to expose the calices, to discover and remove stones, to explore the pelvis for papilloma or aneurysm, as well as to find and operate upon a valvular ureteral orifice. I think I do not exaggerate the present status of this operation when I declare that it is occasionally in the highest degree dangerous, and usually accompanied by more or less serious hemorrhage and subsequent destruction of the renal tissue through infarcts which invariably occur whenever any important vessels are divided. The discovery of the system of vascularization of the two halves of the kidney by Hyrtl, and the rediscovery and application of this fact to surgery by Mr. Broedel, have done much to render safer our methods of exploration. All now know that the irregular dorsal white line marks the plane of maximum vascularization, and must be avoided both on the surface and down in the substance in opening the pelvis of the kidney through its dorsum. Previous to the demonstration of this fact the surgeon was more apt to choose this particular area as likely to afford an avenue of entrance into the kidney through apparently non-vascular fibrous tissue. Now it is universally avoided by an incision made well to one side strictly parallel to the plane of the vessels. Yet, though we follow this salutary rule in opening the kidney, the hemorrhage is still greater than it ought to be, and the reconstruction of the kidney after such an exploration is always followed by more destruction of the kidney tissue than ought to take place after a purely exploratory operation, which, as its name implies, should be both simple and safe, merely a means to an end, and not in itself an aggressive surgical act. For two years past Mr. Broedel has been calling my attention to an important method of entering the pelvis of the kidney through the notch in the lower part of the hilum on its posterior surface at the junction of the overlapping anterior with the posterior vascular trees. If one could penetrate at this juncture in an ideal manner, there would be no bleeding at all, while the inferior calix and the lower portion of the pelvis of the kidney would be perfectly opened to inspection (Fig. 4). Two of my staff, Drs. Ernest F. Cullen and Herman F. Derge, have made experiments on dogs which have been confirmed in man, demonstrating the important fact that we have at last an almost bloodless method of laying open the entire organ from one end to another. The method is as follows: The kidney is brought carefully outside of the body, detached from its surrounding fat; the vessels and the pelvis lie within easy grasp in the incision. In the typical, normal kidney the important vessels pass in front of the pelvis, which lies below and behind. Now, rotating the kidney so as to expose its posterior surface, the notch which lies exposed at the lower part of the hilum marks the limit of vascularization between the vessels which supply the posterior half of the kidney and the vessels which supply the anterior half, together with the entire lower pole. One then takes a well-curved flat, blunt Kousnietzoff-Cullen

liver needle, armed with a silver wire, and passes this up under
the margin of the kidney at the notch, penetrating up inside
the kidney until it encounters the increased resistance of the
calix, which it then perforates. The point is now made to
appear on the surface. The capsule of the kidney between
the points of entrance and emergence is divided when the
wire is drawn up through the kidney substance saw fashion.
This lays open the lower posterior calix. It is important
while severing the kidney tissue to hold the organ firmly,
using counter-traction so as to avoid pulling on the renal
vessels. (See "Use of Silver Wire in Opening the Kidney,"
Johns Hopkins Hospital Bulletin, November, 1909, No. 224,
p. 20.) The opening thus made into the calyx may be
extended down into the pelvis and be used for the extraction
of a stone or for the exploration of the remainder of the pelvis
(Fig. 5). If it is important to explore the entire kidney from
end to end, the blunt curved needle, similarly armed with
silver wire, is passed into the opened lower calix and carried
up to the upper pole into the most distant calix, when it is
brought through onto the dorsum of the kidney. Once
more the capsule of the kidney is divided and the wire used
with a sawing motion, to effect the splitting of the kidney
into its anterior and posterior vascular trees. This operation,
which may appear startling, is in reality often almost bloodless;
indeed, in animals, Drs. Cullen and Derge found it often so
entirely devoid of hemorrhage that they did not find it necessary to put in any renal sutures to control such. All that
was necessary was a few superficial sutures pulling the capsule
together. I show here a sketch of an infarct from a dog's
kidney following the opening made with the knife; also
another of the infarct following the use of the method just
described. Owing to the fact that the wire does not divide
the papillæ at the centre, but slips up to the side of the papilla,
only a short portion of the terminal tubules are severed from
their terminal ducts, while the remaining portions of these
divided tubules still continue to do their work by forming

new openings into the calix, discharging into a rent above the calix, as seen in the pictures. In the average kidney described the hilum is deeper on its posterior surface; in rare cases, in which the reversed condition is found with the vessels in front, the needle is entered also in front at the inferior notch. With a distribution of the vessels, some in front and some behind, it will be best not to open from the pelvis inward as described, but to plunge the needle through the dorsum directly into the substance of the kidney, in the middle of one of the pyramids, and bring it out through one of the upper pyramids, avoiding by keeping parallel to the white line. I emphasize the previous insertion of the ureteral catheter and the distention of the kidney with fluid at the time of the opening as greatly facilitating the entrance of the needle into the calices.

DISCUSSION.

DR. R. C. COFFEY, of Portland, Oregon.—Dr. Kelly's paper is certainly a very instructive one, and practical in its details. The last kidney case I had, which was discharged before I left home, was one of enormous kidney in which I was forced to make an incision similar to the one Dr. Kelly has described, and I thought of Dr. Kelly's T-incision in beginning to do transperitoneal removal of the kidney, and finding I could not do it through a longitudinal incision, I found it necessary to make the T-incision, crossing back toward the spine, and going as far back as the muscles, because it seemed there were lakes of pus in it, necessitating drainage. The question of whether or not such an incision would so disturb the abdominal wall as to render the liability of hernia very great is to be borne in mind. I have had some uneasiness about the case, and I hope Dr. Kelly can give us some idea as to the possible dangers of hernia, or bad results from such an incision.

DR. THOMAS S. CULLEN, of Baltimore.—A thorough exposure in these cases is just as important as it is when we are dealing with a large myoma, with vessels coming from the

upper part of the omentum instead of from the pelvic structures.

A case reported by Braun[1] before the German Surgical
Society in Berlin, in 1908, demonstrated this point very well.
The tumor was situated below the left kidney. The operator
after pushing the ureter to one side found that it was still
difficult to get his bearings and lengthened his incision until
it extended from the back almost to the median line anteriorly,
The aorta lay in a groove on the inner aspect of the tumor.
After a very careful dissection the tumor was removed, but
on account of the intimate attachment to the tumor the outer
coats of the aorta had been injured. The raw area in the
vessel wall was partly turned in by a running suture. A
second suture was necessary. After this had been introduced
the operator noticed that the lower extremities were blue and
cold as a consequence of the partial shutting off of the blood
supply. It was therefore found necessary to remove the two
vessel sutures. The aorta at the point of injury looked so
ragged that nothing remained but to attempt resection of the
injured portion with end to end anastomoses. This was
rendered feasible by the fact that the vessel had been drawn
far to the left and formed an extended curve so that a considerable portion could be removed and the ends still approximated.
After the anastamosis the clamps were removed from the
vessel and the large wound was closed except for a small drain.
The child recovered, and Braun showed the patient at the
German Surgical Society a month later.

I have had the opportunity of following Mr. Brödel's renal
injections which he has been making for the last ten years.
He has clearly shown that the bloodvessels of the kidney are
divisible into two vascular leaves, which can be readily -
rated from each other. The posterior is the larger one.sepa

I have had the opportunity of using silver wire as a means
of opening the human kidney as suggested by Cullen and
Derge,[3] and the results have been just as satisfactory in the
human being as they have proved to be in animals.

[1] Verhand. der Deutsch Gesell. f. Chir., 1908, Band xxxvii, II, 104.
[2] Max Brödel, The Intrinsic Bloodvessels of the Kidney and Their
Significance in Nephrotomy, Johns Hopkins Hospital Bulletin, 1901,
vol. xii, No. 118.
[3] The Use of Silver Wire in Opening the Kidney, Johns Hopkins
Hospital Bulletin, November, 1909.

Dr. Albert Vander Veer, of Albany.—A few years ago Dr. Kelly gave us a paper somewhat along this line in regard to opening the kidney. At that time he spoke of the distribution of the bloodvessels, and of a little white line which he has not mentioned today. Following out that thought, I have operated twice in opening the kidney for the removal of stones, and have been surprised at the small amount of hemorrhage which has ensued. Operating as I did in some cases before, in splitting the kidney, the hemorrhage was quite profuse, but I remembered Dr. Kelly's reference to this distribution of the bloodvessels, and the method of reaching the kidney through the posterior border. I think Dr. Kelly's first incision, to which he called attention, is very useful, and if we follow out the ureter we can extend that kind of incision much better. Dr. Kelly has one illustration of a large free incision, and I made one somewhat like it ten or twelve years ago, and I felt all the while that I was going into the peritoneal cavity, and yet by careful stretching I removed a large diseased kidney in that way. Surely this method of getting in and removing the kidney posteriorly extraperitoneally is one that is very desirable.

May I ask Dr. Wilson whether in his histological description and reference to the description of pathological examinations of these specimens he has found the condition to be a true fibrous structure, with an amount of cell growth, etc., particularly in the class of kidneys he has referred to tonight, when they are exposed? I have had two cases of that kind in which the hardness of the kidney tissue has impressed me each time. This hardness could be felt as one approached the kidney. I would like to ask why we should meet with such a hardness in these cases of hypernephroma, where we have hemorrhage which is so profuse.

Dr. J. Wesley Bovée, of Washington.—I am very glad to see Dr. Kelly come around to the point of adopting the anterior route in making these large incisions. My experience has been that in reaching a large kidney tumor, and removing it, that an incision running toward the median line gives much more space. One can extend this incision by making an incision at an angle from it, which gives an angular flap to lift up, and a larger opening. I have been very much surprised to observe the large working space that is obtained by making an almost transverse incision. I have removed large tumors, some of them weighing as much as eight pounds, and one of these was a hypernephroma, through a small transverse incision, and I have noticed a few times, when we had such large tumors as that, we could get down on the median side of the tumor, catch hold of the bloodvessels, and control them before loosening the tumor along the line. If we can control the circulation there we can more readily deal with the other vessels the same as we can in catching hold of the splenic vessels. If we get hold of the splenic vessels in a large spleen and pick up the arteries first, so that no more blood comes into the organ, and ligate the veins and arteries *en masse* before we remove the tumor, it is a great deal safer procedure.

DR. WM. P. MATTHEWS, of Richmond, Virginia.—I have recently operated on a case which I desire to put on record in connection with this discussion. In doing the operation I followed Dr. Kelly's original method in removing a large stone from the kidney. The patient was a woman, aged thirty-eight years, and the kidney stone was removed on May 28 of this year. She left the hospital July 1. It was found necessary to use a drainage tube in this case, on account of the condition of the interior of the kidney. Drainage was used for several days, which rendered the closing of the wound a little slow. She remained at home until the middle of August, when trouble started again, and on her return to the hospital we removed a second stone without any difficulty through the original incision. The kidney was found to be very much enlarged, and it contained a stone more than one-half the size of the original stone which was removed. This operation was done September 15.

DR. KELLY (closing).—I should be very glad, indeed, if the method I have described will enable us to adopt some uniform practice when making incisions for the purpose of getting at the kidneys, and treating them more intelligently. I put in silkworm-gut stitches an inch apart in the big incision, and nothing between them, and healing took place beautifully with the exception of one little point. I would advise keeping in a good liberal drain.

AN EXPERIMENTAL AND CLINICAL RESEARCH INTO NITROUS OXIDE VERSUS ETHER ANESTHESIA.

AN ABBREVIATED REPORT.

By George W. Crile, [M.D.,
Cleveland, Ohio.

In the hands of skilled surgeons there is at present only a slight immediate mortality in the good risk patient, whatever the operation. This slight risk is made up largely of factors over which we have at present little or no control, *i. e.*, embolism, pneumonia, suppression of urine, etc.

Indeed, the mortality rate can with no inconsiderable accuracy be predetermined by discrimination in advising operation.

In the good risks should we not endeavor to lessen the immediate postoperative discomforts and the postoperative neurasthenia, and in the bad risks should we not only decline to accept defeat, but here search for new methods to reclaim the handicapped patient? I venture to state that foremost among the means of achieving more nearly ideal results in the good risks, and of reclaiming the handicapped, is the anesthetic.

It is quite unnecessary to enumerate the well-known limitations of the anesthetics now in use. Ether still stands first as an all-around general anesthetic.

Local anesthesia has special limitations, and spinal anesthesia is in the midst of its tryout.

In the minds of the public, ether, as given by the usually unprepared interne or the uninitiated, bears a reputation approximately that of a combination of hazing and sea-sickness. Not only has it a popular ill repute, but we shall try to show that it has at least two vital limitations: (a) it contributes to postanesthetic depression, and (b) it impairs immunity. If these points are established, the question that follows is: Is there any general anesthetic that is preferable? I shall hope to show that nitrous oxide is such an anesthetic.

In the laboratory, animals in parallel series were subjected to shock producing experiments of varying severity, and the results obtained were carefully studied by the means of:

1. Observation on the pathological physiology recorded on a smoked drum.

2. By histological study of the central nervous system.

In the laborious task of accumulating the data upon this subject I was largely relieved by Dr. Prendergast in the physiological part, and by Dr. Austin in the pathological. The research has been under active prosecution for more than a year, and the following is but a summary of the results obtained.

In overdose, nitrous oxide causes death by a combination of asphyxia and cardio-inhibition. When the inhibition is controlled by atropine or scopolamine, death may occur by asphyxia alone. Nitrous oxide, too, in overdose may inhibit respiration. Muscular tone is diminished far less under nitrous oxide than under ether anesthesia. The animal comes out of the anesthetic immediately, quite regardless of the duration of the anesthesia. And repeated anesthesia seems to develop no immunity.

Its action being quick and its effect evanescent, nitrous oxide anesthesia runs the entire gamut, from slight to fatal anesthesia, with remarkable celerity. Its best administration is therefore especially difficult, requiring far more alertness and ability than ether; indeed, a number of experiments were sacrificed to the technique of administration.

There is apparently no postanesthetic effect upon either

the lungs or the kidneys, nor, indeed, upon any other part of the body.

Does an animal under nitrous oxide anesthesia endure shock producing trauma better or not so well as under ether anesthesia? Here the difference is so striking that doubt lingered not at all. The nitrous oxide animals resisted shock producing trauma far better than did the ether animals. Then, too, in handicapped animals, *i. e.*, animals reduced by infectious hemorrhage or hyperthyroidism, the nitrous oxide showed a marked advantage over ether.

The composite chart indicates graphically this result.

The changes in the ganglion cells of the central nervous system from the cortex to the cord, as indicated by the newer pathological cytology methods, shows a distinct difference between the cells in the ether and nitrous oxide animals. The cells of the nitrous oxide animals showed much less change than in the ether dogs. This part of the work has important bearings in other directions, and will be reported in full in a later communication.

CLINICAL. My first attention clinically was called to nitrous oxide by the work of Dr. Teter, who had acquired a splendid empyrical knowledge of the administration of nitrous oxide in his dental work, and invented an excellent apparatus bearing his name. A few administrations of this anesthetic by Dr. Teter were sufficient to indicate its clinical possibilities, hence this research.

My general anesthetist, Miss Hodgings, gave the anesthetic in the experimental laboratory, and there acquired an excellent working knowledge of it. Miss Hodgings has administered nitrous oxide in 575 major operations, and has kept careful notes. She had had a large previous ether experience, with which comparisons were made. The following is a summary as to the technique, the phenomena, and the results.

THE TECHNIQUE. It was only after considerable experience that Miss Hodgings was able to so skilfully adjust the dosage as to keep the patient under the anesthetic sufficiently for surgical purposes while maintaining a pink circulation. We soon found that the beneficent quality of inconsequential after effects became a shortcoming, viz.: Postoperative ether cases, like seasick travellers, are quite oblivious to environment and even pain; but postoperative nitrous oxide patients, being at once in possession of all their faculties, have an unimpaired painful appreciation of the operative trauma. This was admirably met by a combination of scopolamine and morphine precedence. This almost ideal combination will be alluded to later.

The principal phenomena of nitrous oxide anesthesia are the state of the circulation, of the respiration, and of the muscular system. In overdose all the blood assumes a venous color, the heart is slowed, and the blood pressure rises, and if excessive the heart is suddenly arrested in over dilatation. The heart is the key to the situation, the warning being too much slowing. Dr. Teter introduced the method of continuous auscultation by means of a unilateral phonendoscope. This we have found practical. In nitrous oxide the longer the anesthetic the better the anesthesia becomes. Unfavorable circulatory phenomena are, we found with added experience, merely expressions of the unskilled administration, and not in the least necessary to the maintenance of surgical anesthesia.

The respiration, like the circulation, is easily overanesthetized, the phenomenon being gradual impairment and finally arrest.

In both the circulatory and respiratory phenomena of danger the remedy is always at hand, and can be instantly applied, viz., turning off the nitrous oxide and turning on fully the oxygen. This maneuver requires but a few seconds.

The muscular system becomes a problem because of the very innocuousness of the anesthetic; the muscles are not so well relaxed as in ether anesthesia.

In women and children, and in anemic or otherwise weakened subjects, relaxation is usually ample. In robust subjects satisfactory relaxation may become difficult and, indeed, sometimes impossible with nitrous oxide alone. The way out of this difficulty was rapidly found, viz.: A saturated ether cone is substituted until sufficient relaxation is obtained, usually in from two to five minutes. The nitrous oxide anesthesia alone will then be found sufficient; that is to say, nitrous oxide may, with certain modifications become a routine anesthetic.

Nitrous oxide as now used costs approximately eight dollars an hour. This may be reduced to about three dollars an hour by manufacturing the gas in the basement of the hospital and having it piped to the operating room. Not only does such a plant reduce the cost, but by providing an even flow makes the administration much simpler and more efficient than by the high-pressure cylinders and bag, with the troublesome freezing high-pressure valves.

CLINICAL RESULTS. In my service we have given nitrous oxide 575 times for major surgical operations. Among these are included many of the hazardous risks in which ether was contra-indicated.

In one of the early cases, an exceptionally bad risk, in which ether was contraindicated, the heart was arrested. The patient was resuscitated, but died six hours later. I attribute the death to the anesthesia, in part to the anesthetic per se, and in part to imperfect technique of administration. This occurred before our laboratory research, and before nitrous oxide was routinely given. I am quite certain that this result would be now very readily obviated by Miss Hodgings.

As to nausea. Comparing the nitrous oxide cases with ether cases, nausea occurred in 17 per cent., as compared with 42 per cent. in ether. This includes all cases. Postoperative nausea is, of course, not wholly due to the anesthetic, *i. e.*, peritonitis and certain visceral operative traumas may, independently of the anesthetic, cause nausea.

Nausea in nitrous oxide cases in which there is no other nausea-producing factor rarely occurs.

In the course of the operation, nausea, in nitrous oxide, as in ether, is usually due to uneven administration. At the conclusion of the operation the patient is fully awake and in unclouded possession of all his faculties in two or three minutes.

There is unmistakably a great diminution in surgical shock. Indeed, the immunity from shock is as striking in the clinic as in the laboratory.

I am well aware that the shock in the routine cases, free from predisposing complications, is rare; but in the cases most urgently demanding surgical relief such predisposing causes are present, and frequently constitute the principal factor of the immediate risk. It is here that nitrous oxide appears at its best. Then, too, in infections, we are equally certain that ether as compared with nitrous oxide impairs the immunity of the patient. The difference is so striking that only a great emergency would now induce us to use ether instead of nitrous oxide in grave infections.

In a parallel series of acute infections consisting of 75 cases operated under nitrous oxide and 75 under ether, the technique and the after treatment being constant factors, careful records were kept at the time of the operation and after. The average pulse observation is here presented. At the time of operation the average pulse of the ether cases was 114; and the average of all the pulse observations during the first twenty-four hours following operation was 117. While in nitrous oxide the average pulse rate at the time of operation was 115, the average of all the counts during the first twenty-four hours following operation was 105. In ether there was an average postoperative *increase* of 8 beats during the first twenty-four hours; in nitrous oxide there was a *decrease* of 10 beats. In every other respect also the patient

MM. of HG	AVERAGE NORMAL BLOOD PRESSURE	AFTER ½ HR TRAUMA	1 HR. TRAUMA	1½ HRS.	2 HRS.	2½ HRS.	3 HRS.

130
125
120
115
110
105
100
95
90
85
80
75
70
65
60
55
50
45
40
35
30
25
20
15
10
5

A
B

PAWS BURNED
PAWS BURNED
PAWS BURNED
PAWS BURNED
PAWS BURNED
PAWS BURNED
PAWS BURNED

showed a more distinctly favorable course after nitrous oxide than after ether. Not a case showed the rapid march to fatality immediately following the operation as occasionally follows ether. Neither has there been any case of pulmonary complication.

The work of Graham, of Chicago, on the phagocytes showed that ether distinctly lowers the phagocytic power.

There are, indeed, many points I should like to discuss. Based upon experimental and clinical observations, I may summarize as follows:

Nitrous oxide as compared with other general anesthetics is technically difficult and expensive. It has certain dangers, which are almost wholly in the control of the skilled anesthetist. The patient should remain *pink throughout the anesthesia.* If nitrous oxide alone will not accomplish this and maintain an efficient anesthesia a sufficient amount of ether must be added. *It is not the anesthetic of choice for the uninitiated, but only for the highly trained anesthetist.* Properly supplemented and skilfully given, it may be used as a routine anesthetic in general surgery. Once the operation is over, the patient is strikingly better off than after ether anesthesia. The role of shock and infection is far less in nitrous oxide than in ether anesthesia, and accumulating evidence seems to show that there is a distinct diminution in postoperative neurasthenia.

In routine operations the combinations of small doses of scopolamine and morphine, given one and one-half to two hours prior to nitrous oxide anesthesia, form so effective a combination that in over 50 per cent. of my patients the day of operation is robbed of all disagreeable operative memory, and in the remainder it dulled the edge of both the physical and the mental distress.

DISCUSSION.

Dr. Charles A. L. Reed, of Cincinnati.—Mr. President: I have only recently come to an appreciation of this method of anesthesia. I was literally forced to take it up because of a patient, a woman, aged fifty-three years, who had the interesting combination of valvular disease of the heart, atheromatous arteries, and chronic interstitial nephritis, with a fifty-four pound ovarian tumor. The cardiac conditions were inhibitory of chloroform; the renal conditions were also inhibitory of ether; and under these circumstances, being totally unfamiliar with the technique of the administration of nitrous oxide and oxygen in combination, we had Dr. Teter come down from Cleveland to administer the anesthetic in this case. The experience was a delight and joy. I said to Dr. Teter, "When you are ready, I will begin." He began, and in two minutes the patient was quiet and sleeping. As I began to close the incision I said to him, "You may let up now;" but Dr. Teter replied, "When you get the last pin in the dressing I will let it out." When we got the last pin in the dressing, and he took the cone away, the good lady began talking with us. She did not have a particle of nausea or shock, and went through convalescence in an entirely normal way.

Dr. Teter administered this anesthetic to a second patient of mine the same day, with equally satisfactory results. I at once installed the method, and we are now using it in a large number of cases with uniformly satisfactory results.

I look upon the advent of nitrous oxide and oxygen anesthesia as a distinct advance in modern surgery.

Dr. J. Shelton Horsley, of Richmond Virginia.—I would like to ask Dr. Crile how he explains the difference in the degree of shock following ether and nitrous oxide anesthesia.

Dr. Howard A. Kelly, of Baltimore.—When I was in Philadelphia twenty-two years ago I bought from F. W. White an apparatus for administering nitrous oxide, and I took it with me to Baltimore, where I secured the services of a dentist who specialized in giving this anesthetic for the purpose of extracting teeth. He administered the anesthetic for me, but found it hard to keep the patient profoundly under its influence. I therefore gave it up for a time, but subsequently took it up again, and since then have given it to patients literally by the thousands in my private hospital and in the Johns Hopkins Hospital, and for the last five years I have given with nitrous oxide a little oxygen, which enhances its effect; mixed with a little ether the anesthetic effect is much more complete. The whole anesthesia is carried on with nitrous oxide, plus a little ether, to get complete relaxation. I use it for all renal work, where I can get complete relaxation with it. I likewise use it for examinations, for dilatations and curettements, and particularly if anything turns up postoperative in the way of an emergency. While I am sure in some cases the patients would die if I used ether again, after having been through a severe operation, I have no fear whatever of the use of nitrous oxide, and give it once or twice to the same patient postoperatively in critical condition, so I can agree with Dr. Crile as to its being an ideal anesthetic. The only difficulty is it takes an anesthetist who is more skilled in its use than in the administration of ether. Some men never learn to administer nitrous oxide as it should be given. They do not get patients completely under its influence. But nitrous oxide with oxygen, and then the addition of a little ether occasionally, in my mind is an ideal anesthetic.

Dr. Warren Buckley has worked out all these problems for me in my private hospital.

Dr. R. C. Coffey, of Portland, Oregon.—Probably the next great thing for the advancement of our statistics in surgery is the improvement in anesthesia. I think the first thing required will be the enaction of a law prohibiting the average doctor or interne from giving anesthetics. I think most every surgeon who has tried expert anesthetizers is opposed to the administration of anesthetics by the average physician who is picked up here and there from time to time. I am satisfied that the great amount of shock we have in our surgical operations today is due more to the anesthetic and the manner in which it is given than to anything else.

This work which Dr. Crile has brought before us today is new to me, to a certain extent, and I predict great things for it. There is one question, however, I would like to ask him, and that is about scopolamin. I have a mortal horror of it.

About a year ago, in the beginning of our animal experiments, we used a series of twenty each of the H. M. C. tablets, and found the mortality was more than twice as great when we used these tablets than when we had not preceded the use of ether with them. Scopolamine, as I understand it, is the same drug practically. When scopolamine-morphine first came out the mortality was great from this combination. Some one looked it up and found the mortality was 1 or 2 per cent., but that is not all. The patients were so greatly depressed after its use that I soon dreaded its employment, and I would like to ask how Dr. Crile did this, to prevent the bad effects of this drug.

Dr. Wm. D. Haggard, of Nashville, Tennessee.—This subject is exceedingly interesting to me, because it fell to my lot to look the matter up for the anesthesia commission a year ago. It was totally new. I had never seen it employed, except by dentists, and these dentists used it principally for extracting teeth. I was obliged to use it myself, in order to make an intelligent report. In the first thirty cases in which it was employed we found it was a method of great usefulness, and we are indebted to Dr. Crile for having presented the method in the manner in which he has. My own experience has been very pleasing with its use in the class of cases in which it is particularly indicated.

The first class would be those persons that have been referred to as bad surgical risks, who cannot take a general anesthetic. They take nitrous oxide beautifully, and I am satisfied, as the essayist has said, that it minimizes shock to a surprising degree. The most delightful experience I have had with this anesthetic has been in the cases of so-called minor surgery in the office, and in the clinic, such as the removal of bone felons, the reduction of dislocations, the opening of pelvic abscesses, etc. It takes but a few moments to anesthetize a patient with nitrous oxide sufficiently for one to do an operation, and the patient wakes up in a minute or two after the cessation of its administration, in a pleasant frame of mind. It looks like a slight-of-hand performance, or an hypnotic exhibition. One lady from whom I removed a forty-pound ovarian cyst woke up at the end of the operation and asked, "Doctor, how much do I owe you?" (Laughter). That is a feature of anesthesia I have not witnessed before.

There are some contra-indications to it. I think we should bear in mind that patients with bad hearts ought not to take nitrous oxide. I hope Dr. Crile in his closing remarks will tell us about that, because when anything does happen, it happens quickly. We have had no fatalities in something over one hundred cases of major surgical work with this anesthetic. With nitrous oxide alone we have only had one bad scare, and that was in the early use of the agent, when we did not understand its technique. It should be distinctly and thoroughly understood that various and sundry persons cannot give it, and in our reports we are accentuating that recommendation. Persons should be thoroughly trained to administer nitrous oxide well, even more so than in giving other general anesthetics.

One of the features of our anesthesia commission is to insist upon personal instruction and teaching of anesthesia in all medical schools, and in Nashville we are doing this. In our hospital work we are giving young men who are to graduate practical training in the administration of ether and other anesthetics.

Another thing I want to call attention to is the safety of nitrous oxide compared with chloroform. Chloroform is undoubtedly the most dangerous of all anesthetics, and those who are the least capable of administering anesthetics usually pick it out. Surgeons will not give chloroform, but the man who has had no particular opportunity for acquiring skill in its administration is the one who invariably gives it. That is why so many deaths from general anesthesia occur. Thirty deaths occurred in England in one year from the administration of chloride of ethyl. Nitrous oxide cannot be used by the general practitioner, and it cannot be used very well in house-to-house operating, because it is cumbersome to carry the apparatus around. It can be used in the office to do minor surgical operations, and in the hospital.

Again, nitrous oxide can be used to the great comfort and delight of patients, in removing dressings, which would otherwise cause a great deal of pain or suffering.

In conclusion, I wish to say that inasmuch as our anesthesia commission is to report on this agent at the St. Louis meeting of the American Medical Association, I shall be deeply obligated to those who may communicate their experience with this anesthetic to us before that meeting.

Dr. CHARLES H. MAYO, of Rochester, Minnesota.—If there is one thing the profession has been anxiously looking for it is an ideal anesthetic. For many, many years we have been looking for some change. In making a change we should not only consider the mortality, but the fact that the general condition of the patient is improved, and the dangerous effects following the anesthetic are greatly minimized. Dr. Crile has brought out these points very clearly.

Jonnesco, as many of you know, has recently arrived in this country, and is not only demonstrating but advocating a modification of the old method of spinal injection. It is to be hoped this constant changing of anesthetics will at no distant date enable some one to develop a method who knows how to give it. We must have in every hospital some one who is trained in the use of it. Take it in the East. Dr. William J. Mayo, while on a recent trip to New York, went with a surgeon to a private house, where a patient was to be operated on. He went to the house with the surgeon the night before, and while they were discussing the case the men drove up with a furniture van and began to unload, and Dr. Mayo said, "What are they doing? Is there somebody moving in?" "No," replied the surgeon, "that is the anesthetizer bringing in his material for tomorrow." (Laughter.) You see the surgical end becomes the smallest end, and the minute you get a real anesthetizer, the surgical end will be the smallest end. (Applause).

Dr. Crile (closing).—Dr. Horsley asked for an explanation as to why there was less surgical shock from nitrous oxide anesthesia than from ether anesthesia. I am unable to answer the qestion. The newer psychopathology that has been developed recently has enabled us with considerable accuracy, I think, to point out changes in the ganglion cells of the central nervous system in surgical shock. With nitrous oxide anesthesia these changes are not so marked as they are under ether anesthesia. Nitrous oxide anesthesia is only possible by the administration of oxygen.

As to the repeated use of anesthetics, in one case we gave nitrous oxide anesthesia thirty times for the making of painful dressings, and neither susceptibility nor immunity were established.

With reference to the question of Dr. Coffey concerning scopolamine, I do not believe that the so-called H. M. C preparation is as reliable as the pure drug alone. We have used scopolamine a great many times. For instance, in a robust young patient, we give $\frac{1}{100}$ grain of scopolamine, with $\frac{1}{6}$ grain of morphine; in older subjects we give $\frac{1}{250}$ grain of scopolamine, but the dose is graded according to the physical condition and age of the patient. We have not seen any unfavorable results.

Dr. Haggard spoke of the heart as a contra-indication to nitrous oxide anesthesia. This is the key to the situation. I do not think that nitrous oxide acts upon the muscle as a poison. An unskilled anesthetist should not be intrusted to give nitrous oxide excepting under supervision. No other anesthetic requires as much skill in its administration as nitrous oxide.

DR. RUFUS B. HALL.—Suppose you had a patient on whom you were doing a prolonged and difficult operation in the abdomen, and the muscles are rigid, as they are oftentimes under gas, how do you overcome that rigidity?

DR. CRILE.—I would give ether until the muscles were relaxed.

DR. HALL.—Will they stay relaxed?

DR. CRILE. If they do not, administer still more ether.

DR. HALL.—I have used for years a combination of gas with ether, and the muscles become relaxed immediately.

SOME OBSERVATIONS ON GALLSTONES, WITH REFERENCE TO CANCER OF THE GALL-BLADDER.

By Albert Vander Veer, M.D.,
Albany, New York.

For some time I have had an impression that cases of carcinoma of the gall-bladder and gall-ducts had gallstones present for a number of years, as an etiological factor, and yet I did not find the condition apparently so frequently as I had expected. In going over 77 cases, somewhat recently, and not previously reported, I am able to present some facts that in themselves are rather interesting. Of these cases there were males, 19; females, 58; illustrating the fact so often observed, that females suffer more than males from gall-bladder complications.

Regarding their ages there were:

	Cases.
26 to 28 years .	3
30 to 39 years .	15
40 to 49 years .	26
50 to 59 years .	22
60 to 69 years .	11

The study of the duration of symptoms is also very valuable and is as follows:

Age.	Cases.
2 to 4 days	2
6 to 11 weeks .	5
2 to 18 months.	13
1 year .	3
2 years .	7
3 years .	9
4 years .	8
5 years .	8

Cases.

6 years 5
7 years 1
8 years 1
10 to 19 years 11
20 to 26 years 4

The diagnosis before operation of the 77 cases was as follows:

Cases.

Gallstones 64
Cholecystitis 10
Gallstones and carcinoma 3

Operation revealed the following conditions:

Cases.

Gangrene of gall-bladder 2
Obliteration of gall-bladder, with many adhesions . . 1
A very contracted gall-bladder with thickened bile . . 1
Stricture of common duct, with distended gall-bladder . 1
Distended gall-bladder with inspissated, dark bile . . 5
Gallstones in common duct 4
Gallstones in cystic duct 2
Gallstones in gall-bladder and cystic duct 2
Exploratory incision revealing carcinoma of gall-bladder
    and no further operative intervention 2
Exploratory incision for carcinoma of gall-bladder and
    ducts and calculi found 2
Exploratory incision for carcinoma of gall-bladder, ducts
    and liver—no calculi found 3
Abdominal section in which gallstones were found and
    removed:—
        Ovarian cysts 2
        Uterine fibroids 6
        Appendectomies 5
One case of cholecystotomy showed no calculi, but an
    enlargement of the head of the pancreas, and was un-
    doubtedly a case of pancreatitis recovering through
    drainage 1
Nephrectomy of right kidney — transperitoneal — also
    cholecystotomy and removal of several calculi . . . 1
Stricture of cystic duct 1
Case of long, serious illness in which patient gave all
    the symptoms of biliary colic, obstruction of bowels
    following about two years after, and laparotomy done.
    A large gallstone found blocking ileus. Removed.
    Death from exhaustion 1

S Surg   21

It will be noted there were but fifty-five in which gallstones were really found, though in the other remaining nine patients all had given the symptoms of having passed them.

After careful analysis of the five remaining cases it is fair to assume they were of the nature of cholecystitis with possible chronic pancreatitis and the operation of chole-cystotomy, with drainage, resulted in their cure.

The mortality immediately following the operation was eight cases, none living to exceed ten days. This mortality list includes the five cases of carcinoma, of whom two died within a few days and three lived sometime later; in fact two of them lived so long a period after the operation it gave me some doubt as to the diagnosis being correct.

Three deaths followed cholecystotomy, in two of which calculi were removed. Two died from shock. In these latter cases there were many adhesions, the stones deeply located, one in the common duct, and the operation very difficult. In the other case there were several stones deep down in a mass of adhesions and persistent hemorrhage followed. In the case of obliteration of the gall-bladder, above reported, death resulted from shock. In the one case of contracted gall-bladder, in which there were several stones, it was found necessary to use the long Murphy button, and death resulted from peritonitis on the tenth day. One death resulted from obstruction of the bowels, due to a large stone found blocking the ileus, and not really to be properly classed as an operation for primary removal of gallstones.

There were three cases of cholecystenterostomy. One was for a biliary fistula following one of the operations for chole-cystotomy, where many calculi had been removed. The fistula persisted for months, but closed quickly with the use of the small Murphy button. The second case was that of stricture of the common duct, where the Murphy button was used and complete recovery followed. The third case was the same as the first.

While there were several cases that developed fistulæ

lasting even as long as a year they ultimately healed. In some cases I have seen good results follow the application of a few drops of carbolic acid into the sinus. One patient is yet living with a fistulous opening of nearly eight years duration. She cares for it very kindly and is content. Whenever it closes she is so uncomfortable she is very anxious to have it reopen.

There were two cases of persistent intermittent discharge with occasional colic so pronounced that the patients submitted to a second operation, one at the end of three, the other at the end of two years.. Recovery followed removal of the gall-bladder in each case.

These, together with the case of non-malignant tumor of the gall-bladder, made three cholecystectomies.

Of the seven cases in which there was malignant disease present, two of carcinoma of the gall-bladder were inoperable; two of carcinoma of the gall-bladder and ducts, in which there were calculi present, were also inoperable; three cases in which there was carcinoma of the gall-bladder, ducts and liver, in which no calculi were found, and inoperable.

The average length of symptoms in the above cases was as follows:

Male, aged 58, symptoms of . . . . 11 months' duration
Male, aged 40, symptoms of . . . . 3 months' duration
Female, aged 52, symptoms of . . . 5 years' duration
Female, aged 53, symptoms of . . . 12 years' duration
Male, aged 49, symptoms of . . . . 7 years' duration
Male, aged 65, symptoms of . . . . 3 years' duration
Female, aged 53, symptoms of . . . 15 years' duration

It will be observed that there was a great discrepancy here in ages and duration of time of symptoms.

No doubt our pathologists are correct in that at some period gallstones produce an irritation that results in the development of malignancy, and when once this period is reached the carcinoma must advance with considerable rapidity, and that we have not been at all in error when advising patients suffering from gallstones to have a prompt operation, for there can be no question that some of these cases of attacks of biliary colic do result in cancer.

It may be proper to state here that these seven cases of carcinoma of the gall-bladder, ducts and liver did not have any evidence of primary carcinoma of the stomach.

It will be noted that there were quite a number of cases in this group that extended over a long period of years without developing malignancy.

In going over these cases it is interesting to observe the symptoms in some of the special ones. For instance, the case that developed marked symptoms in two days was a chauffeur by occupation, and had had symptoms of indigestion, as he supposed, for two years, without consulting a physician. He was taken suddenly ill with great pain in his side, was seen by my son, Dr. James, who readily discovered a tumor in the region of the gall-bladder, and believed it a case of acute abscess associated with gallstones. The patient was taken to the hospital the next morning. Upon operating we found the gall-bladder greatly distended, packed with gallstones, and just approaching a gangrenous condition. The acute symptoms were here very pronounced and an immediate operation was a fortunate procedure for him.

The drainage continued for three months, then closed, and for some three weeks he was quite comfortable, when the gall-bladder again became distended. Another incision was made by my son, Dr. Edgar, and drainage carried out for some time, after which the sinus healed and the patient has remained in excellent health since.

In the two cases of gangrene one, as noted, had had symptoms for a period of twelve years, during which time she had been advised to have an operation, then had her acute attack, which was very pronounced, immediate operation called for, and gall-bladder found in a gangrenous condition.

In the other case the symptoms previous to the acute attack, which resulted in this condition, were not so characteristic.

A case of much interest, now under observation, was operated upon nine years ago. The patient had marked symptoms of biliary colic extending over a period of twelve years, when finally her sufferings were so great that she submitted to an operation. Forty-six, decidedly facetted stones were removed, and no more to be felt in the gall-bladder, but in the course of the drainage in the next four months she passed in this manner forty more calculi, also had some three well-marked attacks of biliary colic. The patient then made an excellent recovery and remained in good health until November of this year, when she had a return of very severe pain, which her physician telephoned me was precisely like her old attacks of biliary colic of years ago. In the course of about a week or ten days the site of the incision became distended, and on consultation we thought we had a case of abscess of the gall-bladder to deal with. The patient was very much exhausted, but under cocaine and a few inhalations of chloroform I made an incision, finding the gall-bladder so attached to the edge of the liver that I finally had to open into the peritoneal cavity, reached the point of distention and removed sixteen gallstones, which were decidedly facetted, then introduced drainage. The patient was critically ill for forty-eight hours, but finally began to rally. In securing movements of the bowels the nurse observed a large gallstone, which, on examination at the laboratory, proved to be that and not a fecal concretion. Possibly this is the stone that gave her her sharp pain in the beginning of the present attack. Had this patient been in any kind of proper condition I would have done a cholecystectomy. Aside from this case I cannot call to mind any in which the gallstones reformed.

In this group there were two interesting cases in this respect: The one in which 1900 calculi were removed, returned to the hospital in six months, stating she had precisely the same symptoms she had before the operation. The patient was kept under close observation. She was in a great state of fear, very nervous and excited, but when assured there was no re-formation of the stones finally realized her sufferings were somewhat imaginary. She ultimately recovered. I have had the case under observation more or less since and she has had no return of her old attacks. The same conditions apply to another case where the patient suffered fear of a return of the trouble.

That stones are sometimes hidden in a dilated duct or sac, and that we fail to always reach the entire number, is illustrated in two cases: One in which the drainage continued, and after four or five months a good-sized stone was found in the lower part of the gall-bladder which required quite an effort to remove.

In the other case several stones made their appearance almost a year after the first operation for drainage in a case of supposed cholecystitis, where no stones were found, although careful search was made at the time.

The skill with which we can now bring together portions of the omentum and place in a drainage tube so as to keep up continuous drainage, in cases where the gall-bladder is so small and impossible to remove or attach to the incision, brings greater success than ten or fifteen years ago, our technique becoming so much more perfect. Drainage down through the peritoneal pouch, opening through the lumbar region, is very satisfactory, and as mentioned so favorably by Mayo Robson at one time.

I am quite sure that death resulted in one of my earlier cases from imperfect drainage.

It is worthy of note that one of the cases of uterine myoma, in which there were gallstones removed, had had her attacks of biliary colic from early girlhood.

The study of the mortality list impresses one with the statement that has been made by other operators that stones of the common duct, of long standing, are very difficult to reach and the percentage of deaths much greater here than in simple cholecystotomy, where there were no such complications. The mortality in the latter cases is very small.

One very impressive case, regarding the courage and confidence of the patient, is as follows: February 18, 1903, she had marked symptoms of endometritis, was curetted and relieved. March 2, 1905, had an operation for a movable right kidney. Her symptoms of cholecystitis continued, with pain over appendix, and she was operated upon April 11, 1905, for removal of the appendix. A gallstone was felt in the bladder and removed by cholecystotomy. The patient made a good recovery and has remained well since.

One case of the group illustrates most forcibly the marked cholemia, which is not always fatal after an operation. For two years the patient had been ill with attacks of pain and jaundice, with bleeding from the gums and lips for two days before the operation. Cholecystotomy was done, calculi removed, and she made a good recovery.

One of the fatal cases was associated with somewhat similar symptoms.

A case that went over twenty-five years was most interesting in its history. The patient had had many attacks and at last, although reaching the age of sixty-two, could bear her sufferings no longer and submitted to an operation. Quite a number of stones were removed, and although she was very ill for a few days she ultimately made a splendid recovery. She returned to full health, and a year after her operation her color and added flesh were so pronounced as to impress her friends very forcibly.

A very unusual case was that of a female, aged fifty-eight, who had given symptoms for a period of twelve years. Has resided for the past three or four years in Cuba. Was quite comfortable up to two years ago, when she began to have more serious and painful symptoms, and during the past year frequent attacks of colic. Six months ago she noticed a circumscribed pain under the edge of the liver and a fulness afterwards. Patient returned home to the United States three months ago and came under my observation, when I could make out a distinct tumor in the region of the gall-bladder, not movable, and with an apparently circumscribed attachment to the abdominal wall. Her general appearance was good, she had not lost in flesh, was not suffering so much, no stomach symptoms, and bowels were moving quite regularly, but the pain was somewhat steady and continuous, although not so markedly the nature of biliary colic. Operation advised, to which she readily consented, and done November 18, 1909. An incision made down to the tumor revealed a condition in which the gall-bladder, with mesenteric attachments, could be felt as a circumscribed mass about like a medium-sized split lemon. Adhesions were loosened up as well as possible, the mass separated from the mesenteric attachments and the ascending and transverse colon and by the thermo-cautery from the under surface of the liver. Hemmorhage not at all severe. A complete cholecystectomy was done, and one large calculus, not at all facetted, was found present.

The material removed had the appearance of true carcinoma of the gall-bladder.

Report from the pathological laboratory, December 6, was as follows: Hypertrophy of gall-bladder. Acute and chronic cholecystitis, and peri-cholecystitis. Acute myositis. Chronic myositis. Marked acute and chronic inflammation. Many large, closely meshed epithelial cells filled with fat. No evidence of malignancy.

DaCosta, *Surgery*, 1903. Gallstones may lead to suppurative inflammation of the gall-bladder or bile passages, ulceration, occlusion of the neck of the gall-bladder, dilatation of the stomach from the formation of adhesions which kink the pylorus, abscess, peritonitis, empyema of the gall-bladder and cancer of the gall-bladder."

Adami, *Pathology.* "Carcinoma, usually of the cylindrical-celled variety, affecting the gall-bladder, may result from the irritation of a calculus. It often spreads to the liver by contiguity."

Keen's *Surgery*, vol. iii, p. 1006, Section written by Wm. J. and Chas. H. Mayo. "(1) Gallstones are almost always present in primary cancer of the gall-bladder, and not in secondary metastasis. (2) The relative disproportion of malignant disease of the gall-bladder and gallstone disease in men and women is practically identical. (3) The pathological lesions actually found are best explained on the irritation theory."

Moynihan, *Gallstones and their Surgical Treatment.* "Malignant Disease. One of the most serious of the sequelæ of cholelithiasis is malignant disease of the gallbladder or of the ducts. The close connection between gallstones and malignant disease has never lacked recognition, though opinions have differed as to which is the cause and which the effect. Opinion is now universally in favor of the view that it is the irritation of the gallstones that determines the incidence of cancer, the view that was first supported by Klebs.

"In his record of cases Courvoisier found the following results: Of 84 cases of primary cancer of the gall-bladder, stone was found in 72; in 2 others stone had passed in motions. In 10 cases no mention of stone made; in 4, certain pathological changes—scarring of duodenal papilla, stricture thereof, and dilatation of all the bile passages, indicating unquestionably, the former presence of calculi.

"In primary cancer gallstones are present in 15 per cent.

"Musser, 1889, had collected notes of 100 cases of primary cancer of the gall-bladder and verified by post-mortem. Gallstones were present in 69. Jayle, in 30 cases collected, entirely from French records, found stone present in 23 cases."

Rolleston, *Diseases of the Liver, Gall-bladder and Bile Ducts*, p. 627. "Relation of Primary Carcinoma of the Gall-Bladder and Gallstones. Special interest attaches to the association of gallstones and carcinoma of the gall-bladder, inasmuch as the calculi are generally thought to be the cause, whether by direct irritation or otherwise, of the neoplasm. That calculi are commonly met with in primary carcinoma of the gall-bladder is shown by numerous statistics. Conversely, it appears that primary carcinoma of the gall-bladder occurs in from 4 to 14 per cent. of all cases of cholelithiasis. Among 242 cases in St. George's Hospital there were ten cases of primary carcinoma of the gall-bladder, or 4.1 per cent. In twenty-one and one-half years in this institution there were 16 cases of primary carcinoma of the gall-bladder; 13, or 81 per cent. of which were associated with gallstones.

"Experimentally, however, it does not appear that bile is more likely to crystallize on stagnation provided the gall-bladder is asceptic. (Mignot).

"There is undoubtedly a very definite relation between cholelithiasis and the development of primary carcinoma of the gall-bladder. But gallstones are so commonly present without carcinoma developing, that though they dispose to its occurrence, some additional factor is necessary. Possibly the part played by calculi is that of preparing the soil for the direct cause, whatever it may be, of carcinoma.

"Malignant disease of the gall-bladder is very much commoner in women. According to Fütterer's figures (202 females, 52 males), it is four times more often seen in women.

"Frereichs described the disease as one of old age. Carcinoma of the gall-bladder is very rare before forty years of age."

Douglass, *Surgical Diseases of the Abdomen*, p. 389. "Gallstones are often found in association with primary malignant disease of the extra-hepatic bile-channels. Clinical evidence altogether favors the conclusion that cholelithiasis exists prior to the development of the neoplasm. The theory of irritation has, therefore, received general acceptance, and primary carcinoma of the bile-channels is commonly regarded as a sequel of gallstones."

Kehr, *Gallstone Disease,* p. 46. "It is an uncontrovertible act that the concretions furnish the stimulus to cancer formation."

A. J. Ochsner, in Kelly and Noble's *Gynecology and Abdominal Surgery,* in summing up the medical treatment of cholelithiasis says, "there is always the danger of carcinoma as a result of the long-continued irritation."

Mayo Robson, *Gall-bladder and Bile Ducts,* p. 122. "Cancer of the gall-bladder is not nearly so uncommon as was once believed, but as a primary affection is somewhat rare. It is usually secondary to gallstones, or to cancer of adjoining organs, and in the latter case is not amenable to surgical treatment." This statement coincides with my cases.

Eisendrath, *Surgical Diagnosis,* p. 341. "Malignant Disease of the Gall-bladder. This frequently follows cholelithiasis and should be suspected if a hard mass is found in the right hypochondriac region following a history of gallstones in an elderly patient with persistent jaundice. The tumor is usually nodulated, rarely smooth, and is very hard in consistency. This induration, the nodular surface, and the rapid appearance of cachexia followed by icterus and ascites, serve to distinguish it from cholelithiasis; but in the latter the organ may be indurated so that a diagnosis is often not made until the abdomen is opened. The pains in cancer are not sharp and colicky, but of a dull character. If fever and colicky pains appear, they indicate an infection of the carcinomatous gall-bladder. The course is a very chronic one."

Hektoen-Riesman, *An American Text-book of Pathology,* p. 818. "One result of the presence of gallstones should not be forgotten—carcinoma, which may spread by continuity to the liver, so that the point of origin may at last be difficult to make out. It is usually of the cylindric-cell type. Sarcomas, fibromas, and myxomas are recorded."

Martin, *Surgical Diagnosis,* p. 523. "Cancer of the gall-bladder, usually due to stone, is characterized, aside from the symptoms of this latter condition, by nodular tumor in the gall-bladder region. Diagnosis should be made by operation, and before a tumor becomes demonstrable.

"Gall-bladder cancer, secondary to infiltration of the liver, usually gives no history of stone, and is of minor moment compared to the primary disease. In either case, if the cystic duct be occluded, acute suppurative cholecystitis, with its characteristic symptoms, may develop and mask the original lesion.

"Occlusion of the common duct by cancer of the papilla cannot be distinguished from that due to stone, since it is usually secondary to this condition, except for the lack of intermittence in obstructive symptoms and the development of ascites from vein involvement. The complicating gastric disturbance, the constitutional manifestations of cholangitis, and the symptoms and signs of pancreatic involvement, are the same in both affections."

Johnson, *Surgical Diagnosis*, vol. ii, p. 163. "Gallstone Disease. The experience of surgeons throughout the world during the past ten years indicates that early diagnosis is of the greatest importance to the affected individual; thus Wm. J. and Chas. H. Mayo, in one of their most illuminating papers on this topic, 'The Diagnosis of Gallstones Disease,' *St. Paul Medical Journal*, February, 1905, write as follows:

"In reviewing the mortality of 1000 operations for gallstone disease we have been impressed with the very fortunate outcome where gallstones were in the gall-bladder and therefore were without complications. In the 1000 cases there were 50 deaths, or an average mortality of 5 per cent. The death rate in 820 cases where the disease was confined to the gall-bladder and for benign conditions was 3 per cent. In 416 cases of simple gallstone disease the mortality was less than 0.5 of 1 per cent. The common duct operations amounted to 14.6 per cent. of the whole. In 137 operations for common duct stones the mortality was 11 per cent. In 40 cases, or 4 per cent., malignant disease was discovered, and the operative mortality was 22 per cent. In practically all of these cases gallstone irritation had been the cause of the development of cancer."

DISCUSSION.

DR. SAMUEL LLOYD, of New York.—Dr. Vander Veer has been telling us about some remarkable cases of gallstones. I would like to report a case of a woman I saw a few days ago, who had been operated for gallstones and drainage of the gall-bladder instituted. The original wound closed, and later she developed a persistent sinus over the greater trochanter of the femur. She also had had symptoms of gallstones a few months before I operated on her. I operated for the purpose of closing this fistula over the trochanter, and removed a gallstone in that region, and followed up the fistula to the gall-bladder.

DR. CHARLES H. MAYO, of Rochester, Minnesota.—This paper of Dr. Vander Veer's certainly covers nearly all the complications which arise in gall-bladder and biliary duct work. The surgeon is compelled very largely to depend upon the diagnostic ability of the physicians of his neighborhood, and in that connection, also, we must consider the price of olive oil, so that I would say he has a somewhat larger per cent. of cases of carcinoma and other troubles than would come if there was a better surrounding group of physicians, who would deliver the cases to the surgeon before some of the complications arose which he reports, so that the percentage of serious cases is greater, and the number of cases of cancer is greater than should appear. Gall-bladder work today, when we get the cases early, with gallstones, is not difficult or serious. The mortality following operations on the gall-bladder is low.

Dr. Vander Veer brought up the question as to whether we should remove the gall-bladder. Of course, there are some surgeons who have insisted that the gall-bladder should be removed every time because of the fear of cancer, and gall-stones, cholecystitis, and pancreatitis, and other conditions which may happen if we leave the gall-bladder, because it is so simple to remove it. Leaving out the first four days following operation, the patient gets along quicker with gall-bladder out than with drainage, but drainage is an important thing, and it is my belief that we should not remove the gall-bladder unless there are some positive indications. During this summer, in three months we had three cases of cancer of the gall-bladder, none of them diagnosticated previously as cancer, but as gallstones. In one of them a large amount of material loose in the gall-bladder came out preceding the stone. In the other two toward the pelvis the carcinomas were small. It is all right to remove the gall-bladder where there are positive indications of its lining having been destroyed by chronic disease, and where you often find a hard nodule in which you fear malignancy. The reports showed that about 15 per cent. of cancers of the liver are primary, and the rest of them are secondary metastatic growths. Of the primary growths, considerably over 90 per cent. develop around the gallstone, so that we should take the individual while we believe he has a gallstone present, or cholecystitis, and operate on him. And some of these cases really need operation more on account of the cholecystitis which exists than for other gallstone conditions, such as infectious conditions of the biliary tract. We can tell these individuals that they have a simple pathological condition, which can be operated on with as much safety as chronic appendicitis, but that if they keep on postponing operation, no matter how many attacks they have, these attacks will lead to future and more deeply seated complications. Patients with such conditions as I have described should be urged to undergo operation, because repeated attacks lead to disease of the ducts and pancreas, and then comes cancer, of which they stand the chance of one in twenty-five. Many of these patients come to us with a history of chronic irritation from stones or stone. When they come to us with a history and with symptoms of gall-bladder disease, instead of shouldering the responsibility ourselves, we should give them what facts we possess, which will enable them to decide whether they want to submit to operation or not, and if they postpone operation, they should assume the risk themselves.

Dr. J. Garland Sherrill, of Louisville Kentucky.— This subject is of extreme interest to the entire body and to the entire profession. It is true, however, that the education of the general practitioner is largely at fault for the late time we see these gall-bladder cases.

Some years ago I had occasion to look up the subject

because I became impressed with the frequency with which I was seeing cancers of the gall-bladdr. At that time 14 per cent. of the cases were showing primary cancer of the gall-bladder. In looking up the literature I was forcibly impressed by the statement made by G. R. Slade, of England, who stated that 33 per cent. of cases examined microscopically, taken from the postmortem rooms, showed cancer of the gall-bladder. That was a surprising number, and seemed to emphasize to me the importance of early diagnosis, and the early relief of these patients by operative measures. In some of these cases, as you all know, the gall-bladder will appear thickened, indurated, and hard at the time of the operation, and even if you do not remove the gall-bladder, but simply drain, this induration and hardening will disappear in many cases.

I agree with Dr. Mayo in the statement that cholecystotomy in many of these cases is sufficient treatment. In some, where the gall-bladder is extensively indurated, where its mucosa is interfered with, where drainage is going to be imperfect, we should resort to extirpation of the sac.

Dr. O. H. Elbrecht, of St. Louis.—What I am about to say is not entirely germane to the subject under discussion but enough so to justify its being brought out in connection with this valuable analysis of cases. Dr. Vander Veer tells us that these patients are all easily shocked, and I feel sure that all are agreed, for all who have operated on the common duct for the removal of stones recognize its dangers. One of our esteemed fellows, Dr. Ransohoff, has proved by experimental work on rabbits, that any traction put upon the common duct will cause almost an immediate lowering of the pulse rate. His work may be found in an article in the *Annals of Surgery*. I have verified his observation in at least 50 clean abdominal cases where the operation was in the pelvis or some other region, and in which I instructed the anesthetist to count the pulse before I put traction on the common duct and to watch the change brought about when sufficient traction is put upon the common duct, and in almost every case the pulse will drop from 20 to 30 or 40 beats, which demonstrates sufficiently the importance of avoiding as much traction as possible while working in this region. This, of course, does not apply when we simply open a gall-bladder to drain, as it only pertains to the common duct cases.

I would suggest to those who have not made the observation to try it in the next suitable case, and thus glean the value of handling these structures gently and with more respect for the bad inflnence of unnecessary traction.

DR. GEORGE W. CRILE, of Cleveland.—In over three hundred operations on the gall-bladder I have not infrequently encountered similar results. The cases in which I succeeded least well were those in which I should have done cholecystectomy. So far as I am personally concerned, I have adopted at present this guide: Whenever the gall-bladder is itself, at the time of operation, physiologically removed from the body, I make the anatomical removal. If the cystic duct is closed, I know of no way of opening it. In these cases it is my practice to follow the physiological excision with the anatomical one.

DR. VANDER VEER (closing).—In regard to the remarks made by Dr. Lloyd, with reference to the location of a gallstone in a sinus, several years ago I reported a series of cases of gall-bladder work, in which I removed a number of stones from the umbilicus. That patient suffered a long time from gallstone colic.

I remember a case in the practice of Dr. McDonald in which he began an operation for the removal of the appendix with a good deal of earnestness, and came upon an elongated gall-bladder containing seven good-sized stones, which made an impression upon us. I have also seen two cases, one in my practice and one in that of another surgeon, where we opened an abscess associated with the kidney, in each one of which we found gallstones. These cases are interesting, but they are not coming to us of late years. They are being attended to earlier now. When beginning work upon the gall-bladder a number of years ago and in some of my earliest operations done in our territory, my greatest difficulty was to convince the old practitioners of the necessity of operation, and such practitioners always brought up the point which Dr. Mayo has referred to, namely, "Doctor, this patient has never been jaundiced." They do not offer this objection now. The patient may have been jaundiced, but the jaundice has gradually disappeared and not returned in succeeding attacks. Some twelve years ago through our section of the country practitioners used large doses of olive oil in their gallstone cases. Some of them became great believers in the olive oil treatment for these troubles, and with this treatment many patients were tided over for a period of a year or more, some of them thinking that they were well. We had in our county society a very remarkable case. The patient, a physician, suffered severely from gallstone colic. He came to one of our meetings and was asked, "Doctor, how are you getting on with gall-stone trouble?" He replied, "I am well, and have been for a year. I have taken large doses of bicarbonate of soda, and I feel that I am cured." The next night he was taken with a severe attack, the gall-bladder ruptured, and he was in a condition of profound shock. He was a man, aged sixty years, and died within a few hours after rupture. At the autopsy over three hundred calculi were found.

I recall another case not unlike this. The patient came from Plattsburg. I saw her two or three times, and urged operation. She had a severe attack, and finally said, "Well, I had better go to Albany; I ought to have an operation." She was put on a sleeper at 11 P.M. She reached Albany at 4. A.M., and when I saw her she was in profound shock, and died toward evening. We have these cases to bring up to illustrate to the practitioners in our section the necessity of prompt operation, and results are being produced. We are getting these cases early, and those that have no complications are easy to deal with. We are approaching these cases in precisely the same way Dr. Mayo has referred to. We say to them, you have all the symptoms of gallstones. We believe you have them. Occasionally gallstones pass without operation, but I believe many of these patients suffer from a single stone, while the smaller stones may have passed. We give them every reason for believing that they have gallstones, and if they have them there is more or less inflammation of the gall-bladder, and recently we have said to them, you have trouble with the pancreas, or sweetbread. We are understanding better these cases of pancreatitis, so admirably referred to in this discussion here, and we say to these patients the gall-bladder ought to be drained anyway, and we believe you have gallstones. Such remarks have saved me from embarrassment in my last series of cases. In the first series of cases I was confident the patients had gallstones, but in operating gall-stones were not found in some of them, but they got well with drainage, and were pleased afterward. I approach these cases by saying that there is undoubtedly cholecystitis, and drainage

S Surg   22

is desirable. Drainage is the saving factor in the treatment of our cases.

All of you who have looked up the subject and have studied it carefully recognize that the operation of cholecystectomy has carried with it a larger mortality than cholecystotomy and drainage. Cholecystectomy is an easy operation to do in many instances, and from what Dr. Crile has said, it is appropriate in some cases, and I feel that if I had my work to do over again—and I say this to my young surgeons—I should be justified in doing the operation of cholecystectomy more often in the future than in the past.

The other points referred to are exceedingly interesting. Reference was made by Dr. Elbrecht to traction upon the common duct. That is a point which should attract our attention in doing this kind of surgery. It is something like the reference we used to make as far back as the time of Peasley, when he said very emphatically, in operating for the removal of ovarian tumors, I am careful not to bring any traction upon the other ovary, and this was said more than thirty-five years ago, and what he said then holds good in our work upon the common duct today.

The remarks of Dr. Sherrill have an important bearing upon this class of work.

While the group of cases I have presented to you is exceedingly small as compared with the enormous work done by the Mayo brothers, yet it has in it some points that are of interest, and I feel I have received some instruction in studying my own cases.

ACUTE DIFFUSE SUPPURATIVE PERITONITIS FROM A RUPTURED PUS TUBE.

By J. Wesley Bovée, M.D.,
Washington, D. C.

Perhaps to many gynecologists, who for a considerable number of years have been assisting to definitely decide upon the proper treatment of suppurative infections of the uterine appendages in women, the title of this contribution may recall memories. But the condition of a patient who from a ruptured pyosalpinx has a general suppurative peritonitis rapidly becoming fatal is one that does occasionally occur, and its gravity demands rare surgical judgment and skill. It is quite probable that when the purulent contents of a Fallopian tube have become sterile rupture of that structure with escape of its contents into the peritoneal cavity may occur, with little or no harm to the individual of which it is a part. Not uncommonly are the fimbriated ends of such tubes found permeable and without macroscopic appearances of inflammation in their vicinity, though pus may be coaxed or kneaded from the lumen of them. Again, localized peritonitis about suppurating tubes is quite the usual condition noticed. It is to another and very different condition I would invite attention, which is, Fallopian tubes distended to a considerable degree by infected fluids, to which is added the phenomena of sudden and notable rupture of the tube, with escape of the contents into the general peritoneal cavity.

An experience of this character has been mine, and I will

detail it as follows: During the early morning of May 7, 1909, I saw, in consultation with Dr. Ramsburgh, a woman aged thirty-eight years, who apparently weighed about two hundred and thirty pounds. Dr. Ramsburgh stated he had attended the patient professionally for a few years and had delivered her of her third baby in January, 1909. During coitus early in the morning of May 4 she had experienced very severe pain in the right iliac region. He saw her promptly, and at 6.45 A.M. found her in some pain, but a pulse rate of 76 and temperature of 98.4° he noted in his minutes. By enemata her bowels were freely moved, and at 11.30 A.M. the temperature was 103.6° and the pulse rate 120. The following morning (9.30 A.M.) the temperature was 100.6° and the pulse 84. During the night the bowels had moved six times. At 4 P.M. temperature was 101.2° and pulse 106. The following day the temperature ranged from 101.6° in the morning to 103.2° at 8 P.M. Her condition was little changed. The pulse reached 120 that evening. At my first visit we found her temperature was 101.6° and the pulse 100. She was complaining of having a severe pain in the right inguinal region. A quite careful examination failed to find an unusual mass at any place, and on bimanual examination I could find no evidence of a pathological appendage. To place her in a hospital for careful observation and, possibly, operation seemed advisable, and she was at 10.30 A.M. admitted to Columbia Hospital for Women. At 4 P.M. her temperature was elevated to 102.4°, while the pulse remained at 88. A leukocyte count was made and a report of 23,100 returned. She seemed brighter, and operation was deferred, yet considerable gaseous distention of the intestine was troubling her. On the 8th she was progressing toward recovery, apparently, when late in the afternoon, after freedom from pain since morning; the temperature at noon being 101° and the pulse 84 to 90, she was again attacked by pain, now very violent, in the right inguinal region, with a chill followed promptly by collapse. The abdomen rapidly increased in tension, and in the evening an operation was done. An incision was made a little to the right of the right linea semilunaris, its upper end being opposite the umbilicus. When the peritoneum was incised a considerable quantity of thin seropurulent material poured out through the opening. The cecum and vermiform appendix were found much nearer the diaphragm than they are usually placed and macroscopically normal. The right Fallopian tube was from one to one and one-half inches in diameter and ruptured. It was exceedingly friable and removed in pieces, the stump being whipped over by catgut. Several intestinal loops were adherent to this tube, but easily separated. The pelvis was lightly packed with gauze, one end of which was carried through vagina and vulva. At the end of the operation her temperature was 99.2° and pulse 120. At noon the day after operation the temperature, rising gradually, had reached 103.4°, but twelve hours later had dropped to 101.8°and the pulse to 100. The drop method of instilling salt solution into the rectum had been employed quite faithfully since her admission to the hospital. The bowels were at noon moved well with a purgative enema. On the 10th the condition was worse; vomiting was an additional symptom, and the end seemed near. It came at 3 A.M. on the 11th, nearly seven days after the first severe pain and about fifty-four hours after the operation.

That the condition is a rare one is suggested by the small number of cases reported, that the largest number reported from the experience of one man is six (Boldt), and that several have reported one or two. Bonney states he wrote fifty surgeons asking for reports of their experience with such cases. Of the forty who replied, but fourteen had seen the condition. He received in this way notes on 14 cases. In a moderately careful review of medical literature I have found 55 cases, which, added to the one I herein report, makes a total of 56 cases. It is quite probable a careful perusal of all reports and tables of series of surgical treatment of pyosalpinx and of acute peritonitis would disclose a few more. But I think the infrequency of the condition must be apparent. The gravity of such a calamity is shown in the high mortality attending it, 32 (58 + per cent.) having died either with or without operation. In 1 (Anderson's) the result was not given and the case was reported the day of the operation.

Etiology. An inquiry into the causes of pyosalpinx rupture into the peritoneal cavity, with resulting acute peritonitis, carries with it the presumption that the infecting organism in the tube was permitted to pass through the rupture in sufficient strength to immediately involve the whole peritoneal surface in the same process as existed in the tube. The larger part of tubal infections producing suppuration is caused by the gonococcus. Yet in no instance in this series of cases was that organism found in the abdominal contents. In but a few were bacteriological reports made. Frank found the Staphylococcus pyogenes aureus, and the colon bacillus was recognized by another. I will not here enter into a discussion of the various pathogenic organisms that produce suppuration of the Fallopian tube. We are informed by some careful observers that the gonococcus is not capable of extensively injuring the peritoneum, and, *per contra*, others insist peritonitis of a fatal character may be produced by this organism unassisted. But those of us accustomed to treat extensively tubal infections and to await an innocuous state of the pus before operation are impressed by the very large proportion in which but a few days or weeks are required for that state to be reached. In these the gonococcus is probably acting alone. But can all these temporarily quiescent cases be thus produced? If so, can the gonorrhœal tube contents be suddenly aroused to fury when allowed in liberal quantities to reach the peritoneum, or is the infection of the tube of a mixed character, all the varieties remaining quiescent until rupture occurs, a period of months in some of the cases reported? In most cases violence of some sort was reported. Perhaps it was not more than transportation to a hospital for treatment for pelvic inflammation (Ingalls, Vance, Mann), and during the following day or two the acute and striking symptoms would ensue; ofttimes the patient had not been out of bed for several days just preceding the rupture. In several instances the traumatic element was childbirth. In this respect the experience of Oleson, of the Cook County Hospital, Chicago, was unique. He had at one time two cases in which this accident caused death in the puerperium. In one the labor at eight months was rapid, and death occurred five days later. In the other the labor was of so short duration that he had not time to get into the ward before the birth, and she also died in five days (see table). A few quickly followed curettage, and Legueu reports two that were noticed as soon as the accident occurred, which was during a bimanual examination of the pelvic contents. Two occurred during coitus, and another was probably a direct result of the woman lifting a heavy child.

Symptomatology. In the cases that ruptured during labor the symptoms of this grave accident were clouded by those of labor, and in them usually an autopsy revealed the first knowledge of the real pathology. Fabricius' case is a bold exception, and the only one that recovered. In the others the symptoms are quite like those of ruptured tubal pregnancy or tubal abortion. Usually, however, the patient is ill with pelvic inflammation, but perhaps does not remain in bed. While at her duties, after recovery from an attack of infection of the uterine appendages, or resting comfortably in bed, perhaps in a hospital preparatory to surgical operation, she suddenly experiences excruciating localized pain, perhaps a chill and collapse. Fever and high thready pulse promptly follow, if death does not soon supervene, and distention of the abdomen together with the general symptoms of diffuse peritonitis are not long delayed. Sometimes the surgeon, being familiar with the pelvic contents before rupture, has readily discovered after it that the tube was collapsed and flaccid instead of full and tense as before rupture.

TABLE OF CASES OF ACUTE GENERAL PERITONITIS FROM RUPTURE
OF PYOSALPINX.

Reported by	Duration or stage of peritonitis.	Notes.	Result.
1. Chipault, Bull. Soc. Anat. de Paris, 1861, xxxvi, 149	Acute, general	No operation. Autopsy findings: Right tube distended with pus; left tube contained some pus and had a small rupture. Cancer of uterine cervix was advanced	Death.
2. MacLaren (see Bonney)	Acute, general	Second day of attack, incision with flushing and drainage. Autopsy findings: A ruptured, distended pus tube and general peritonitis	Death two days after operation.
3. Almagro, Bull. Soc. Anat. de Paris, 1862, xxxvii, 171	Acute, general	No operation. Autopsy findings: Pus in abdominal cavity; right tube enormously distended by pus and has a rupture 4 cm. long; left tube also distended, but not ruptured	Death second day in hospital.
4. Rochet, J. d'accouch., 1892, xiii, 195	Acute and general	Five days after admission to hospital abdominal and vaginal sections were made, drainage employed. Autopsy findings: General purulent peritonitis, with tubes enlarged and the right ruptured and containing pus	Death promptly followed.
5. C. S. Wood, Trans. N. Y. Med. Assoc., 1890, vi, 49	Acute, general	Operation during the first twenty-four hours by W. Gill Wylie, during collapse; abdominal section; right pyosalpinx had ruptured	Recovery.
6. E. G. Janeway, N. Y. Med. Jour., 1880, xxxii, 522	Admission on fourteenth day of attack	No operation. Autopsy findings: General peritonitis, patches of fibrinous lymph on liver, intestine, and uterus: 12 ounces of pus in pelvis, right pus tube ruptured, left pyosalpinx unruptured	Death four days after admission.
7. Spehl (reported by Wicot), Clinique, Brux.,1893, vii, 529	Ill with the attack of pelvic peritonitis fourteen days before admission	No operation. Autopsy findings: Pus pocket in right inferior lobe of lung; pus very abundant in peritoneal cavity; intestinal loops covered by fibrinous, thick, and very adherent exudate; circular rupture in left tube 2 cm. in diameter	Died twelve days after admission to hospital.
8 and 9. Legueu, Compt.-rend, Soc. d'Obst., de Gynec., et de Péd., Paris, 1903, v, 83	Both acute	Operation was done at once. Both were ruptured by examination and abdominal section one and one-half hours later in one and one hour in the other; ruptured tube found in each	Both recovered.
10 Peuch, Compt.-rend Soc. de Biol., Paris, 1860, 3 s, i, 27	Subacute	No operation. Autopsy findings: Cystic left ovary; inflammation and abscess of both tubes, one ruptured, and abdominal cavity deluged	Died three and one-half months after admission to hospital.
11. Cerné, Bull Soc. Anat. de Paris, 1880, viii, 37	Acute, suddenly seized three days before admission	Autopsy findings: Ruptured left tube and general acute peritonitis; intestinal coils adherent	Died three days after admission.

Reported by	Duration or stage of peritonitis.	Notes.	Result.
12. P r o u s t and Mascarenhas, Bull. et mém. Soc. Anat. de Paris, 1909, lxxxiv, 294	Admitted on sixth day of attack	Operated upon at once upon admission. Large quantity of fetid, purulent fluid escaped from the abdominal incision; rupture found in lower posterior surface of the right pus tube, the latter removed; left tube normal; drainage	Recovery.
13. Fabricius, Wien. klin. W o c h., 1897, x, 1056	Acute, ruptured during labor	Prompt operation with removal of the ruptured tube	Recovery.
14. B o l d t, American Jour. Obstet., 1889, xxii, 262	Acute, general	Operation done on the sixth day; pus found in peritoneal cavity; intestines matted together; both tubes ruptured	Death in sixty hours.
15. B o l d t, ibid.	Acute, general	On second day abdomen was opened and right tube found ruptured	Died.
16. B o l d t, ibid.	Acute	Operation a few hours after rupture of right tube; perforation 2 cm. in diameter; free fluid in peritoneal cavity and the peritoneum considerably congested	Recovery.
17. B o l d t, ibid.	Three days' duration	Operation refused. Autopsy findings: Peritoneal cavity full of pus, intestines matted, double pyosalpinx—the right ruptured	Died.
18. B o l d t, ibid.	Acute	Operated upon three hours after onset and in collapse; free fluid in the peritoneal cavity, and the left pus tube ruptured	Recovery.
19. B o l d t, ibid.	Acute	Operation deferred too long because of apparent improvement; operation was not done at all. No autopsy	Death in thirty-six hours.
20 and 21. H. Brin. Arch. méd. d'Angers, 1900, iv, 556	Both acute	Autopsies disclosed ruptured pus tubes and acute general peritonitis	Both died.
22. Cotte and Cha l i e r, R e v . d e gyn. et de chir. abd., 1907, x i, 579	Admitted two days after beginning of attack of acute perforative peritonitis	Operation a few hours after admission. Peritoneal cavity found full of seropurulent fluid; intestines not adherent. Nothing but insertion of drainage tube into pelvis was done. Autopsy: Perforation in a right pyosalpinx large enough to admit little finger	Died forty hours after operation.
23. Cotte and Cha l i e r, ibid.	Acute, general, of two days duration	Operation day of admission, free fluid in peritoneal cavity and pus in pelvis. Left pyosalpinx found ruptured, collapsed, and nearly empty; perforation in middle of a gangrenous arch near ampulla; appendage removed and drainage through abdomen and vagina	Death three days after operation.
24. Cotte and Cha l i e r, ibid.	A d v a n c e d, general	No history obtainable; condition very grave, precluding operation. Autopsy showed rupture of right pyosalpinx	Death a few hours after admission.
25. Cotte and Cha l i e r, ibid.	Admitted sixth day of attack of general peritonitis	Operation a few hours after admission; free fluid in peritoneal cavity and pus in pelvis; perforation ½ cm. long found in anterior surface of a right pyosalpinx, tube not removed; abdominal and vaginal drainage; condition precarious; repeated operations during the following three months ended the condition	Recovery.

Reported by	Duration or stage of peritonitis.	Notes.	Result.
26. Cotte and Cha l i e r, ibid.	Admitted third day of attack of general peritonitis	Operation one hour after admission; large quantity purulent fluid in peritoneal cavity. Two perforations found in large right tuboövarian abscess — one as large as a franc piece	Died twenty-four hours after operation.
27. Bu l l i t t, Louis v i l l e J o u r. of Me d. and Surg., 1900-1901,vii, 471	Acute, general	Admitted for operation for chronic salpingitis and pelvic peritonitis; no urgent symptoms, though abdomen distended and painful; operation deferred; suddenly became worse; died forty-eight hours after admission. Autopsy revealed general peritonitis and a large perforation in a left pyosalpinx	Death.
28. Cartledge, Louis v i l l e J o u r. of Me d. and Surg., 1900-01, vii, 472	Acute, general	Moribund when first seen; perforation of left tube found as cause of peritonitis at operation	Death
29. V a n c e, Louis v i l l e J o u r. of Me d. and Surg., ibid.	Acute	Admitted to hospital for minor gynecological treatment; next day suddenly became shocked and abdomen opened in three hours. A ruptured pus tube was found	Recovery.
30. A b e l l, ibid., 1906-07, xiii, 403	Acute	Operation third day of illness; a ruptured right pyosalpinx found	Recovery.
31. A n d e r-son, i b i d., 153	Acute	Operation and both tubes contained pus and ruptured and general peritonitis; patient was living at time of report, which was made on day of operation	Not known.
32. L e i t h, African Med. Rec., Cap e Town, 1907, v, 230	Acute, general	Operation first day of attack; parietal peritoneum thickened and congested and lymph on intestines; left pyosalpinx ruptured	Recovery.
33. Y o u n g, Boston Med and S u r g. Jour., 1905, clii, 551	Acute, general	Admitted third day of attack of pelvic suppurative inflammation. The following day had excruciating abdominal pain, vomiting, collapse, and rapidly developing peritonitis. Operation without delay; pus found in all parts of peritoneal cavity; a ruptured pyosalpinx was found and exsected	Recovery.
34. Fenwi c k, L a n c e t, Lond., 1897, ii, 1385	General suppurative operation	Died two days after admission and without operation. Autopsy showed general suppurative peritonitis; evidence of old pelvic inflammation and a ruptured pus tube discovered	Death.
35. Ol e s o n, C h i c a g o Med. R e c., 1 8 9 4, v i, 324	Acute, general suppurative	Died five days after labor, at which pus tube probably ruptured. Autopsy showed a pus tube ruptured near fimbriated end and general acute suppurative peritonitis; rapid labor at eight months	Death.
36. Ol e s o n, ibld.	Same as in 35	Rapid and sudden delivery before arrival of obstetrician in ward; two days later chill and temperature 103.2°; died five days after labor. Autopsy findings the same as in Case 35	Death

Reported by	Duration or stage of peritonitis.	Notes.	Result.
37. M. Price, A., Jour. of Obst., 1889, xxii, 925	Acute suppurative and general	Operation fifteen days after apparent rupture of a pyosalpinx in a case of incomplete abortion; both tubes had ruptured	Death.
38. Louis Frank, Med. News, Phila., 1895, lxvi, 609	General, acute suppurative peritonitis	Admitted to hospital in midst of an attack, and next morning was in collapse; laparotomy a few hours later; the patient died in nine hours. Autopsy revealed rupture of a right tuboovarian abscess	Death.
39. M a n n, Amer. Jour. Obst., 1907, lvi, 461	Acute, general	Patient in hospital for pelvic suppuration; sudden onset of alarming symptoms on second evening after; next morning operation showed right pus tube ruptured an inch from fimbriæ and general peritonitis	Recovery.
40. M a n n, ibid.	Acute suppurative, general	Two days after an examination by a physician, who diagnosticated tuboövarian abscess, was suddenly attacked by illness, and collapse promptly ensued. Operation done at once; a large tuboövarian abscess, ruptured, was found, the opening being the size of a ten cent piece	Recovery.
41. Cushing (see B o n- ney), Surg., Gyn., and Obst., 1909, ix, 542	Acute suppurative	Operation day of rupture of a tuboövarian abscess into peritoneal cavity	Death.
42. D u d l e y (see Bonney)	Acute suppurative	Operation a few hours after rupture of a pyosalpinx into the peritoneal cavity, complicated by rupture of vermiform appendix	Recovery.
43. F i n d l e y (see Bonney)	Acute, general suppurative	Induced criminal abortion, followed in three weeks by curettage for infection of uterus and appendages; three days later evidence of general peritonitis; operation refused, and death four days later. Autopsy: Double pus tubes; the left contained a large perforation causing diffuse suppurative peritonitis	Death.
44 and 45. G a r d n e r (see Bonney)	Acute, general suppurative	Two cases practically alike. Both admitted during attack. Operation, both tubes found to be enormously distended with pus, and one had ruptured; contents free in peritoneal cavity. Neither had acute fulminating peritonitis	Recovery in both cases.
46. I n g a l l s (see Bonney)	Acute suppurative	Patient in hospital and treated for acute salpingitis. Late one afternoon found in collapse; abdominal distention rapidly followed. Operation in a few hours. A ruptured pyosalpinx removed, abdominal drainage	Recovery.
47. I n g a l l s (see Bonney)	Acute suppurative	Admitted to hospital six hours after rupture, and three hours later operation; general peritonitis, and a ruptured pyosalpinx removed. Vaginal and abdominal drainage; fever continued	Death in three months.

Reported by	Duration or stage of peritonitis.	Notes.	Result.
48. MacMonagle (see Bonney)	Acute septic	Patient apparently ruptured pus tube in labor, and had acute septic peritonitis, dying on the fourth day. Autopsy: Left tube had ruptured and discharged pus into peritoneal cavity	Death.
49. MacMonagle (see Bonney)	Acute, general suppurative	Young woman on whom an abortion had been attempted; acute peritonitis followed. Operation immediate, when first seen, and right tube found ruptured	Recovery
50. Smith (see Bonney)	Acute suppurative	Patient seen one hour after rupture; operated on at once; pyosalpinx had ruptured in the middle and deluged peritoneal cavity	Recovery.
51 and 52. Webster (see Bonney)	Acute fulminating	In both a pyosalpinx had ruptured into the general peritoneal cavity and gave rise to an acute fulminating peritonitis. Both made stormy recoveries. Operation done during first few hours.	Both recovered.
53. C. W. Bonney, Surg., Gyn., and Obst., 1909, ix, 542	Acute	Suppurative inflammation of the appendages had probably existed three weeks before very alarming abdominal symptoms, and apparent imminent death induced her removal to hospital at night and operation five hours after first alarming symptoms; an abundant outflow of seropurulent fluid from abdomen; intestines injected and distended; a partly collapsed right. large pus tube was found perforated. Appendage removed, peritoneal cavity flushed out, abdominal drainage	Recovery.
54. A Thielhaber, Münch. med. Woch., 1905, lii, 69, 122		This author, in an article of six pages on "The Pathology and Therapy of Chronic Salpingitis," merely mentions a case in which perforation was followed by an unsuccessful operation	Death.
55. A. Mary, Sur un cas de rupture de pyosalpinx pendant l'accouchement, Thèse de Paris., 1908	Acute	A girl, aged sixteen years, died six days after labor. Temperature was never normal afterward. Two days post partum curettage was done, as the pulse was 125 and temperature 102.4°. Autopsy revealed general peritonitis and a large right pyosalpinx ruptured midway in the length of the tube	Death.
56. Author's	Acute diffuse	Severe pain through iliac region during coitus; under observation by me from early in fourth day; symptoms of rupture on fifth day of illness; operation done a few hours later; tube had ruptured and inundated the peritoneum with pus	Death third day after.

Diagnosis. When rupture occurs during labor the accoucheur should discover a considerable softening in a mass existing at the side of the uterus before labor, and symptoms of peritonitis appear so promptly that they should be readily recognized. The cause of the peritonitis would then have to be learned by a process of exclusion and a knowledge of the antepartum symptoms, and tubal conditions will markedly assist in reaching a correct diagnosis. In non-puerperal cases the previous history of pelvic infection accompanied by suppuration, the absence of evidence of pregnancy, especially tubal, together with the rapid appearance of the symptoms of diffuse peritonitis, should be sufficient for a diagnosis. When the right tube has thus ruptured it has been mistaken for fulminating appendicitis. The previous history will be an important element in making differentiation. In those cases in which the vermiform appendix is simultaneously markedly involved the differentiation or possibility of diagnosticating both conditions is not always present.

Prognosis. What can be said of the prospect of recovery? It requires no comment when the death rate in all cases is 58 per cent. and 100 per cent. without operation. Much depends upon whether a previous severe attack of pelvic infection has left the patient with little or much resistance; whether the total of virulence of the invading tubal contents be great or slight; the general condition of the patient independent of these features, and the form of treatment instituted. At the best these patients must be considered as in a critical condition, and whatever the plan of surgical treatment employed, it must be instituted with the least possible delay.

Treatment. All of the 18 that were not operated upon died. The time they lived after rupture varied from a few hours to three and one-half months. Two patients admitted to hospitals on the fourteenth day after rupture lived, respectively, four and twelve days. Of the 12 others that died without operation of which data is obtainable, the average number of hours they lived was fifty-nine.

Thirty-eight were operated upon, and 14 of them died, a mortality rate of 37 per cent. One of this series (Ingalls) lingered along for three months in the hospital, and yet her operation was but nine hours after rupture. But three of the postoperative fatalities were in patients operated on during the first twenty-four hours after rupture. The other deaths occurred in cases in which rupture preceded the operation by from two to fifteen days. One operation was done during the first few hours (Anderson) and reported the same day without the result being mentioned. Of the 23 in which successful operations were done, in 20 it was performed during the first twenty-four hours. Such expressions as "immediately," "at once," and "a few hours" are used in the reports of them. The other 3 successful operations were done, 1 on the third and 2 on the sixth day. Twenty-five of the operations were done during the first twenty-four hours. In one of these no result was given. In the other 24 operations 5 were unsuccessful. One of the 5 deaths occurred in nine hours, 1 in fifty-four hours, and 1 in three months. The 3 patients operated on during the second day all died. Of 3 operated on the third day, 1 recovered. Of the 7 operated on more than three days after rupture had occurred, 4 died. We find the mortality rate, then, for operations during the first day after rupture was (excluding Anderson's case) nearly 21 per cent.; for those done during the second day, 100 per cent.; for those done during the third day, 67 per cent., and for those done after the third day, 57 per cent. It would seem, then, that if possible all cases should be operated upon, since in all of the 18 reported in which no operation was done death resulted. The comparatively small mortality rate of the first-day operations would seem to demonstrate the decided urgency of operating the first day and without delay. While but 1 of the 6 operations done on the second and third days was successful, 3 of the 7 done at more remote periods were successful and we should be encouraged to operate even if considerable time has elapsed since rupture, although moribund patients do not present a hopeful spectacle to the abdominal surgeon. The late lamented Cartledge states in the report of his fatal case of this kind that enthusiasm and ignorance of early experience led him to operate, but that greater experience and better judgment would form an opposite decision.

DISCUSSION.

DR. O. H. ELBRECHT, of St. Louis.—I have had a rather unique case in this line of work, which has led me to about the same conclusions at which Dr. Bovée has arrived. I reported it fully before the American Association of Obstetricians and Gynecologists at its New York meeting in 1905. The case was exceedingly interesting in several respects: first of all, it was a twin-pregnancy that went to full term, without any complications and was delivered without any trouble, but a few days after delivery she presented a picture typical of sapremia and was treated for this. The lochia being very profuse and offensive and tenderness that existed in the pelvis was thought to be a salpingitis due to the infection being transmitted to the tubes. The pulse and temperature remained low for the first few days and there was no distention of the abdomen, and she did not present the alarming picture which is usually presented in those cases in which we have more marked symptoms of peritonitis. Her condition, however, grew worse and within the last twenty-four hours of her life her abdomen distended rather suddenly and the pulse mounted to a very high rate. She was then a moribund case and it was thought advisable not to operate. The autopsy showed double pyosalpinx, very marked on one side, the unruptured tube being about the size of a good sized lemon, and the other being a ruptured pyosalpinx and its contents having escaped, it was collapsed so that it was hard to judge its size before rupture took place. The rupture was the result of a combination of circumstances, the first being that the omentum had been firmly attached to the tube on this side and as soon as delivery occurred, unquestionably the omentum was put on a stretch and whether this in itself was sufficient to rupture the tube or whether it was the expulsion of the placenta by Crede's method is not known, but it seemed more probable that the tube was ruptured during the manual expulsion of the placenta. There was a diffuse gonorrhœal peritonitis, which was demonstrated positively by making numerous smears from the intestinal surfaces in all portions of the abdomen from the diaphram to the pelvis. They were stained by the method of Gram and found to be gonococci, pure and simple. Dr. Bovée mentioned that gonococci was not usually demonstrated in these cases: This, too, has been my observation in studying the literature, and it seems unfortunate that this is not resorted to more often to bring out the importance and a better idea of the frequency of a diffuse gonorrhœal peritonitis, for many cases are called gonorrhœal peritonitis without subsequent verification.

There is an interesting biological factor in this case, which I have thought of many times since, and that is, did both pus tubes exist at the time of impregnation or was only one side affected at that time, and did the other tube become infected by transmission of the infection from a leaking pus tube on one side during pregnancy, being carried to the other tube by way of the fimbriated extremity instead of by the intrauterine route?

Another case that I operated on gave about the same pathology, in that the patient had had the tubal trouble for some time and had quite a severe fall the day before I saw her, being operated upon immediately by reason of the gravity of her symptoms, and in this case also it was found that the omentum was attached and had been torn from the ostium, allowing pus to escape, which produced a localized infection, which incidentally involved the appendix. Patient made a nice recovery, the infection remaining confined to the area involved at the time of operation.

As Dr. Bovée has brought out, that leaking pus tubes are common as compared to the ruptured variety, the literature being full of the latter class, and I have seen several others in which a leaking pus tube brought about severe disturbances during the puerperium, several of which I operated upon and was able to demonstrate the cause.

Dr. Lewis S. McMurtry, of Louisville.—All phases of disease of the tubes, both pathological and clinical, have been so thoroughly gone over in this and other special societies that very little is left for discussion. But I think Dr. Bovée has rendered distinct service in collecting these cases, and treating the subject in relation to their management, and the way to recognize the condition early.

I want to add one case to those Dr. Bovée has reported It is interesting to note how rarely this accident occurs. I saw a woman in the country, seventy-two miles from Louisville, at home on a farm, who had symptoms suggestive of ruptured tubal pregnancy. On opening the abdomen I found the left Fallopian tube was ruptured, with extravasation of pus all around, without any protection whatever; she was in profound shock at the time of operation and died.

Dr. I. S. Stone, of Washington.—The subject is one of great interest, on account of its rarity, and Dr. Bovée has shown its fatal character. I remarked to him before leaving Washington that I recollect only one case, and I am sorry, in some respects, to report it, because I have not had time to look over the records carefully before leaving for this meeting. I was called about ten days after the patient had been exposed to inclement weather, followed in a few days by a severe chill and fever. She had been married for fifteen or eighteen years without having children. There was no history of any conception having taken place. She was sterile, and it is possible she had a salpingitis. When I was called in consultation I found that she was taking treatment from a so-called "Viavi" specialist. The diagnosis rested between salpingitis and appendicitis with acute peritonitis. She was sent to the hospital the next day, and an operation was performed. The patient was much alarmed because of pain following the treatment administered by this woman, who really was giving massage. The operation was done fifteen hours after the rupture of an abscess in the right Fallopian tube. I cannot state positively that there was no tuboövarian abscess, but surely the tube was ruptured and the appendix was somewhat involved in adhesions round about, but was not diseased in itself. There could not have been an appendiceal abscess. I was fortunate enough, by making through-and-through drainage, to save this patient. Her recovery for six or eight days after the operation was almost uninterrupted, when she developed a violent attack of pneumonia, which nearly proved fatal. Nevertheless, she recovered, and is quite well today. During the time she had pneumonia we had her blood pressure taken at intervals along during the attack, and after she recovered she asked me what I thought had cured her, or to what she owed her restoration to health, and especially during the attack of pneumonia. I told her that

I thought it was a combination of circumstances. "Well " she said, "doctor, I will tell you what I think. I think it was due to the apparatus they put on my arm. I believe that did it."

DR. HENRY T. BYFORD, of Chicago.—I do not think we ought to include the splitting of the tube in the class of cases under discussion, because that is a comparatively common condition, and these patients get well, as was mentioned in one case. Dr. Bovée referred to the more severe cases, and there are more of them than we have heretofore thought. I have seen quite a number of them. I recall one case in which rupture of the tube occurred in a prostitute (during coitus), and who died in three or four days with peritonitis. Recently I was called to see a doctor's wife in whom the attack came on suddenly, and when I saw her she was already pulseless. I recall a case in which there was evidence of rupture of the tube, and operation revealed not only a ruptured tube, but its entire destruction. The patient finally got well. I have seen many cases after labor similar to those that have been reported. I mention them, not to add to Dr. Bovée's statistics, but to show that these cases occur more fequently than a great many writers have supposed. and that many of them are not reported. Undoubtedly there are severe cases of rupture of the tube that have recovered without operation and were not understood. We cannot say that all of those bad cases of ruptured tubes are fatal.

DR. J. GARLAND SHERRILL, of Louisville.—We are all aware that these chronic cases of tubal disease have frequent exacerbations, and some of these exacerbations are due to a leak in the tube. I take it that Dr. Bovée's paper meant to include these acute cases, where there is a distinct rupture, and extravasation of a great deal of the material into the peritoneal cavity. I have had one such case in my own experience. The patient was a young girl, who had acute infection of the vagina from the gonococcus. She was removed to the infirmary with a view of treating her sufficiently long to get a good interval for operation. As the result of the transportation, or from some other cause, she developed immediate and very severe symptoms. Already a diagnosis of tubal infection had been made. The symptoms became so severe that I was compelled to open her abdomen, and at the operation found a ruptured tube, with the abdomen containing a large quantity of serum, with very little lymph formation in it. The diagnosis of the case was clear. The vaginal secretion had been examined, and in it was found the gonococcus. The wound at the end of the third day began to discharge this same serum, which was present at the time of the operation in the abdomen, and this discharge kept up for a number of days, and from it was obtained a pure culture of gonococcus, making it clear that the case was one of gonorrheal infection. In our opinion this is a class of cases which gets well faster than some of the other infections, either with the staphylococcus or with the streptococcus, when the attack is acute.

DR. S. M. D. CLARK, of New Orleans —The paper of Dr. Bovée has been extremely instructive to me from the fact that from having had a large experience in the colored clinics of New Orleans, I find pus tubes rarely ever rupture. I have never seen a case of spontaneous ruptured pus tube in a colored woman, and Dr. Ernest Lewis tells me that in his extensive experience in his clinic he has never witnessed an actual rupture of a pus tube. Hence to have heard Dr. Bovée's paper causes me to alter my views on this subject. I recall one case of acute pelvic infection with suppuration where the temperature went up to 103°, and I decided to drain through the vagina. In my efforts to introduce my finger through the mass, with counterpressure on the abdomen, I felt the tube rupture very distinctly. I was uneasy for awhile as to whether to open and remove that tube, or to content myself with establishing drainage. I instituted liberal drainage through the vagina, and the woman made an uninterrupted recovery. This is the only case that I have positively recognized as a ruptured pus tube.

DR. LEWIS C. MORRIS, of Birmingham.—I believe ruptured tube is more frequent than Dr. Bovée's paper would indicate. In my experience I have seen and operated on three cases of ruptured tube, but all of them occurred in white women. Just as with Dr. Clark, I see many cases of pus tubes among negroes in my clinic in Birmingham, but have never seen a rupture. This occurs less frequently in negroes than in white women. I have operated on three cases of pus tubes in negroes to one in white women. I have seen three cases of acute rupture of the tube, with beginning peritonitis, two in prostitutes, and one in a woman who had gonorrheal salpingitis.

Dr. Bovée (closing).—I am very glad my paper has brought out reports of so many cases. When you go over the literature and find only 56 cases on record, considering the vast experience of so many men, it infers that there must be a great many more cases which probably have not been reported.

The class of cases I referred to are cases of distinct acute peritonitis, and not merely rupture of the tube. There are lots of cases of ruptured tubes where the pus was sterile, in which the patients get well without any alarming symptoms, and without operation, but I dealt with cases in which we had a ruptured tube, whose contents consisted of highly infectious material, and the nature of that material was not made manifest by elevation of temperature and pulse rate previous to the occurrence of rupture. Some of them are acute cases. We see that in some of our section cases.

As regards the possibility of pregnancy during double pus tubes, when the tube is glued upon the ovary there is no reason why the ovule should not rupture and open out through sterile pus and get into the uterus. The pus is not always blocked, and this was one point made in Dr. Goodell's introduction to Keating's and Coe's work on "Clinical Gynecology." In the great onslaught he made he expressed himself as being bitterly opposed to frequent operations for pus in the Fallopian tube. He referred to cases in which he found double pus tubes, and the women later became pregnant. I have removed, myself, double pus tubes in pregnancy. One of the women was two months pregnant. I removed the tubes, and she went on to full term. Pregnancy, therefore, is possible in the presence of double pus tubes.

SOME THERAPEUTIC ADAPTATIONS OF CECOS-TOMY AND APPENDICOSTOMY.

By CHARLES A. L. REED, M.D.,
Cincinnati, Ohio.

My own experience for some time and that of other surgeons for longer periods indicate not only that ostiomatic operations on the intestinum cecum and the appendix vermiformis have already attained a considerable range of application, but that they are destined to be even more extensively employed as adjuncts of medical treatment in several very important diseased conditions. The application of these strictly surgical measures, now being undertaken with increasing frequency at the instance of strictly medical men, for the purpose of assisting them in the treatment of hitherto intractable cases, seems, indeed, to be based upon very logical considerations. The practice is based primarily upon a recognition of the fact that there are certain conditions that are strictly local to the colon and that are, consequently, better treated by measures addressed exclusively to the colon—the word "colon" being here employed to designate the whole of the large bowel from the ileocecal juncture to the rectum. This conception takes into account two additional facts of great practical importance, viz., first, that the attempt to medicate the colon locally by way of the rectum is painful, tedious, and generally unsatisfactory, and, so far as the upper colon and cecum are concerned, wholly impracticable; and, second, that the attempt to medicate the colon by way of the stomach is fraught with uncertainties due to chemical change of medicaments in the stomach and upper intestines, interference with digestion, and consequent impairment of the general health. It is recognized, furthermore, that by direct access through the cecum by an entirely safe operation, not only are these objections entirely obviated, but certain signal advantages obtained, among them being the hygienic control of the large intestine and the ability to apply treatment, medicinal, bacterial, or dietetic, directly to the viscus, and, by absorption therefrom, to the general system without reference to the condition of the stomach or of the upper intestines.

SOME ANATOMICAL FACTS. But before I take up the various conditions for which this relatively new surgical measure is being employed, I ask attention to a few anatomical facts that have a particular bearing on the choice of operation, that is, as between cecostomy and appendicostomy. Thus, it is a matter of some significance that the large pouch or convolution of the intestinum cecum is the part that lies in direct contact with the anterior abdominal wall; that, consequently, when in *locus naturalis* it is from an inch to two inches nearer the parietal peritoneum than is the base of the meso-appendix, and that it occupies a position on the side of the cecum directly opposite the valvula coli. Relative to the appendix vermiformis, it is of some importance to remember that its lumen is of variable diameter, and in certain cases it is entirely obliterated; that the sickle-shaped fold of mucous membrane, the valvula processus vermiformis at its cecal orifice is sometimes absent; that the meso-appendix is of variable length and is inelastic; and, finally, that the walls of the appendix proper are of variable thickness and are but poorly supplied with elastic tissue. Then, too, it should be kept in mind that the autonomic algesic areas of the cecum and appendix veriformis correspond to the distribution of the twelfth dorsal and first lumbar nerves to the integument and to the underlying obliquus internus, obliquus externus, and transversus abdominis muscles, and, in exceptional cases, to the distribution of the iliohypogastric nerve in the groin— all, of course, on the right side.

THE CHOICE OF OPERATION.—I have mentioned these usually disregarded facts, first, because they have more or less bearing upon certain phenomena both preceding and following operation. With respect to the choice of operation, I fear that I shall seem a trifle heterodox when I state that, all things being equal, and in consideration of the anatomical facts that I have given, I prefer the older procedure of cecostomy to the newer one of appendicostomy. If my colloquialism of "all things being equal" shall be interpreted to mean the average normal conformation of, respectively, the cecum and the appendix and the absence of pathological states that make the appendix the logical avenues of ingress— and I confess I do not know which pathological states should be so regarded—then I believe the force of the anatomical features to which I have called attention will incline to a decision on the side of cecostomy. The proximity of the presenting pouch of the cecum to the peritoneum permits of its fixation in the operation wound practically *in situ naturalis;* it can be utilized for either a small opening or a larger one, as may be indicated; it permits an opening through which a catheter may be passed at any time through the valvula coli into the small intestine; it is free from undue tension after fixation, thus avoiding the possibility of prematurely breaking up the anchorage or causing painful adhesions following the operation; and, if properly managed, it is no more liable to be the source of fecal extravasation than is the appendix.

On the other hand, the relative remoteness of the appendiceal base makes its fixation not infrequently a source of painful tension, which, with the pressure on its walls by a catheter, causes the latter to perish. As a matter of fact, the majority of appendices do perish within a few days after operation, leaving the condition of cecostomy with an opening at an undesirable point. The adhesions resulting from appendiceal implantation are frequently very painful owing to the constant traction which likewise has a tendency to induce closure of the fistula earlier than may be desired.

The relation of both the cecum and the appendix to the autonomical nervous system has been demonstrated by Langley. Through the dorsolumbar division of this system hyperalegesias are given definite and recognizable expression in the abdominal wall. In this way we are enabled to reduce conditions involving these strictures to a more definite basis for diagnosis and to control the pain originating in them, either before or after operation, without overwhelming the sensorium with powerful narcotics. And now having said this much by way of introduction, permit me to leave the application of my observations to a consideration of the following conditions:

IN AMEBIC DYSENTERY. The necessity of bringing the entire colon within the range of local medication, and the futility of doing so by injections through the rectum in cases of amebic dysentery, was the indication that first prompted the opening of the cecum as an elective operation. The names of Skene, Keith, White, and Murray are associated with the earliest development of this practice, which, however, dated back only to 1895. Since that time the operation of cecostomy has been done for this purpose many hundreds of times, especially in the tropical countries, in which the disease is prevalent. It has also been employed by John Bell, at the Government Civil Hospital, Hong Kong, for the treatment of dysentery caused by another but unnamed parasite peculiar to New Guiana. It was in a case of dysentery of possibly amebic variety that prompted Weir, in 1901, to attempt a cecostomy when, according to his own account, "as the cecum was exposed the appendix rose so naturally I determined to employ it to make the desired fistula." This was the beginning of appendicostomy, subsequently so called by Willy Meyer, of New York. The case did not prove to be amebic, but one of chronic mucous colitis, which was cured by the subsequent medication applied through the appendiceal tube. The results achieved by this method of treatment in the strictly amebic variety of the disease stamps it as the treatment of choice for an otherwise practically hopeless malady.

IN CHRONIC CATARRHAL, OR MUCOUS, COLITIS.—The natural history of chronic catarrhal colitis and its resistance to all other forms of treatment, and the comparative uniformity with which it yields to colonic lavage when applied through the cecum and kept up for several months, points to it as the one disease occurring in our climate that demands this form of intervention. This holds true whether the disease is simple or ulcerative. Some of the most satisfactory results have been realized in cases such as one that recently occurred in my own practice, in which large mucous casts were shed and in which, on examination by the sigmoidoscope, the whole surface of the descending colon and of the sigmoid seemed to be granular. Keetley reports a successful case in which no evidence of disease could be seen through the sigmoidoscope, but in which pain was experienced and mucous casts were shed from a localization of the disease evidently farther up than the splenic flexure of the colon. The value of the surgical treatment as compared with the former medical and dietetic treatment, unassisted by surgical access to the colon, in the ulcerative variety of the disease is strikingly shown by two very contrasting reports. Wm. Murrell reported five cases of ulcerative colitis, with four deaths and an average duration of ten months, under polymedication. Holton C. Curl, quoted by Keetley, reported eleven cases, with eight recoveries and three deaths (one from chronic nephritis and the other moribund at time of operation), the average duration much less than Murrell's cases, all having been treated by lavage through the cecum.

Keetley himself reports ten cases, with nine cures. My own experience has been limited to four cases, with three cures, the fourth case having voluntarily discontinued the treatment before results were realized. I have not had time to collect the statistics of the operation of these cases, but from other data at hand I am sure that the figures given are fairly representative of the whole.   There ought to be no mortality from this operation in favorable cases, and I have seen no record of fatality attributable to it.

IN CHRONIC CONSTIPATION.   Constipation, especially of the atonic type and not complicated with enteroptosis, has yielded excellent results to colonic lavage through cecal irrigation.   I may be pardoned if I refer briefly to a typical case in my own practice.

A woman, aged forty-two years, was sent to the Good Samaritan Annex in April, 1909, with symptoms of internal obstruction.   She gave a history of constipation extending nearly over her whole lifetime, the intervals between spontaneous defecations being sometimes as long as twelve days. The sigmoid was obviously heavy laden, but the unloading of it by enemata and instrumental means did not relieve the symptoms of obstruction.   I accordingly did an exploratory incision, and found another focus of fecal accumulation in the transverse colon near the splenic flexure.   This was moved on into the decending colon by manual manipulation. Scybalous deposits could be felt in practically every convolution of the gut.   I thereupon opened the cecum and began the infusion of a very weak solution, consisting of one ounce of magnesium sulphate to one gallon of water at 105° F.   This was very slowly infused at intervals of every six hours, until by the end of the second day the incredible amount of fecal discharge indicated that the colon had been thoroughly unloaded.   The treatment was then continued by flushing the colon once daily with hot normal salt solution, the heat acting as a stimulus to provoke vigorous contractions of the bowel.   This was the central feature of a more comprehensive treatment, chiefly dietetic, that was continued for the next two months.   The patient, with the tube *in situ*, went about her usual tasks after the second week following the operation.   Reports by other operators, notably Keetley, indicate that my experience is not unique.

IN ACUTE SEPTIC PERITONITIS. The adaptation of a cecal opening for postoperative treatment of acute septic peritonitis is accomplished by the method that I have termed *coloclysis*, and is illustrated by two cases that occurred in my service in the Cincinnati Hospital in May of this year, and recently reported to the Cincinnati Obstetrical Society. One, refered to the service by my colleague, Dr. E. W. Mitchell, was admitted five days after cordent rupture of a pus tube, with temperature, 103.5°; pulse, 130; respirations, 26; tympanites; white count, 17,000. She was operated on immediately by incision on the right side and a leaking pus tube removed, as was the appendix vermiformis. The other tube was not involved. The patient required an intravenous salt infusion during the course of the operation, which I concluded by fixing the cecum in the incision and placing in it a large sized catheter. The patient was hurriedly returned to bed, a thick but short rectal tube was inserted, and the cecal tube was attached to a reservoir of water at 105° F. In this way the colon was speedily filled, with the effect of having an effective hot water bottle on the inside of the abdomen. As soon as reaction was thus induced and the colon had been thoroughly washed out the treatment was kept up by the continuous infusion of normal salt solution through the cecal tube by the drop method. Later the patient was nourished through the tube. The case made a prompt recovery. A second case occurred the week following, and in all essential points as to condition, operation, and results was sufficiently like the preceding one to make a longer reference unnecessary in this connection.

The eligibility of coloclysis as compared with rectalysis is, I believe, apparent. I may, however, emphasize the following points: (1) Coloclysis permits the immediate application of heat on the inside of the abdomen precisely at the place and at the time it is most needed; (2) it at the same time thoroughly washes out the colon, thus removing not only the fecal content, but the toxins with which it is laden; (3) it permits the immediate and indefinitely sustained infusion of normal saline solution into the colon at a point whence it must traverse the entire absorbent area before it escapes at the anus; (4) it permits the nourishment of the patient—administration of nutritive enemata under precisely the same conditions and entirely independent of the tolerance of the rectum or the condition of the stomach; (5) it makes possible the catheterization of the small intestine through the valvula coli and the consequent flushing of the upper bowel when necessary for the relief of either tympany or volvulus, either idiopathic or postoperative.

INTUSSUSCEPTION. The association of ideas prompts me next to mention the eligibility of ostiomatic operations on the cecum in cases of intussusception. That this is the correct form of intervention in many, if not a majority, of these cases seems to be indicated by the phenomenal experience of Mr. Charles Clubbe, of Melbourne, in 144 operations performed in fourteen years. In the majority of the cases the trouble began in ileocecal connection. The beneficial influence of the direct application of heat to a bowel wall that is injured on both its mucous and serous surfaces and that may be near the perishing point from long interference with its circulation is too obvious to require discussion. It is known, furthermore, that there is a tendency to early if not immediate recurrence in these cases and this tendency, it would seem, can be materially controlled by irrigating the cecum at will with considerable volumes of water. This contention has been resisted by Mr. Cardwine. As his objection is based on a single case of recurrence six months after the operation and presumably almost as long after the closure of the appendiceal fistula, I cannot concede that his point is well taken, except in so far as it shows that fixation of the cecum is not a guarantee against recurrence of the intussusception at some more or less remote period. On the other hand, that the tendency of such an anchorage of the cecum, in the event of recurrence, is to reduce the invagination to the minimum and to keep the trouble in the right lower quadrant where it can be more easily reached is certainly a fair deduction from the plain principles of physics that are involved. This, is, furthermore, confirmed by the fact that the cases so far treated by this method point to its high efficiency.

IN DEFECTIVE FLORA OF THE COLON. This caption is used because it is believed that bacterial deficiencies in the colon are sometimes responsible for the impairment of its functions. This was shown in a case in which I did an appendicostomy in January, 1909, and in which the study of the flora of the colon was begun by Dr. W. H. Strietmann, of the bacteriological department of the University of Cincinnati. Standardization bouillon and agar-agar were used, and inoculations were made from the feces, both through the wound in the cecum and as they were discharged by the rectum. After the cultures were incubated plates were poured. These observations showed no anaërobes, while the plates revealed only a pure culture of a bacillus with rounded ends, non-motile, which produced acid and gas and coagulated milk, and was probably *Bacillus lactis aërogenes*.

Ten days later it was found that one of the plates revealed a single colony of *Bacillus coli communis*. Later cultures modified this finding but slightly. Those from February 3 to 6 showed greenish colorization in the bouillon, while the hanging-drop revealed a motile bacillus and a non-motile one of different size. Agar plates showed the same green color and this same bacterium in gram positive. It was probably *Bacillus pyocyaneus*, which may have reached the colon through the appendicostomy wound.

These revelations, indicating the practically complete absence of the usual flora of the colon, suggested a change of treatment. Milk cultures of the *Bacillus lactis aërogenes*, *Bacillus bulgaricus*, and the *Streptococcus lacticus*, derived from lactic bacillary tablets (Fairchild) and from lacteol (Boucard), were accordingly thrown through the tube directly into the colon.   This on two occasions was fortified with the *Saccharomyces cerevisiæ.*   The trend of the case was in the direction of a more normal average flora according to the standard established by Herter, when the patient discontinued the treatment.   I urge these observations as suggestions for a further trial at the hands of other operators.

IN AUTO-INTOXICATION OF INTESTINAL ORIGIN.   The series of facts established by Herter, namely, (1) that oxygen exists only in the small intestines; (2) that bacteria in the large intestines must therefore be anaërobic; (3) that these anaërobes elaborate a toxin; and (4) that this toxin is absorbed from the colon into the system, is a logical explanation of many abnormal conditions effecting the general system.   Hollis, Ditmar, and Burch, accepting this theory of causation of pernicious anemia, have successfully treated these cases by colonic lavage through the cecum.   Laplace has reported the cure of a case of idiopathic epilepsy that had existed from childhood in a patient aged twenty-three years and that had developed into daily seizures of great severity.   The patient had no seizure after the first day following operation for the establishment of lavage through the cecum.   The irrigations were continued for ten months.   Armstrong has reported the successful treatment of rheumatoid arthritis by the application of the same principle.   Bennett, Ewart, and Maunsell have called attention to the advantage of dealing in this way with the toxins elaborated in the course of enteric fever, and Dr. R. W. Thomas, of the Cincinnati Hospital, to whom I am indebted for much research on this question, has elaborated the physics involved in the application of this method to the irrigation of the small intestines in typhoid.

CONCLUSIONS.   I wish to emphasize a few facts which I believe have become apparent from this brief survey of an extensive subject as follows:

1. The establishment of colonic irrigation through the cecum, whether by cecostomy or appendicostomy, is a proceedure attended with the minimum of surgical risk.

2. The application of the operation as an adjunct of medical treatment, under the conditions indicated, is based upon the principle of direct treatment of the colon for conditions that are local to the colon.

3. The operations of (*a*) coloclysis in septic peritonitis; cecal access to the colon (*b*) for purposes of nutrition following operation, (*c*) for irrigation and medication in amebic dysentery, (*d*) for chronic mucous colitis and (*e*) for other conditions of the mucosa of the colon not amenable to other treatment, stand on a basis of logical and clinically demonstrated value.

4. The treatment of various toxemias due to auto-intoxication of intestinal origin offers a field for the legitimate trial of ostiomatic operation on the cecum as a means of bringing the colon under control and eliminating its toxic content.

5. The results so far realized justify the continued use of the operation and the more extended application of the principle that it embodies.

BIBLIOGRAPHY.

1. Hale W. White. Lancet, London, March 2, 1895, p. 537.
2. John Bell. Lancet, London, Jan. 16, 1909.
3. Robert *F.* Weir. Med. Rec., New York, Aug. 9, 1902.
4. Willy Meyer. Med. News, Aug. 26, 1905.
5. *C.* B. Keetley. Brit. Med. Jour., Oct. 7, 1905.
6. Holton *C.* Curl. Ann. Surg., 1906, p. 543.
7. Charles Clubbe. Brit. Med. Jour., June 15, 1907.
8. S. Cardwine. Brit. Med. Jour., June 16, 1909.
9. Charles A. L. Reed. Direct Bacterial Treatment of the Colon through the Vermiform Appendix, Jour. Amer. Med. Asso., Feb. 22, 1909, lii, 636.
10. Dr. J. *M.* T. Finney, Baltimore, in the discussion of this paper, urged that this method of treatment deserved more serious consideration as the treatment of election in cases of neurasthenia dependent, of course, on auto-intoxication of intestinal origin, and alluded to some successful experiences at his own hands.
11. Lucius E. Burch. Appendicostomy in Pernicious Anemia, Jour. Amer. Med. Asso., March 13, 1909, lii, 888.

12. Earnest Laplace. *Preliminary* Report of the Treatment of Idiopathic Epilepsy by Appendicostomy for Colonic Irrigation, Jour. Amer. Med. Asso., June 2, 1906, xivi, 1678.

13. W. Armstrong. Lancet, London, Feb. 13, 1909.

14. Sir W. H. Bennett. Lancet, London, Feb. 17, 1906, p. 419.

15. William Ewart. Lancet, London, May 12, 1906.

16. Personal letter to the author.

17. Dr. W. *M.* Polk, New York, in the discussion of this method as applied to the treatment of "typhoid reservoirs," *i. e.*, persons who having had typhoid fever and having thus become immune and in whom the typhoid bacillus has become a permanent feature of their intestinal flora, continue to disseminate the disease through their dejecta. He instanced "Typhoid *Mary*," a somewhat notorious example of this form of pestilential centre, to whom many cases of typhoid had been traced, and who had finally been quarantined for the protection of the community.

18. Additional contributions to which, in a general way, I am indebted for my conclusions on this sublect, are:

R. W. Allen. Brit. Med. Jour., Nov. 28, 1908.

C. C. Barry. Indian Med. Gazette, June, 1908.

Percy R. Bolton. Ann. Surg., May, 1901.

F. Bushnell. Brit. Med. Jour., Nov. 28, 1908.

Robert H. *M.* Dawbarn. Ann. Surg., 1903, p. 613.

J. B. Dawson. Brit. Med. Jour., Jan. 9, 1909.

S. Gant. New York Med. Jour., Sept. 8, 1906.

S. G. Glover. Lancet, London, Jan. 9, 1909.

H. *M.* W. Gray. Brit. Med. Jour., March 3, 1906, p. 596.

Oscar Gray. Tr. Ark. State Med. Assn., 1908.

J. A. Pottenger. Lancet, London, Dec. 28, 1907.

J. L. Stritton. Lancet, London, March 14, 1908.

W. *Morley* Willis. Lancet, London, April 26, 1906.

James P. Tuttle. Appendicostomy, Jour. Amer. Med. Asso., Aug. 11, 1906, xivii, 426.

19. Dr. G. S. Hanes, in discussing this paper, stated that he had treated many cases of amebic dysentery by irrigating the colon through the rectum, but that he had been unable to do so satisfactorily without opening the cecum—I think by appendicostomy—for the purpose of permitting the displacement of the gas always present in the colon.

DISCUSSION.

DR. LEWIS S. McMURTRY, of Louisville.—Dr. Reed has presented a subject of great practical importance. It is now generally conceded by surgeons that so-called high enemata, long regarded of intestimable value in the treatment of colonic diseases and postoperative conditions, do not reach higher than the sigmoid flexure; that is, the soft flexible colon tube will rarely pass beyond the sigmoid but turns upon itself, and with the patient upon the bed in a horizontal position the fluid does not reach the transverse colon. With an opening in the appendix or *caput coli*, so that gas can pass out, and with the pelvis elevated, fluid can readily be made to traverse the entire colon from the rectum to the cecum.

My colleague, Dr. G. S. Hames, who I trust will contribute to this discussion, has made some original investigations, both clinical and experimental, that are of the utmost value in this connection. That the soft flexible tube does not reach higher than the sigmoid, and that lavage of the colon as generally practiced is deceptive, he has demonstrated by repeated *x*-ray observations. In several cases of appendicostomy for the treatment of amebic dysentery I have been associated with Dr. Hanes, and have observed how readily the entire colon can be irrigated from below after an outlet has been established by opening the appendix.

About a year ago Dr. Dock, of Tulane University, in an address on tropical diseases, stated that amebic dysentery is indigenous in this country as far north as Cincinnati.

Dr. Hanes has demonstrated within the past two years that this disease exists all over this country, having had cases from Maine, Iowa, and Illinois as well as the Southern States, and the disease was undoubtedly contracted in the residential locality of the patient. The idea that this disease is limited to tropical and semitropical countries is erroneous. A large proportion, perhaps the majority, of cases of so-called ulcerative colitis are in reality cases of amebic dysentery. Hanes has shown that the vitality of the amebæ is impaired by altered temperature, and that they will be overlooked unless their temperature is maintained; hence examination of the feces is misleading. The patient should be placed in Hanes' inverted position and scrapings taken from the ulcerated surface and examined immediately under the microscope. A large number of these cases·are treated for tuberculosis, and especially in advanced and neglected cases such error of diagnosis is apt to occur. I have opened the appendix in a number of these cases, and lavage can then be directed both from above and below and reach every' fold of the mucous surface of the colon. Dr. Hanes has demonstrated that the amebæ are destroyed and the disease cured by freely injecting coal oil (petroleum); also that this substance can safely be injected undiluted without being absorbed and without injury to the mucous surface of the intestine.

As Dr. Reed has indicated, this operation opens a new access to the large intestine for the treatment of numerous diseases hitherto among the opprobria of medicine and surgery.

DR. R. C. COFFEY, of Portland, Oregon.—I want to mention a method which I have. applied very successfully in cases of intestinal obstruction. When we stop to consider the cause of fatality in many cases of intestinal obstruction we find it is not sepsis, but in some cases at least it is a matter of starvation. An intestine which has become distended for a considerable length of time has paralysis of its vessels, so that it becomes practically as inactive as a rubber tube. These cases come in with vomiting of fecal matter, and enemata have been used until the colon is so distended that the sphincter has finally become paralyzed. We find after opening and draining this intestine, especially high up in the small intestine, that even then the patient will die from what seems to be largely water starvation in the cases I have seen. It has been taught by those who have investigated this matter, that probably less than 20 per cent. of the water taken into the mouth is absorbed before it reaches the cecum, and especially high up. If the small intestine has been widely dilated we find the stomach and small intestine absorb practically nothing. If we take, in addition to this, the fact that the rectum has become so paralyzed that enemata of salt solutions cannot be retained, we have practically water starvation. After having some experience of this kind I decided to use appendicostomy with this method, and have accordingly employed it in these particular cases, and have used the drop method of infusing salt solution, after opening the intestine in these gangrenous cases, and drop by drop have had the patients fed with salt solution with what seems to me a marked improvement over any other method of introducing fluids into the patient's bowel.

Dr. J. Garland Sherrill, of Louisville.—My friend, Dr. Hanes, is very modest, and I hope the President will call on him to get his ideas upon this subject.

There is one point in Dr. Reed's paper which differs from my experience in working with Dr. Hanes, and that is the impossibility or the great difficulty of reaching the head of the colon through the anus. This can be accomplished by the method that has been devised by Dr. Hanes of inverting the patient. I have seen Dr. Hanes put the patient over the edge of the table, with head down, then the anus falls partly open, and pass his instrument into the rectum and fill the patient's bowel with as much petroleum as he desired. By this method he can reach all the way to the ileocecal valve, and it is the only known way we can reach that part of the anatomy in my opinion.

I wish the Chair would call on Dr. Hanes to take part in this discussion and give us his ideas on the subject.

Dr. J. M. T. Finney, of Baltimore.—I have been very much interested in this paper, because it opens up an important question. With the conclusions of the reporter I should be in most hearty accord, but with some of the statements that he has made I cannot quite agree. In the first place, as to the anatomy of the colon. If I understood the essayist rightly, he said that the colon lends itself better to this operation than the appendix. This does not appear to me to be the case. I would call your attention to the variability in the anatomy of the large intestine, particularly of the ascending colon, including the cecum and the sigmoid flexure. It seems to me that, of all structures in the body, the large intestine is the one which is subject to the greatest anatomical variations. The appendix, of course, as the reporter said, is subject to wide anatomical variation. The same objection, it seems to me, would apply to one as to the other; the colon, being the larger structure, is easier found, and of course it is always a guide to the appendix.

Personally, in opening the abdomen, in doing an appendix operation, I never look for the appendix at first, but find the cecum and you have the appendix. So in this operation, if you look at the cecum, and examine it thoroughly, and then if the appendix lends itself best to this particular operation, use it.

So far as the indications for the operation are concerned,

they are also wide. I want to suggest one more condition, which, in my experience, has been satisfactorily treated by this method, namely, that large class of cases which our President so happily referred to last evening in his Presidential address—the surgical neurotic. I have somehow associated a great many of these with these operations on the large intestine. Many times we are forced by the patient's importunities and the existence of pain to make an exploratory incision, sometimes against our better judgment, and we may not find anything to account for this pain except an excessively long large intestine. I have so many times felt that that explains—how, I do not know—in some way these symptoms. In these cases there is always, owing to the faulty position of the large intestine, a chronic catarrhal condition, an excessive mucous discharge. For want of something better to do lately I have performed appendicostomy, and have flushed out the colon systematically in these cases with most satisfactory results. Only recently one of the most confirmed neurotics that it has been my misfortune to meet with was signally benefited by this procedure. I believe she has been cured by simply performing appendicostomy and systematically flushing the colon.

I have treated in this way one or two cases of chronic infection of the bowel. In one of them the infection was due to streptococcus, following directly after an attack of scarlet fever, and which had persisted uninterruptedly for thirty-odd years. The patient was a woman, whom I had known as a boy, and always heard her spoken of as a chronic invalid. She came to me some years ago, and on bacteriological examination of her intestinal content it was found that streptococci were present in large numbers. We used a solution of permanganate of potash, beginning with 1 to 10,000, and gradually increasing the strength up to 1 to 1000. The transformation in that case has been extraordinary. I have used the same solution in all similar cases, and the results have been satisfactory.

I saw in one of the German medical journals recently a report of several cases, where the same solution was used in similar cases, with satisfactory results.

I have in all my cases made it a practice to wash back and forth with this permanganate of potash solution. We introduce a tube into the rectum, with the hips of the patient elevated, and let the solution run in until it comes out through the appendicostomy opening. I have never failed to see the solution come out through the appendicostomy opening.

Another thing: not infrequently when the abdomen has been opened, for one cause or another, I have passed a rectal tube and felt the tube pass up through the sigmoid flexure into the transverse colon.

DR. WILLIAM M. POLK, of New York City.—As to the extension of this principle advocated by Dr. Reed, I do not think it would be unwise to extend it to cases of "typhoid reservoirs," so to speak. We are now beginning to discover in various parts of the world, more particularly in the last month or two in the City of New York, an extremely difficult class of cases to handle. We find that ordinary measures of treatment in no way mitigate the situation, so far as they are concerned; and as an illustration of the danger which resides in these cases, I will simply narrate certain facts that have come recently to our attention, and which have been demonstrated by Dr. Biggs in connection with our Board of Health.

Typhoid fever broke out on the East side last summer, with one hundred or more cases. The Board of Health traced the infection to the milk supply which came from a certain part of the State back of the Catskills. Further investigation showed that the milk supply of the dairies was short, and one man secured a reinforcement from the dairy of his father-in-law some twenty miles away. This man and his dairy were investigated. Typhoid was discovered there, and he himself was put under investigation, as it is now the habit in typhoid epidemics to bring under investigation every individual connected with a suspected milk supply. This man thirty years ago had an attack of typhoid fever, and from that time up to the present has been carrying typhoid bacilli with him, and his excreta were found to be loaded with them. You perhaps recall the case of what is known as Typhoid Mary. This poor woman carried typhoid bacilli around to different locations about New York. She was treated somewhat as this man was, but was not completely relieved of the germs of this disease. It seems to me, in the work outlined by Dr. Reed, we have to a large extent an answer to that question. It is true that in many of these cases the bacilli rest in the gall-bladder, but I take it they cannot remain long there without producing certain symptoms which would lead to operation upon that organ. In a large proportion of these cases the difficulty appears to lie in the large intestine. I would suggest that Dr. Reed add that as one of the indications to the performance of this operation, which I think we have now come to accept as a most desirable procedure in the class of cases he has designated.

Dr. GRANVILLE S. HANES, of Louisville (by invitation).— Dr. Reed's essay and the discussion it has inspired have interested me intensely. The subject is broad in its application and therefore intimately related to many surgical and medical questions.

Within the past twenty months I have treated 46 cases of amebic dysentery, and it is for this reason that this subject appeals to me with such interest. Only six of the total number were infected in tropical or semitropical countries. They were from various parts of our own country, the majority being from Kentucky and adjacent States. I have under treatment now, however, five cases, one residing as far east as Maine and another from Idaho. There can no longer be any doubt about the amebic type of dysentery being indigenous to temperate climates. Internal medication may aid in the treatment of amebic dysentery, but one must rely chiefly upon local methods. It is along this line that I have had occasion to do considerable experimental work. By completely inverting the patient, allowing him to hang on his thighs over the end of an office table and resting his head on his folded arms, I observed marked advantages in making proctoscopic examinations. It was not a great while until I became convinced that no kind of instruments, flexible or inflexible, could be introduced through the normal rectum and sigmoid into the descending and transverse colon as we have hitherto been taught. To prove this point I introduced soft rubber colon tubes, Wales' bougies and proctoscopes, into the rectum of living subjects in various positions, and while these instruments were thus introduced radiographs were taken by Dr. Edwin T. Bruce, an expert radiographer, and not one instrument had passed into the colon. The flexible tubes had turned and coiled upon themselves in various ways, while the proctoscopes had raised the floating sigmoid up into the abdomen until the sigmoidal mesentery was stretched its full length. The proctoscope was thus shown to occupy the lumen of the first or lower half of the sigmoid. I then went to the surgical laboratory and opened the abdomens of ten bodies and observed the position and anatomical relations of the entire large intestine.

The descending colon was bound down closely, no mesentery appearing until it had reached a point near the brim of the true pelvis, when the sigmoid began, and this loop of gut was found to vary in length from seven to twenty-eight inches. About the third sacral vertebra the mesentery ceased to exist, the gut again being bound down closely, which established the beginning of the upper extremity of the rectum. I observed that the lower end of the colon and the upper extremity of the rectum, which are fixed portions of gut, were not more than three or four inches apart. Intervening between these two fixed points is the sigmoid loop of gut. When it is lifted up and its mesentery spread out free from folds it has the form of an open fan.

It requires no further argument to prove the impossibility of an instrument entering the sigmoid from below, lifting it up into the abdomen its full length, then, turning acutely upon itself, descending along the second or upper half of the sigmoid till it reaches the lower extremity of the colon, to again turn acutely upon itself and ascend along the lumen of the descending colon.

My next effort was to pass fluids through the rectum to the cecum if possible. It was obvious that tubes could not be introduced high into the gut and aid obtained in that way. It was only a short time till I found it was easy to pour large quantities of liquids into the gut through the proctoscope with the patient in the inverted position (Hanes' position). I observed next that on account of the outlet of the rectum remaining open by the presence of the proctoscope the natural accumulation of gases in the gut escaped through the proctoscope as the column of water pressed upon it. The escape of gas can be facilitated very much by the patient breathing deeply and manipulating the surface of the abdomen. The gas can easily be heard and seen to bubble up through the column of water as it escapes from the bowel. There are a number of factors that play an important part in determining the amount of fluids the large gut may receive and retain. The large bowel cannot be filled with solutions until the natural gases retained therein have been eliminated. Dr.

Finney's success in passing liquids through the rectum around the large gut and out at the appendicostomy opening was not because he passed a soft rubber tube through the large bowel, for the tube must have coiled, but the gas in the bowel was forced in advance of the fluid and escaped through the appendicostomy opening. This allowed the water to follow and also escape through this opening.

I have inverted patients and filled the bowel as above described and forced coal oil out through the appendicostomy opening as described by Dr. Finney.

The next observation I made was that plain water is an irritant to the mucous membrane of the bowel, and excited peristalsis, which caused an expulsion of the fluid. Ordinary commercial coal oil was found to be a sedative to the inflamed or ulcerated mucosa. It can be introduced in larger quantities than aqueous solutions and retained for much longer periods. Coal oil does not harm the mucous membrane, and is not absorbed by the bowel; patients often retain a part of the oil for twenty-four hours or longer without any discomfort. I have treated more than a hundred cases by pouring into the large bowel unlimited quantities of coal oil with no untoward symptoms. A little less than half of this number were cases of amebic infection. Patients are always directed to remain in the recumbent posture after treatment for an hour or two if possible. When it is necessary to relieve the bowel on account of fulness, patients are advised to pass as small quantities of the oil as possible. The object of this method of treatment is to fill the large bowel with oil and retain it as long as possible. By this means the folds and pockets in the mucous membrane are obliterated by distention and the coal oil brought in contact with the entire mucous surface. The solutions should be introduced very slowly, allowing the bowel to fill to its utmost capacity, due consideration being given to overdistention when ulcers are present. Never insert a tube in the rectum to aid in passing fluids unless absolutely necessary.

No one can speak dogmatically concerning recurrence in cases of amebic dysentery. Patients are treated, and they apparently recover; treatment is discontinued, and in a few weeks, months, or even longer there is a recurrence. One little ulcer secreted in a fold of mucous membrane is sufficient cause for reinfection months later. The almost continuous presence of the coal oil renders the habitat of the ameba intolerable, causing extermination.

Dr. McMurtry has referred to the necessity of curetting the amebic ulcers and searching for motile ameba. Examination of the fecal discharges cannot be reliable, as I have proved many times. I desire to emphasize the statement that I have never seen a case of amebic dysentery without ulceration of the rectum and sigmoid. This portion of the bowel is occupied by the concentrated accumulation of infectious material from above.

In conclusion, I wish to say that the treatment of amebic dysentery requires the most careful scientific application of every factor and influence that is available.

Dr. REED (closing).—The method mentioned by Dr. Finney is interesting in that he says he looks for the colon and cecum first, and these serve as a guide to the appendix. That being true, it strikes me that under the circumstances that becomes the logical method of ingress into the colon. I'do not pretend to say that this is a hard and fast rule, and that a wise eclecticism should not be exercised. In either event, the thing winds up with an appendicostomy, because these appendices practically all perish from the tube pressure and from traction. In other words, they nearly all break down. I grant that there is a variability in the conformation of the colon, and hence a wise eclecticism ought to be exercised in this regard.

With reference to the question of neurasthenia as an indication for operation, that phase of the subject was embraced in the latter division of my paper, in which I took up the subject of autointoxications of intestinal origin, but the suggestion made by Dr. Finney is well worthy of consideration, that is, operating in an elective way upon certain of these cases, because it did not occur to me, and I believe it will come in as a valuable adjunct to the therapeutics in handling a number of these cases.

The observation of Dr. Polk is a good one, but it is embraced in the general proposition of washing out toxins from the colon; but certainly these typhoid reservoirs, these walking propagationists of the typhoid bacillus, ought to be subjected to some such treatment, and I can see an additional application for the method I have described to you.

As to the method of flushing the colon, I think possibly my

technique may have been faulty in the light of what has been said this morning. I have been very faithful in my efforts to wash out the colon through the cecal opening, and have never succeeded, but Dr. Finney succeeds all the time.

It is very evident that my method of application is defective. I have put the patient in the Trendelenburg position and in the extreme Trendelenburg position, and the water has not come around to the cecal opening. I have not inverted these patients, as suggested by Dr. Hanes, but I shall try this method of inversion at the very first opportunity.

SUCCESSFUL ENUCLEATION OF A MENINGEAL ENDOTHELIOMA INVOLVING THE MOTOR CORTEX.

By Stephen H. Watts, M.D.,
Charlottesville, Virginia.

———

While with better powers of diagnosis and better operative methods the number of successful cases of extirpation of brain tumors is constantly increasing, nevertheless they are still of sufficient rarity to justify the reporting of individual cases.

The meningeal tumors are of especial interest since they represent the most favorable cases for surgical treatment. This is due to the fact that they are usually benign, are well encapsulated, grow slowly, and owing to their superficial situation, are apt to give rise to localizing symptoms.

The following case is one of meningeal endothelioma, a type of tumor which is especially prone to occur in the cerebello-pontine region, though here it involved the motor cortex.

Mrs. S. K., aged thirty-three years, housewife, was admitted to the University of Virginia Hospital, September 27, 1909, complaining of headache, vomiting and dimness of ision.

Family History. Father, mother, three brothers and one sister living and well. Two brothers and one sister died of acute illnesses. No history of tuberculosis, tumor or nervous trouble in the family.

Personal History. The patient had mumps, measles, whooping-cough and diphtheria when young. She has never had typhoid, pneumonia, malaria or scarlet fever; has never suffered to any great extent with headache before the present illness and eyesight has been good. No history of injury to the head. No history of chronic cough, shortness of breath, bronchitis or hemoptysis. No history of genito-urinary disease. No disorders of menstruation.

Marital History. Has been married twice. Had one child by the first husband and three by the second. Youngest child is three months old.

Present Illness. Began about two years ago. While sitting in a chair one day she fell forward and remained unconscious for some time. These "fits" recurred almost once a month up to three months ago, since which time they have been more frequent. She describes the convulsions as beginning with a twitching of the right corner of the mouth, passing to the right arm and then to the right leg, when she would become unconscious and remain so for perhaps half an hour. She does not remember when the headaches first began, but for the last three months they have been very severe and she thinks the pain is worse on the left side of the head. She says she has had vomiting spells since she first noticed any trouble, though recently they have been more frequent, in fact of almost daily occurrence. The trouble with her eyesight was first noticed about four months ago, found that she could not see to sew. Weakness of the right arm and leg was first noticed three or four months ago. She thinks her memory has not been so good since her trouble first began.

Examination. Patient is fairly well nourished. Expression is rather dull and does not change when she is spoken to, but when she is suffering with her head the face shows pain and the left hand is held to the left side of the head. The pupils are somewhat dilated, are equal, and react to light and accomodation. She can distinguish colors, and count one's fingers when held in front of her, but she cannot make out printed matter. Movements of the eyes are apparently normal.

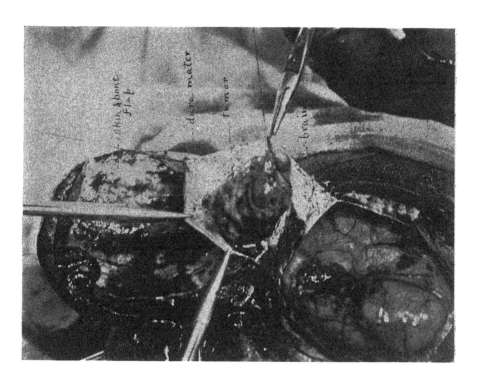

FIG. 1.—Photograph of tumor during operation.

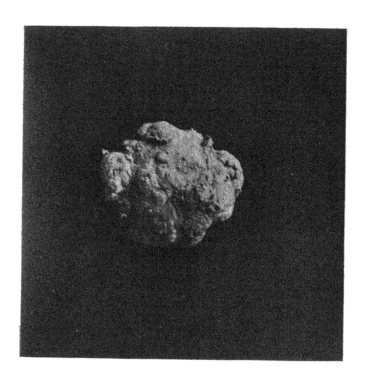

Fig. 2.—Brain tumor, actual size.

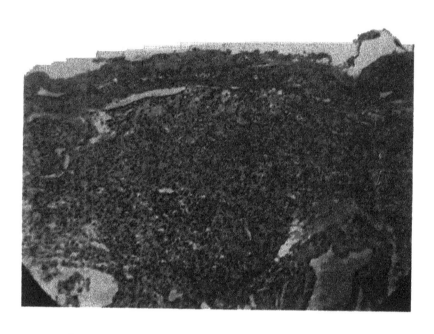

FIG. 3. Photomicrograph of section of tumor. × 90.

Both optic disks markedly choked, elevated fully × 4 diopters in each eye; vessels are clear after getting well away from the swollen disk; no hemorrhages.

When the patient is spoken to, it takes a long time for her to answer; she apparently knows what she wishes to say, but cannot express it (motor aphasia). Hearing is apparently equal in both ears. The right facial nerve is weak, but is not completely paralyzed. The tongue deviates somewhat to the right when protruded. The pulse is of fair volume and good tension, 60 per minute; has been as slow as 50 per minute.

The right arm is distinctly weaker than the left and there is distinct atrophy of the muscles of the right shoulder girdle, arm and hand. The right leg is perhaps somewhat weaker than the left, but there is no atrophy of the muscles.

Perception of touch, pain, heat and cold is present everywhere, but seems somewhat diminished on the right side, particularly in the arm. The patella reflex on the right seems a trifle more marked than on the left. No ankle clonus. No Babinski reflex. There is no ataxia, no nystagmus, no astereognoses.

Examination of heart, lungs, abdomen and urine negative.

Diagnosis. The symptoms and physical signs seemed to point definitely to a growth in the lower portion of the left precentral gyrus. The absence of any history of syphilis or other evidence of tuberculosis tended to exclude syphiloma or tuberculoma, and the long duration of the symptoms seemed to indicate a slow-growing neoplasm, probably benign.

Operation. October 5, 1909. A large bone flap was turned down on the left side of the head over the Rolandic area after the usual method, with trephine openings, DeVilbis forceps and Gigli saw. The dura bulged somewhat, seemed very tense and there was no visible pulsation. In the centre of the area of exposed dura there was a small reddened area about 4 to 5 cm. in diameter, which seemed to indicate that something was adherent to the dura in this region. A flap of dura, corresponding to the opening in the skull, was reflected and the convolutions of the brain found to be considerably flattened by the intracerebral pressure. In the middle of the area of brain thus exposed a tumor, about 3 by 4 cm. in diameter, was discovered, which was adherent to the dura and embedded in the precentral gyrus apparently between the arm and the face areas. The growth was well encapsulated and was peeled out without difficulty, being lifted up with the dura to which it was adherent. It was then easily separated from the dura itself by blunt dissection, it being unnecessary to do any cutting. The tumor lay apparently between the arm and face areas of the motor cortex, making pressure upon these areas and upon the posterior portion of the inferior frontal convolution, thus causing the partial paralysis of the right side of the face and the right arm, and a certain amount of motor aphasia. The growth extended down to the lateral ventricle, which was opened when the tumor was shelled out, a small amount of fluid escaping. The dura was closed with interrupted fine silk sutures and the skin with the same material, small protective drains being placed down to the trephine openings. A photograph was taken during the operation showing the growth adherent to the dura, Fig. 1.

Pathology. The tumor, which is about 3 by 4 cm. in diameter, is fairly firm, smooth, somewhat lobulated and of a reddish color (Fig. 2). It is enclosed in a capsule containing numerous small bloodvessels and on section it presents a uniform, slightly granular appearance. On microscopic examination (Fig. 3) the capsule is found to be composed of fairly dense connective tissue while the body of the tumor is composed of a richly cellular tissue, containing numerous complex spaces. Some of these have a lining of flat endothelium separating the space from the surrounding cellular tissue, while in others there is no lining, the spaces being surrounded by the cellular tissue. This tissue is composed of fairly uniform cells, the nuclei of which average about

15 microns in size and are round or oval. The nuclear material is moderately coarse and is as a rule uniformly distributed. The individual cells, whose outlines are rather indistinct, take a pale blue stain, are often vacuolated and sometimes finely granular. No definite mitotic figures are seen, the only evidence of cell division being the variation in the density of the chromatin material in the nuclei and the variation in the size of the nuclei. It seems undoubtedly a meningeal endothelioma.

Postoperative Course. The patient made an excellent recovery from the operation and the wound healed per primam, the sutures being removed on the third day. There was no return of the headache or vomiting and when she was discharged on December 1, 1909, the paralysis of the face and arm had almost entirely cleared up, though there was still some atrophy of the muscles of the arm and hand. The most disappointing feature of the case was the failure of improvement in the sight. This seemed to improve slightly for a time, but then became worse, if anything, and when she was discharged she could count the figures at a distance of three feet but found it difficult to recognize persons. Examination of the eyes at this time showed that the swelling of the disks had entirely disappeared, but there was a distinct postneuritic atrophy, more marked in the left eye. This is another illustration of the importance of earlier operation in cases of brain tumor, for so many, even after a successful removal of the growth, become blind or have greatly impaired vision as a result of the postneuritic atrophy.

DISCUSSION.

DR. WALTER C. G. KIRCHNER, of St. Louis.—Strange to say, about a year and a half ago I had a case the history of which was almost identical with the one just recited. The case occurred in a man who also came from the South, and while at work in St. Louis he was taken with an epileptic seizure. A careful neurological examination was made by Dr. Graves, and definite localization of this tumor was made. It was thought best at this time to remove the overlying bone, and this was done, and a tumor identical with the one that has been described, but perhaps a little larger in diameter and a little flatter, was removed from the cortex in the same region. The symptoms were the same in this particular case. The dura was slightly adherent to the tumor, but the greatest adhesions were found at the cortex. The cortex was attached to the tumor and a portion of it was removed with the tumor. The patient made a nice recovery, but at about the end of six months some of the symptoms returned. Recently he has fallen into the hands of Dr. Cushing, and I shall be interested to know the ultimate results. It is rather strange to have two cases with identically the same history. This tumor was also an endothelioma.

DR. JOHN C. MUNRO, of Boston.—There are one or two points which will help us very materially in our work in connection with these tumors. One of these points I have learned indirectly from MacEwen, namely, that in subcortical tumors, as soon as the cortex is opened down to the tumor, the surgeon can sit down and wait a little while, when the tumor will deliver itself. I had noticed this fact in my early surgical work, but did not have enough brains to see the importance of its practical application.

Another point: For a number of years in some tumors— and Dr. Cushing has since then spoken of it—we have done the operation in two stages, that is, we have exposed the dura first, and then a few days later we have turned down the flap, without any anesthesia, exposed the area, and located the lesion. These patients are absolutely without any sensation. There is no shock connected with the operation, and it is a very easy and simple way of attacking certain cortical lesions.

The case of Dr. Watts is unusually interesting, and I want to congratulate him on the results.

A FURTHER REPORT ON THE SURGICAL TREATMENT OF EPILEPSY; NEW METHODS AND POSSIBILITIES OF BRAIN SURGERY.

By W. P. CARR, M.D.,
Washington, D. C.

———

At our last meeting I reported the results of twenty operations for epilepsy; nearly all cases of long standing, not traumatic, and having several seizures a day at the time of operation. All but one were benefited, and at that time five of them had been cured for three or more years. I may now add that none of the five have relapsed, though one died of pneumonia nearly eight years after operation, and they have now been free from epilepsy four or more years; the longest period being ten years. Another case has now gone three years without recurrence, making six cases out of twenty that may be called cured.

Another case overlooked and accidentally omitted from my first report recently came to my office for some minor trouble, and reported herself well after more than two years. One extremely bad case remained well for one year and five days; then had a few mild seizures, and has since been well, two months to date. During the past year I operated upon two more, and refused to operate upon about twenty mild cases that I did not feel warranted in exposing to operation in the present state of our knowledge. These cases will be reported later. One I will briefly sketch. A colored boy, aged twelve years, developed epilepsy after an attack of typhoid fever. He had been treated medically in a hospital, and circumcised without benefit. He was rapidly getting worse. At the operation he was found to have a well-marked and very extensive chronic meningitis, with adhesions between the pia and dura as far as could be seen. These adhesions were separated with the finger, over most of the left cortex and in the longitudinal fissure. Last Thanksgiving day, three weeks after operation, he ate a very heavy turkey dinner and then stuffed himself with oranges and bananas. He promptly went into status epilepticus for twenty-four hours, but recovered and had no more seizures for the two weeks more that he remained in the hospital. Since going home he has relapsed, and this case must go as a failure. And yet he showed so much temporary improvement that I feel he might have been cured could he have had a long course of proper diet and hygiene.

When we remember the advanced stage and severe type of these twenty cases, that they were with few exceptions not traumatic, that six out of twenty may be called cured, and at least six more greatly improved, it seems almost too great to be true. I can only say that these are facts that will be vouched for by many of my associates who saw the cases before and after operation. It may be mere coincidence or it may be, as a distinguished alienist said to me after personally examining some of these cases, that there is something in it. At least I think these results justify a further trial of exploratory craniotomy *when other measures have been found inefficient.*

There is still a very general belief that idiopathic epilepsy cannot be cured nor even improved by such operations. But this belief is not founded upon any extensive observation, since improved surgery has made such operations safe.

It is only within the last few years that anything more than simple trephining was safe, and few surgeons have attempted these operations since then, because they have regarded them as hopeless except in recent traumatic cases.

The epileptic habit has been a serious stumbling block, but is one that ought now to be removed. There is no such thing as the epileptic habit *per se.* The continued attacks are the result of a lesion. And if the lesion can be cured or removed, the attacks will cease. The length of time that seizures have been occurring has nothing to do with the prognosis in cases coming to operation, except that the lesion may be more extensive. This may seem heretical, but several excellent authorities now entertain this belief. In conversation last winter with Dr. Spratling I found that his ideas coincided with my own in this respect, and there is probably no one better qualified than he to express an opinion upon the subject.

Whether epilepsy be caused originally by a brain condition, or by absorption of toxins from the alimentary tract, or by some peripheral irritation, the brain finally suffers, and becomes distinctly abnormal even in its appearance to the naked eye. In *all* my cases marked lesions, *gross* and *microscopic,* were found.

Even after removal of a peripheral cause, if it has existed long enough to produce a brain lesion, the seizures will continue. Hence the so-called epileptic habit. It would appear also that simple exploration of the brain in many cases benefits or cures the cerebral lesion; but if a peripheral cause be still active a cure of the epilepsy will not result. If both conditions, however, can be cured, we may expect brilliant results. And this may possibly be done in a considerable proportion of cases even where two or three causes are operating. I consider the subject still *sub judice,* but my own experience has been so encouraging that I wish to stimulate others, who are competent, to take up this work—some whose opportunities for doing it are greater than my own.

Leaving the subject of epilepsy, let us consider some of

the possibilities of brain surgery with the improved methods of the present time. The method of making large osteoplastic flaps has done for brain surgery what the Sims' speculum did for gynecology.

My own experience has taught me to enlarge the flap from time to time, until there are now few parts of the brain not accessible to safe examination. I have found it comparatively easy to examine nearly a whole hemisphere. I do not wish to encourage reckless exploration, nor brain operations by inexperienced men. In no branch of surgery is a thorough knowledge more essential, not only of anatomy and physiology, but of pathology. One should be especially familiar with the touch and appearance of living brains, both normal and abnormal. And both touch and appearance of the living brain are very different from those of the cadaver. One not familiar with these things is likely to overlook serious lesions or mistake their significance. And one not particularly familiar with safe methods of examination is likely to fail in discovering even such gross lesions as tumors, abscesses, or clots; or, on the other hand, to do serious damage to some vital part. While one soon learns the appearance of the normal brain in trephining for fractures and similar work, it is only by comparing gross appearances with microscopic sections that diseased conditions may be familiarized. I have found it of the greatest value in all abnormal conditions to remove small portions for microscopic examination. And it was only after numerous examinations of this kind of living brains that I began to feel any assurance of recognizing the true significance of the abnormalities most commonly found, and learned to appreciate differences in the feel of normal and some abnormal conditions, both to the finger and to the probe or grooved director, which is the best instrument for exploring the brain. The osteoplastic flap is the method *par excellence* of opening the skull. Much loss of bone is to be deplored.

With increased experience I am making flaps larger than ever, especially where no definite location of a lesion has been made, and I have gradually developed a method of opening the skull, and some instruments that I believe are of value in saving time and preventing shock and hemorrhage. My plan is to place the patient upon the operating table before anesthesia is complete, make the final preparations, and mark out the proposed flap upon the skin while it is being completed. The base of the flap should always be toward the blood supply and considerably narrower than the middle. A small incision is then made in the skin and one blade of a long clamp passed under the base of the flap in the loose tissue between the skin and the periosteum and closed tight enough to check bleeding from the flap. The outer blade of this clamp should be covered with rubber. It must not crush the scalp nor remain on too long. Safety pins may be used, or a long pin with a rubber figure of eight.

The flap is then cut with one sweep of the knife through skin and periosteum—one careful sweep, not a slash. The concave edge of the incision is rapidly loosened and special clamps applied to stop bleeding. These clamps are an invention of my own, and by a glance at the accompanying diagram their structure and use will be easily understood.

They are easily applied, effective, out of the way, clear of the operative field, and not dangling across it, as does the ordinary hemostat. A hemostat or clamps may be required on the flap proper, as the clamp across the base does not perfectly control hemorrhage without too much pressure and crushing. After the bone flap is turned down this pin had better be removed, and any number of hemostats required may then be applied to the edge of the flap and will be out of the way.

For boring the skull I use a small trephine fitted with a handle like a brace, and protected by a guide which regulates the depth to which it will cut. This trephine may be fitted to any brace, cuts very rapidly and safely a hole $\frac{5}{16}$ inch in diameter. There is advantage in the small opening and the rapidity of boring, as several openings may be made and the cutting of the flap with a De Vilbis craniotome facilitated.

I have found no instrument that will do the cutting so rapidly and satisfactorily as a good De Vilbis, provided we do not try to cut too far away from the trephine hole. Two holes will do, but three or four are better in a large flap. The base of the bone flap is made narrow, so that it will be certain to break in the proper line and break easily.

The saving in time by the use of these instruments is very considerable, and the control of hemorrhage almost perfect. These are important factors; more important, I believe, than is generally thought to be the case.

With a large flap in the parietal region the greater part of the motor sensory area is exposed to view, and a finger can be passed under the skull and carefully swept over the surface of the brain from the anterior frontal to the postoccipital lobes, and down under the base in the middle fossa and over the tentorium. The falx cerebri may be palpated almost from end to end, and all this may be done without injury, because the large opening allows a partial displacement of the brain and makes room in the skull cavity for the finger.

No cortical clot of any size on the side of the opening can escape detection by such exploration, and deep-seated clots in the brain substance or ventricles can often be detected by the tension which they cause and by the lack of pulsation over them. I have even been able to detect a tumor situated half an inch from the surface by the sense of resistance to touch. Careful exploration of the brain substance with a grooved director does no harm if properly done, and may be used with considerable freedom. The blunt end of the director will not tear bloodvessels nor

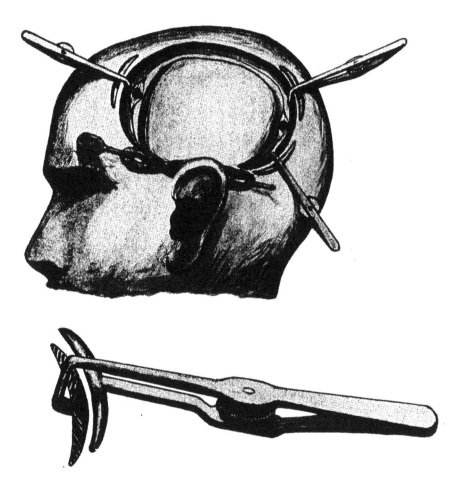

Surgical treatment of epilepsy.

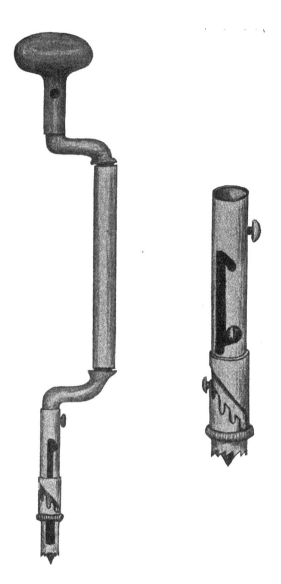

Surgical treatment of epilepsy.

cause much laceration of nerve fibers or cells, but will push these structures aside and separate them without injury.

The exploratory needle with a sharp point is dangerous. It may puncture large vessels, and is useless because it does not evacuate thick pus nor give an altered sense of resistance in meeting abnormal tissues. Even the finger may be introduced into any part of the lateral ventricle with little damage to brain tissue if it is carefully worked in through one of the deep fissures that reach nearly to the ventricle after making a small opening with some blunt instrument such as a hemostat. I have done all these things in a considerable number of cases and had the patients recover, and recover easily without symptoms of shock or other serious disturbance, and with less nausea and general discomfort than follows an ordinary laparotomy.

Quite recently I removed a large clot from the middle fossa which was lying against the side of the pons. The patient regained consciousness, recovered from his paralysis, was comfortable, and apparently well on the way to recovery two days later. Unfortunately, he then developed a rapidly fatal double pneumonia. Leaving out cases of severe injury to the head, I have had no deaths following this extensive exploration, and in a dozen cases done several years ago there have been no sequelæ. None of my epileptics died, none appeared dangerously ill after operation, and in at least three of them the most extensive exploration was made.

It may be said that cerebral lesions should be located before operating, but in practice this is often impossible. The most careful localizations by skilled neurologists have often gone wrong, and in cases of severe traumatic hemorrhage there is no time for elaborate methods. But even when we feel sure that a lesion is pretty definitely located it is necessary to recognize it by touch or sight before it can be removed, and this often requires experience and thorough knowledge of pathology as well as of technique.

Many lesions become practically accessible and discoverable only by a large opening and the thorough training of the operator. With the possibilities before us, however, that we now have, there seems no reason why the field of brain surgery should not be much enlarged. There is now no reason or excuse for allowing patients to die of large clots following injury or following fractures of the base of the skull. Even if these clots cannot be located, they cannot often escape detection at the operation; and if not complicated by multiple lacerations and multiple small hemorrhages, recovery will usually follow their removal. The same thing is true in large measure of cysts, abscesses, and tumors. Further experience may show us that many insanities and epilepsies and certain types of meningitis may be cured by cerebral surgery. Certainly it would seem that purulent meningitis not benefited by serum, spinal puncture, or other means now in use should be directly drained through the skull; and it is not impossible that some cases of tuberculous meningitis may be cured by simple opening and draining, as are some peritoneal infections of the same kind. With more knowledge much may be done that is now considered impossible, and even now I think exploratory craniotomy by competent operators is as justifiable as exploratory laparotomy in many obscure cases.

DISCUSSION.

Dr. J. Shelton Horsley, of Richmond.—Dr. Carr's paper is an exceedingly interesting one. In regard to the technique of the osteoplastic flap, I have adopted the tourniquet as described by Cushing and others, and find it answers very well. An ordinary rubber tube is placed around the base of the skull, just above the ear and eyebrow, and secured by a hemostat. It is made tight enough to control bleeding from the scalp. In this way the incision, which is quite bloody, as a rule, is as bloodless as an amputation of the leg. It does not control the diploë. In the last brain case which I operated upon there was only one vessel toward the median line which required a hemostat. In closing these flaps I sew the scalp, without removing the tourniquet, using rather fine No. 1 catgut in a continuous suture, closing the wound fairly tight to get the hemostatic effect of the sutures. The tourniquet is then taken off and there is usually no bleeding point. If there is, a suture will control it. This procedure shortens the time of operation materially, lessens the staining of the field with blood, and decreases the loss of blood.

The drill exhibited by Dr. Carr is very ingenious and has much to recommend it.

A MEMBER.—I wish to report the case of a male child, aged eight years, that had several epileptic convulsions a day. Between the convulsions the child would play as other children. I resorted to trephining, and seemingly there was nothing abnormal about the meninges, but there was an abnormal amount of cerebrospinal fluid. For three or four days after the operation the child had convulsions, but they decreased in frequency for about eight months, at the end of which time they recurred with varying frequency and intensity for a period of nearly a year. I wanted to operate again, but the parents objected to it. Shortly after this the convulsions entirely ceased, and the patient has not had a convulsion since. It occurs to me that possibly many of these cases may be cured whenever the convulsions are due, as in my case, to an abnormal amount of cerebrospinal fluid, by withdrawing a certain amount of this fluid.

DR. CHARLES H. MAYO, of Rochester, Minnesota.—I have been very much interested in the paper of Dr. Carr, and particularly in what he has said with reference to the treatment of epilepsy. He tells us that he cured six cases in twenty. If that be the case, then brain surgery is not so discouraging after all; but personally I feel that if I could cure six cases in a hundred of epilepsy, I would be greatly pleased. There has been an enormous amount of surgical work done in connection with the treatment of epilepsy. I have operated on a great many cases for epilepsy, but my results have not been as favorable as those which Dr. Carr reports. I operated on one patient who said I had cured him; at any rate, he went through the Philippine war, and six years after the operation was performed he said he had not had any trouble. There is a field for legitimate work on the brain, and so I feel encouraged by the results given in this paper.

As to the question of relieving tension in the head, just now I feel a sense of relief, since some men claim to be curing epilepsy by the removal of the turbinates. They may have my cases.

DR. WALTER C. G. KIRCHNER, of St. Louis.—I think Dr. Carr has called attention to a very important subject, and those who have had experience with surgery of the head will certainly appreciate his devices for controlling hemorrhage.

In the matter of diagnosis spinal puncture has been suggested as a means in making this, and I wish to caution the members about this procedure when there is hemorrhage at the cortex of the brain. In certain cases where fracture at the base of the skull is suspected, and for diagnosis spinal puncture is made, the patient will sometimes suddenly die. In trying to relieve the internal pressure you may have sudden collapse of the patient and sudden death. This has happened more than once, and it is a matter to be considered in all these serious cases, and I do not think we should resort to spinal puncture until the external or cortical pressure has been removed or relieved.

DR. CARR (closing).—I have been asked what the operation was. In the earlier cases I operated with the belief that there was some tumor or abscess or lesion I could probably remove, and made a very large exploration in hunting for it, and did not find it, and I simply found that these patients got better. Later I began to do that intentionally. I simply open the skull widely, and explore the brain thoroughly and drain off fluids, and in almost every case I found large quantities of it. The brain is almost always under great tension, and these patients have what I call a chronic edematous encephalitis, and in some cases there are other lesions. In a few cases I have found the dura very much thickened. In one case I found a small cyst the size of a partridge's egg.

The method mentioned by Dr. Horsley of putting a rubber band around the base of the skull is certainly an excellent one if it will do. I had not supposed, however, that we could get enough pressure in that way to stop hemorrhage. I will try it.

I feel, like Dr. Mayo, that if we can cure one case in twenty or six in a hundred, or one in a hundred, it is well to operate on them, and if some of them die on the operating table, it would not make much difference. When a man goes through life having from five to six or even fifteen or twenty attacks of epilepsy a day, I feel that we are justified in trying to do something for him, even though operation is attended with more or less risk. We certainly cannot make him any worse. He is as bad as he can be, and if he should die, there would not be any great loss. I feel that a little more experimentation along this line ought to be done.

THE SYMPTOMS AND ULTIMATE TREATMENT OF HYDATIDIFORM DEGENERATION OF THE CHORION, WITH REPORT OF A CASE.

By J. E. Stokes, *M.D.*,
Salisbury, North Carolina.

As the process of hydatidiform degeneration of the chorion is a rare condition, and followed not infrequently by a most malignant and rapidly growing neoplasm, the immediate recognition of which is essential to the relief of the patient, this report of a single isolated case may not be without clinical value and a pathological interest.

Report of Case. Patient, G. S., aged nineteen years, white, married, nullipara, no miscarriages.

Family History. Good; father and mother living, both well and strong; one brother and one sister died in infancy; no history of tuberculosis or malignancy.

Past History. The patient suffered all the diseases incident to childhood, from which no unpleasant sequelæ noted. Patient had no illness during early adolescence, save sharp attacks of malaria about twelfth year. About one year previous to first menstruation she complains of having had pain, sharp cutting in character, in right side, unaccompanied by any fever, vomiting, tenderness, or abdominal distention. The pain would require her to go to bed for a day or more, followed by more or less constant hurting in right side. As the periods became established, this pain became more acute and frequent, with distinct increase in severity at the menstrual period, up to two years ago, when finally these attacks of pain ceased.

Menstrual History. First menstruated at fourteen; flow was regular every twenty-eight days, free, lasting five to seven days; some clots, pain dull in character through lower abdomen, necessitating patient to remain in bed for a day Patient menstruated last in March, regular time, period same as previous ones.

Present Illness. Patient married in October, nine months previous to present illness. For first six months after marriage she had her periods regularly, which were same in character as previous ones. In April, May, and June patient missed her periods. There were no especial symptoms except that the last of April she noticed an escape of watery blcod-stained fluid from the vagina. There was also frequent painful micturition, patient being required to get up as often as a dozen times a night. This condition ceased about three weeks ago. Patient also had considerable headache and some nausea with vomiting following shortly after she missed her first period. Has ached all over for past week and has felt weak and languid, bowels constipated. After the first escape of fluid in April, patient had no more signs of it until about five weeks ago. She then began to have the same watery blood-stained fluid, which was of slightly darker color than at first. This would pass from her a few drops at a time, though oftentimes it would be much freer, and especially so at nights, becoming of late of a brighter red color. Two weeks ago patient had a sudden profuse flow of bloody fluid from the uterus. This stopped in about one hour, and she did fairly well until the night of June 11, when she had a very profuse flooding which came on her suddenly during that night. At this time the patient passed a pint or so of blood. During these bleeding spells she would suffer considerable pain of a bearing-down, expulsive character in back and lower abdomen. At no time has she noticed passing any solid particles or firm clots.

Present Examination. Patient is extremely pale and colorless, nervous, and anemic; pulse, 140, weak and irregular; temperature, 99.4°; external surface cold and clammy.

Vaginal Examination. On inspection there is a slight stream of blood flowing from the vagina. Digital examination shows the outlet nulliparous. Cervix low in vagina, small, extremely firm; will not admit tip of finger. Fundus is enlarged beyond the size of four months' pregnancy, extending more than a hand's breadth above the pubes. Walls of the uterus do not appear unduly soft or yielding. The adnexæ cannot be distinctly made out. Owing to the unusual size of the uterus for the period of gestation, the profuse hemorrhage following a previous watery, blood-stained fluid, the pain immediately over the uterus and the elevation of the temperature, it was deemed advisable to empty the uterus.

First Operation. Under ether anesthesia, owing to the firmness of the cervix, the external os was forcibly dilated to admit finger. Uterine cavity was then explored and found filled with soft mushy-like substance presenting at internal os. This substance was thoroughly removed most cautiously with blunt curette and finger, and the walls of the uterus carefully explored. The mucous membrane appeared smooth and free from any elevations. There was a moderate hemorrhage, and the uterus gradually contracted firmly to within just above the symphysis. The cavity was next irrigated and lightly packed with sterilized gauze.

Specimen. On gross appearance the specimen consists of myriads of glistening cysts of varying size, from 1 mm. to 6 mm. These vesicles are oval or elongated and hang in bunches, grape-like in appearance, and are connected each with the other by fine threads of tissue, grayish brown in color. Each vesicle is free except where attached to its pedicle. Most of the external surface of the cysts is smooth and glistening. A few of them are partly colored by thin, gray, fleshy substance, of the same appearance as the connecting strands. The cysts are firmly distended with a clear viscid fluid.

The entire structure gives the typical grape-like appearance. There are no traces of an embryo to be found. There is a small section of pink, smooth, soft tissue of a different character from the remaining portion of the specimen (endometrium).

Histological Examination (First Specimen). The chorionic villi are, on the whole, of degenerate appearance, the Langhans and syncytial layers of epithelium of many villi being absent, and the stroma of a myxomatous character, with many small degenerate nuclei. Other villi have normal stroma with both the two layers of Langhans and syncytial cells well defined; elsewhere there is marked proliferation of both layers, but especially of the syncytial layer, which in places is from 15 to 20 cells deep. Here and there these form bud-like outgrowths with vacuoles and giant cells. There is no invasion of the stroma of the villi by the Langhans or syncytial cells.

Diagnosis. Hydatidiform mole.

Subsequent History. Immediately following the emptying of the uterus the patient reacted satisfactorily. The pulse dropped to 108 and hemorrhage ceased. However, the patient did not improve beyond this. The pulse remained rapid and weak. There was some elevation of temperature, accompanied by sharp pain through lower abdomen, also in a short time there was a return of a light blood-stained fluid from the vagina. This fluid was always freer during the night than the day. The patient continued anemic, weak, pale, and extremely nervous. After a week or so, the escape of a more deeply colored blood-stained fluid from the vagina increased in amount and became more marked during the nights. There was no escape of solid clots or particles in the discharge. At the same time, the patient became emaciated and weaker. Owing to not only the continuation but the apparent increase of the symptoms, a second curettement was decided on.

Second Operation. This was done under ether anesthesia six weeks following the first operation, and consisted in a thorough but cautious curettement. The vagina was first thoroughly examined for any nodular growths. Not any were noted. The cervix was found to be soft and dilated, the fundus enlarged, slightly irregular in contour, and distinctly soft in consistency. On curettement an ounce or so of polypoid-looking material was brought away, but no vesicle-like masses were found in the specimen. The uterine cavity was then thoroughly irrigated and palpated with the finger. The wall was found free from any elevations or masses, and appeared normal to the touch. The cavity was then lightly packed with gauze. The patient quickly reacted, and convalesence was without interruption save a slight show at intervals of blood-stained fluid from the vagina. This, however, completely subsided, and patient has gone on steadily to gain in weight and strength.

Histological Examination (Second Specimen). Pathological No. 203. On gross appearance specimen shows a dozen or more soft, vascular, nodular masses, covered by endometrium of normal thickness, and filled with blood-vessels, while others were filled with thick tenacious mucus. Microscopically, one finds a few portions of the endometrium of a fairly normal appearance present. The stroma cells are large and of an œdematous appearance, while the entire stroma is infiltrated with inflammatory cells, chiefly polynuclear leukocytes, with considerable blood. In at least two places there are islands of chorio-epithelial cells, with large, vesicular, very granular nuclei. These lie embedded in the stroma of the endometrium, with a few large cells lying scattered about in the surrounding stroma.

Remaining sections show chorionic villi with ordinary-looking chorionic stroma. The epithelium shows more marked and active proliferation than in section of mole.

Notwithstanding the fact that this histological examination of the specimen from the second curettement not only showed the presence, but also showed a generally more active proliferation of the Langhans and syncytial cells than in the first specimen examined, and again that in at least two places these proliferating cells penetrated deeply into the endometrium, both of which facts are indicative of the malignant nature of the vesicular mole, get the patient under close observation showed steady improvement, gained in weight, uterus contracted, the bleeding ceased, and there were no indications of metastatic formations, so that the more radical operation of hysterectomy was not advised.

Final Examination. Four months following the first operation final examination was made. The cervix was found in the axis of the vagina, firm and normal in consistency. The fundus of the uterus is small, contracted, and regular in contour. The right ovary is normal, the left ovary is enlarged and cystic and adherent to the wall of the uterus. The patient's general condition is now excellent. She has gained a number of pounds in flesh and has just passed through a normal menstrual period (first since operation) without inconvenience. Urinary analysis, normal. Blood count: Hemoglobin, 95 per cent.; reds, 4,900,000; whites, 8700.

HISTORY OF HYDATIDIFORM MOLE. The process of mole formation within the uterus has been designated under various terms; those most frequently employed being vesicular mole, hydatidiform mole, hydatidiform degeneration of the chorion, uterine hydatids, myxoma uteri.

In Findley's review of Kossman's *Historical Sketch of Mole Formation*, the earlier theories concerning this condition are succinctly given, all of which relate more to the clinical picture than to its true etiology. It is noted that Hippocrates wrote of the cotyledons becoming filled with mucus, followed later by abortion should pregnancy then be present. It was during the early part of the sixth century that Etius of Amida wrote concerning the hydropic uterus, and to him is accredited the earliest intelligent mention of the occurrence of a hydatidiform mole. He first describes the appearance of certain bodies in the uterus with their accompanying symptoms. He then continues that if the separation is especially violent, the small bodies which resemble cysts at times rupture, and from them escapes a water-colored tough fluid. For this condition and occurrence he advises rest in bed, emetics, and powerful enemata. Among the other 'theories following is an interesting one by Percy, who noted the presence of the vesicles and claimed that when they were treated with salt and vinegar they would move like animals, while Goeze, in 1782, believed the origin of the vesicular mole to be parasitic. The first suggestion, however, that the lesion was distinctly fetal, or at least directly connected with some process within the ovum, was not made until 1827, when Madame Boivin and Velpeau recognized the true nature of the affection. The former, however, considered the vesicles to be due to the degeneration of unimpregnated ova, and therefore she does not appear to have recognized that conception was first essential. Finally, in the beginning of the latter half of the nineteenth century, Virchow initiated the histological study of hydatidiform moles and advanced the theory that their formation resulted from a myxomatous degeneration of the chorionic villi. This theory, some years later, was confuted by the now universally accepted explanation of Marchand, who in 1895 explained that the lesion was not a myxomatous degeneration of the connective tissue of the villi, but was a distinct proliferation of the two layers of epithelial cells covering the villi, viz., the inner layer, or Langhans cells, and the outer layer, or syncytium. He claims that as these cells proliferate they penetrate into the decidua, and even then at times on through to the uterine substance, followed by a mechanical dropsy of the stroma of the villi and subsequent formation of vesicles containing fluid.

ETIOLOGY. Even though this theory of Marchand is now accepted that the formation of a hydatidiform mole is due to cell proliferation of the villi, the exact origin of the exciting cause, or what influence brings about the process of mole formation, has never been accurately determined. The question whether the cause for the cystic degeneration of the villi is due to some radical change either in the ovum or in the body of the uterus itself remains yet unsettled. Ouory is of the opinion that the mole seems to be due to a primitive change of the ovum; but the cause of the disease of the ovum is unknown. The question as to whether the death of the embryo is to be regarded as the cause or consequence of the cystic degeneration has been very thoroughly considered. On the one hand, the theory advanced is that degeneration of the chorion does lead to death of the embryo; while others hold the opposite view, and contend that the death of the embryo occurs first and degeneration of the chorion follows as a direct consequence. Concerning this debatable point, Williamson believes that the death of the embryo before formation of the true placenta is a common occurrence; hydatidiform mole is a rare occurrence, and in those cases of blighted ovum which he has examined, even after retention in the uterus for considerable periods, he has nevertheless not found the least trace of anything like cystic degeneration. It still remains, then, to be explained why in 99 cases these conditions do not lead to cyst formation and in the 100th they do. In favor of the view that the degeneration of the chorion occurs first, he continues that many cases have been recorded in which portions of the placenta have shown hydatidiform degeneration and still a living child born at full time. Chalensky suggests that the lesion follows death of the embryo and that the chorion receives in consequence increased nutrition formerly intended for the fetus, thus causing the proliferation of the chorio-epithelium. Marchand, on the other hand, answers that were this the case molar pregnancy would occur more frequently. Among other investigators, Frankel and Pick consider cystic disease of the ovary should be considered a factor in the production of hydatidiform mole, though they differ materially as regards how the influence is brought about. The former claims that the ovum suffers from a lack of lutein secretion, while the latter asserts that in a cystic disease of the ovary there is an excessive production of this secretion (Bland).

In 1853 Virchow was the first to suggest that the condition is due to changes in the endometrium, while Marchand, on the other hand, asserts that when the degenerative process occurs in early fetal life, it is due primarily to changes in the ovum, and that the endometritic changes are only secondary. Regarding this point of the fetal or maternal origin of the occurrence of vesicular mole, Findley gives the following résumé: In favor of the maternal origin may be mentioned the recurrence of the mole in the same individual and by different husbands; the common occurrence late in life; the partial vesicular degeneration of the chorion in the presence of a perfectly healthy fetus; common occurrence of cystic degeneration of the ovary associated with hydatidiform mole; and lastly, that endometritis and nephritis commonly precede the development of hydatidiform mole. In favor of the fetal origin is the fact that in twin pregnancy one mole alone may be involved in a cystic degeneration of the chorionic villi.

RELATION OF HYDATIDIFORM MOLE TO MALIGNANCY. The frequency with which malignancy follows the occurrence of the rare condition of the vesicular formation within the uterus has greatly interested and has held the closest attention of many pathologists. Notwithstanding this, just what the relationship is, or just what the existing association between the two conditions depends upon, remains yet undetermined. Two theories have been advanced regarding the malignancy of the vesicular mole. One is that there are two distinct forms of mole, malignant and benign; while the other theory is that all moles are malignant and that the malignancy manifests itself through a portion of the mole being left behind in the uterus. Ouory draws the following conclusions: (1) Clinically and histologically the hydatidiform mole may behave like a malignant tumor, and must be considered as such; (2) but this special, unique tumor of fetal origin can live a certain time in the maternal organism as a parasite, as a stranger, and can be driven out without leaving the epithelial elements, which are an integral part of its malignity. The mole in this case is called benign, because the consequences of its presence for the mother are absent.

Findley finds from his 210 collated cases that 16 per cent. of hydatidiform mole becomes malignant, but he is rather of the opinion that this percentage is too high, owing to the fact that the occurrence of non-complicated moles is seldom reported in proportion to those undergoing malignant degeneration. Regarding this process of malignant degeneration, Marchand says: "If one now asks in what the malignant nature consists, we can only answer that the most important thing is the unlimited tendency of the cells to proliferate; in the second place, we must also consider the conditions of the surroundings which make proliferation possible or favor it. The unlimited capability of proliferation is an inherent property of fetal tissues, especially of the epithelium of the chorion; but the proliferation is kept in check as long as the ovum develops normally; it may, however, manifest itself in an unlimited manner if the embryo dies early or parts are separated off." He also considers the second necessary requirement, a suitable condition of the maternal tissue in which the newgrowth arises, the so-called diminished power of resistance is most easily explained in the newgrowths in question by the enormous transportation of blood and nutritive material to the parts, by loosening of the tissues, and the serous permeation of the tissues of the uterus in pregnancy. It is clearly recognized by observers that a definite percentage of cases of deciduoma malignum follow the occurrence of a vesicular mole; that a close relation exists between at least the occurrence of these conditions is not denied.

Hart and Barbour, in fifty-five collected cases of deciduoma malignum, found twenty-four followed upon an hydatid pregnancy; while Dorland found that over forty per cent. in his collection of cases were preceded by the history of the expulsion of a vesicular mole some time prior to the appearance of the disease. Regarding this point, Williams in his monograph was unable to note any particular difference in those cases of deciduoma malignum which were preceded by moles and those following ordinary pregnancy, and he considers with our present state of knowledge it would be unwise to attempt to prove that the mole gives rise to the deciduoma or the reverse. The appearance of small masses in the structures remote from the uterus, as in the vagina and upon the vulva, occasionally following the expulsion of a vesicular mole has been noted. Here again is a wide divergence of opinion among investigators as regards the association of these masses to malignancy. These nodules show a certain amount of discoloration, and on histological examination present chorio-epithelium undergoing various changes. On the other hand, some observers regard the occurrence of these tumors as direct evidence of malignancy, and are therefore considered true metastases; while, on the other hand, such observers as Findley and many others quoted by him do not accept the occurrence as positive evidence of malignancy, but rather incline to the opinion that the invasion of remote structure by the chorionic epithelium is merely due to the accidental transportation of particles of a benign growth. Along this line Williams states that his own observation with those of others concerning the transportation of villi in normal pregnancy lends a certain probability to the latter theory, though our present knowledge is not yet sufficient to warrant a positive conclusion.

FREQUENCY OF OCCURRENCE. According to Williamson's statistics, hydatidiform mole is a rare disease. He found that among 24,500 cases of pregnancy occurring in St. Bartholomew's Hospital there were ten instances of vesicular mole; *i. e.*, one mole formation in about 2400 pregnancies; while the ratio has been placed as low as once in 20,000 cases (Madame Boivin).

AGE. In Findley's collection of 210 cases the average age of patient is twenty-seven years; extreme ages are thirteen and fifty-eight years. Dorland found a percentage of 41 occurring in the third decade of life, while Williamson found the greatest number occurred between twenty and twenty-five years, though the second most fruitful age was from forty to forty-five years. He continues the only deduction to be drawn is that hydatidiform mole may occur any time during the child-bearing period, the age of women having very little influence. Two cases occurring in the negro race have been reported.

THE RATIO OF FORMER PREGNANCIES TO MOLE FORMATION. It is interesting to note that the occurrence of preceding pregnancies does not appear to have any predisposing influence upon the appearance of hydatidiform mole. In 178 instances of Findley's 210 cases, in which the history of preceding pregnancies is recorded, we note that vesicular mole occurred much more frequently in nulliparæ than in those women who had had one or more pregnancies; thus, in 178 cases of mole formation, 41 occurred in nulliparæ, or 23 per cent.; 25 occurred in primiparæ, or slightly over 14 per cent., as compared with 24 per cent. of Dorland's and 10 per cent. of Kehrer's cases respectively; while 23, or 12.9 per cent., and 19, or 10.6 per cent., occurred in multiparæ who had borne two and three children respectively. It is to be noted that this percentage steadily decreases as the number of children born increases from nine to even as high as twenty.

SYMPTOMS. As a rule, the occurrence of the vesicular mole is accompanied by most of the cardinal symptoms of pregnancy. The only constant one, however, is the enlargement of the uterus; while the appearance of hemorrhage, one of the most constant symptoms of the presence of vesicular mole, may mislead the patient and be mistaken for the usual menstrual period. It has been noted that nausea and vomiting may be excessive and prolonged. The four most distinct symptoms in their order of positiveness, though not always constantly present, are: (1) The discharge; (2) enlargement in contour of uterus; (3) hemorrhage; (4) tenderness over the uterus (Williamson); (5) presence of the mole by internal palpation.

With the presence of the discharge a positive diagnosis may be made if it contains any of the vesicles. The discharge is watery, blood-stained in character, and when the vesicles are discharged with it the picture has been aptly likened to "white currants floating in red currant juice." Though the discharge may occur within a few weeks following conception, as in the writer's case, the vesicles are rarely seen until the expulsion of the mole is at hand (four times in 210 cases). It may be scant in amount, with slight pain, and appear at irregular prolonged periods, or, again, profuse and painful at frequent intervals. The enlargement of the uterus is a very constant symptom; it may increase with marked rapidity and attain a size far in excess of what one would expect for the corresponiding period of gestation; "be soft, fluctuating, and elastic;" while again cases have been reported in which the uterus was hard, dense, and irregular. It has also been noted that this rapidity of growth may be most pronounced just previous to the expulsion of the mole.

HEMORRHAGE. Though so frequently associated with other complications of gestation, hemorrhage becomes a most significant symptom, and should always suggest the presence of a vesicular mole when occurring in a uterus whose size is larger than expected for the period of gestation, or in which the rate of growth has been noticeably rapid. The second and third months are the most frequent ones in which the hemorrhage occurs, as in the writer's case, and at times it has been noted that the hemorrhage is very profuse during the night, while lessening greatly during the day.

TENDERNESS OVER THE UTERUS. This has been demonstrated by Williamson in 6 cases out of 13, and at times the uterus in shape and consistency differed markedly from that of normal pregnancy.

DIAGNOSIS. The presence of a vesicular mole should always be suspected at least on the appearance of a vaginal discharge, watery, blood-stained in character; or in the appearance of hemorrhage following a period of amenorrhea in conjunction with a rapidly grown uterus; while the vaginal examination may show the uterus to be of an unexpected size, soft and elastic, or again of a peculiar doughy, mushy feel, more or less irregular in contour. Should the cervix be soft and patulous, and dilated sufficiently to admit the finger, the vesicular formation may be plainly felt.

PROGNOSIS. The prognosis should always be guarded, and it is well to bear in mind that in a certain number of cases an early diagnosis following the onset of symptoms is absolutely essential for the permanent relief of the patient. For it should be remembered that from 10 to 16 per cent. of hydatidiform mole undergo malignant degeneration; that over 40 per cent. of the cases of deciduomata are preceded by the occurrence of a vesicular mole (Dorland); and that the percentage of immediate mortality varies from 10 to 30 per cent., according to different observers. Thus, in Dorland's 100 cases the mortality was 10 per cent.; in Findley's 210 cases it was 25 per cent.;

and Williamson's 10 consecutive cases showed a mortality of 30 per cent.

In the above tables, among the causes of deaths recorded were hemorrhage at time of operation, general sepsis, perforation of the uterus, septic peritonitis, uremia, nephritis, endocarditis, and meningitis. In the cases where the question of the presence of vesicular mole arises late in the period of gestation, or where it is probable the condition has been going on for a prolonged duration of time, it should be borne in mind that the serious complication of rupture or sloughing of the uterus may occur.

TREATMENT. The treatment may be divided into the immediate and ultimate. Under the first head will come those cases in which a positive diagnosis of the presence of a vesicular mole has been made. In these cases it is agreed that the immediate removal of the mole should be brought about, and the uterus thoroughly explored by the finger for any particle cleaving to the internal surface of the cavity. In emptying the uterus the greatest care and caution must be exercised. The cervix should be well but cautiously dilated and the mass removed, when possible, by digital manipulation. The sharp curette should not be employed, as perforation of the uterine wall is likely to occur. If the mass cannot be peeled off by the fingers, or all the material lying loose in the uterus cannot be brought away, then the dull spoon curette or placental forceps may be employed cautiously. This is an important suggestion, for it is not possible to say from the gross appearance of the specimen whether malignancy is present or not; how deep the invasion into the uterine wall may be; nor how thin the wall has become. The uterus should next be thoroughly irrigated and gauze placed loosely into the cavity. Where much caution is demanded in the technique of the first operation, equally as much caution and watchfulness for indications of malignancy are to be exercised in the ultimate treatment of the patient. After the removal or expulsion of the vesicular mole the patient should be most carefully watched and examined at intervals, irrespective of her improved condition or freedom from all symptoms. If any invasion of the vagina or vulva should take place, the nodule should be removed and a histological examination made. Williams advises, in case the characteristic lesions of deciduoma be found to be present in a vaginal nodule, immediate removal of the uterus is indicated. At least once following the expulsion of a vesicular mole, some months or so, the uterus should be thoroughly examined and cautiously curetted and the scrapings examined microscopically. Whenever the specimen thus obtained from the uterus even suggests, by an active proliferation of the chorio-epithelium, a malignant invasion, the uterus should be removed on "suspicion."

Findley has formulated the dictum that hemorrhage recurring weeks or months after the expulsion of a hydatidiform mole is suggestive of malignancy, and demands immediate and thorough investigation into the cause. L. Fraenkel considers that the hydatidiform mole is not an undoubtedly benign tumor, and that from his histological findings we are very much justified in doubting its harmlessness.

I am indebted to my associate, Dr. Solon A. Dodds, for the histological examinations made in the reported case of this article.

LITERATURE.

Bland. Chorio-epithelioma Malignum. Journal American Medical Association, vol. xliv, No. 23, p. 1827.

Dorland and Gerson. Cystic Disease of the Chorion, with Tabulation of 100 Cases. University Med. Magazine, 1895–96, viii, 565 to 590.

Findley. Hydatidiform Mole, with Report of Two Cases and Clinical Deductions from Two Hundred and Ten Reported Cases. American Journal of the Medical Sciences, March, 1903, cxxv, 486.

L. Fraenkel. Die Histologie der Blasenmole, Arch. f. Gynäk., 1895, xlix, 481 to 507.

Madame Boivin. Quoted by Williams.

Marchand. Ueber den Bau der Blasenmole. Zeischr. f. Geb. u. Gyn., 1895, xxxii, 405 to 472.

Marchand. Die Blasenmole, Ztschr. f. Geburtsh. u. Gynäk., Stuttgart, 1898, xxxix, 206 to 216.

Kehrer. Quoted by Dorland.

P. Ouory. Etude de la *Mole* hydatidiforme (thesis), 1897.

Williams. Text-book of Obstetrics, 1906, chapter xxxviii; Johns Hopkins Hospital Reports, 1895, iv, 9.

Williamson. The *Pathology* and Symptoms of Hydatidiform *Degeneration* of the *Chorion.* Trans. Obst. Soc., London, 1900, xli, 303 to 338.

Zweifel. Lehrbuch der Geburtshülfe, 1895, p. 306.

DISCUSSION.

DR. THOMAS S. CULLEN, of Baltimore.—We are particularly fortunate in having this subject brought before us at frequent intervals. Hydatidiform mole is not very rare. Chorioepithelioma is relatively uncommon. We have had three cases in the gynecological department of the Johns Hopkins Hospital in the last seventeen years. The clinical diagnosis is uncertain. Hydatidiform moles have been quite frequently mistaken for myomata of the uterus. I know of a case occurring in the last year in which the uterus was removed on the supposition that the condition was myomatous. The uterus with the mole intact was removed. It is impossible for the pathologist to tell from scrapings whether a given case is one of hydatidiform mole or of chorio-epithelioma. Some of the best pathologists have time and again mistaken the one for the other histologically.

Occasionally at autopsy metastases are found in the vagina, lungs, and elsewhere, while the uterus shows no evidence of a malignant growth. In these cases the growth in the placenta has not prior to labor extended to the uterine wall by continuity, and with expulsion of the placenta all trace of the primary growth has been removed. Prior to labor, however, portions of the growth have been carried either by the bloodvessels or lymphatics to distant organs.

Metastases from chorio-epithelioma are prone to develop in the lungs, and occasionally hemoptysis is one of the early signs.

I thoroughly agree with Dr. Stokes in urging the advisability of watching patients who have had a hydatidiform mole, and if there is the slightest evidence of bleeding they should be again thoroughly curetted and watched. If there are any irregularities on the surface of the uterus, if myomata can be excluded, extension of the growth to the outer surface has probably taken place, and in these cases the uterus should at once be extirpated.

DR. WILLIAM D. HAGGARD, of Nashville, Tennessee.—I wish to report one case that came under my observation quite recently. The patient was a woman, aged twenty-four years, who had borne two children, the younger sixteen months. She menstruated normally on August 14 last, but skipped September and October. She stated that after she had skipped about two months she began to flow slightly, following a pain one night, and the pain and hemorrhage confined her to bed. Within three weeks she had developed an elastic, fluctuant tumor of the abdomen of considerable size. While she was only three and one-half months pregnant, according to her count, she was the size of a woman six months in pregnancy. As the tumor was globular and fluctuant, we thought of ovarian cystoma, but she did not have enough pain to account for twisted pedicle, and ectopic gestation was out of the question, although she did have one bad spell of pain. On account of the fluctuation and hemorrhage and the tremendous increase in the size of the growth within such a short period, we felt sure of our diagnosis, and accordingly we removed the product of degeneration, and, contrary to the essayist, it would hardly have been possible to have removed this enormous quantity of degenerated hydatid with the finger or gauze. I tried it faithfully, and after I thought I had succeeded in doing so, I resorted to a large, dull curette, which, if used with gauze, would not cause perforation. This patient did well, and we shall bear in mind the essayist's suggestion to keep her under future observation on account of the great danger of malignant degeneration.

DR. HOWARD A. KELLY, of Baltimore.—Dr. Stokes has drawn our attention to the extreme importance of being prompt in dealing with every case of uterine hemorrhage. I have had many instances of disasters from waiting. One of my last patients, who is still in the hospital, if she is not now dead, has a chorio-epithelioma, and if we had gotten at it earlier, we could have cured her, but it is now too late. We took out an enormous uterus in spite of the fact that the disease had extended into the vaginal vault and beyond. We got rid of the disagreeable discharges, turned out the cervix, improved her condition, but she is beyond hope of being entirely relieved. When these married women have hemorrhages, the only way to relieve them and to determine the true nature of their condition is the prompt use of the curette.

Dr. G. A. Hendon, of Louisville, Kentucky.—I merely wish to amplify the record on this subject by reporting four additional cases. Although I do not do an obstetric practice, I have attended four cases in consultation like the one described by the essayist within the last two and one-half years. The four cases occurred in young women during their first pregnancies. One of them has borne two children since. There were no features in connection with these cases of special interest, all of them being of the type which conforms very closely to that presented by the essayist. All four of the cases made satisfactory and uncomplicated recoveries.

Dr. Reuben Peterson, of Ann Arbor, Michigan.—It is well-known to those who have large consultation practices in obstetrics that this condition is not recognized by the general practitioner, as a rule. The latter often fails to note the abnormal size of the uterus, and unless the vesicles have come away he ascribes the hemorrhage to low implantation of the placenta. I have been called in a number of cases where the diagnosis was not made and the practitioner was in the dark. I do not think, in spite of all the work that has been published along this line, the tendency toward malignancy in these cases is sufficiently appreciated, and I think the paper Dr. Stokes has given us is very timely in again calling attention to this fact.

SOME ACUTE ABDOMINAL CONDITIONS IN INFANTS UNDER ONE YEAR OF AGE.

By RANDOLPH WINSLOW, *M.D.*,
Baltimore, Maryland.

INTUSSUSCEPTION.

THE first few months of life of the human infant are full of peril, but this is from diseases and conditions of a medical rather than of a surgical character. Exceptionally, however, conditions occur that can only be combated by surgical means, and without which death is almost sure to follow. Among these conditions intussusception of the bowels occupies a very prominent position. While this disease occurs in adults, it is especially an affection of infancy and childhood. It is one of the maladies that may occur almost at the time of birth, and certainly does occur in some cases in the first weeks of life. It is said that nearly one-third of all cases of intestinal obstruction are due to intussusception, and while this is certainly not the case in adults, it is the form of obstruction that is found generally in the case of children. My attention has been called to this affection, especially, by the fact that within a short time three cases of this trouble have come under my observation in children under twelve months of age. Kerley, in his book on *Diseases of Children*, reports a case of intussusception in a previously healthy baby two weeks of age. I have not seen a case of as tender age as this, but have met several recently in the first year of life. Generally the attack begins suddenly in previously healthy infants with colicky pain, occurring paroxysmally, and vomiting ensues speedily and is repeated frequently. There may at first have been movements of the bowels, but soon absolute constipation takes place, with the exception that blood and mucus or pure blood are discharged from the anus. This is a very important sign, and one which should always be sought for in cases of pain and vomiting with constipation occurring in children. A tumor often may be felt in some portion of the abdominal cavity, more frequently, perhaps, in the right iliac region, but by no means confined to this area. This tumor is hard, elongated, often sausage-shape, and is more or less tender upon pressure. It is said that a tumor can be felt during life in 86 per cent. of cases. In many cases a finger introduced into the rectum can feel a protrusion of the invaginated bowel in the rectum. Holt says the bowel can be felt in the rectum or it protrudes through the anus in 50 per cent. of cases, and that it may be felt in the rectum within twelve hours of the onset of the first symptoms. There is pallor of the countenance, feeble pulse, mental apathy, and for a time, relaxed abdominal walls. After twenty-four to forty-eight hours, tympanites sets in with, usually, marked distention of the abdomen, progressive depression, and at last elevation of temperature and acceleration of the pulse, which may be due to toxic absorption from the intestines, or to the occurrence of gangrene of the bowels. The pain in this condition is of great severity, causing the child to shriek in many cases in a very characteristic manner. Vomiting is almost always present, is projectile in character, and consists of the bile stained contents of the stomach, and later of stercoraceous matter. In some cases convulsions occur, but not always, the countenance becomes pinched and anxious, the surface of the body cool and cyanotic, the child becomes unconscious, and dies in profound collapse. Death usually occurs within a week, and the larger number die on the third day, and one-half of all cases by the fifth day. In some cases life is prolonged for some weeks, and in a small number spontaneous recovery takes place. Cure sometimes results from spontaneous reduction. The telescoped bowel in some manner becomes reduced; in other cases recovery results from the sloughing of the intussusceptum, which is, however, not to be expected in infants, nor, indeed, in adults, but does occur at times in both. Of 52 cases recorded by J. Lewis Smith, 7 were cured spontaneously in this manner.

The most frequent variety of intussusception is the ileocecal, in which the ileum forces its way through the ileocecal valve, and in some cases traverses the whole length of the large intestine. Next in frequency is the colic variety, when the colon becomes invaginated, and lastly the enteric form, in which the intussusception is confined entirely to the small intestine. Sometimes intussusception is due to the presence of a Meckel's diverticulum. I had a case of this kind not long ago, but it occurred in an older child, a boy of about six years of age. Other cases of intussusception might be due to the presence of indigestible matter, which, by causing irregular contraction of the intestines, might eventuate in invagination. The prognosis, then, of these conditions is very serious; cases do occasionally recover, but we can in no manner foretell which cases will recover, and as most of them terminate fatally, it is necessary that they should be recognized early and treated promptly. The symptoms which call our attention to this condition are sudden, violent, spasmodic pain, vomiting, constipation, the discharge of bloody mucus or blood from the rectum, and the presence in many cases of an elongated tumor in some part of the abdominal cavity. Where these symptoms are present treatment should be prompt and thorough. One of the most important factors in the treatment of the disease is the avoidance of purgatives. If intussusception is present, purgatives can only do harm. An attempt to effect reduction of the intussusception may be made by the injection of lukewarm water or air into the rectum. The buttocks should be elevated to an angle of 45 degrees, or even more, and water from a fountain syringe or other douche held at an elevation should be allowed to run slowly into the rectum. Some remarkable cures have been obtained by the employment of these methods, even after the lapse of some days. Dr. Kerley in cases of this character sends at once for a surgeon, but in the meanwhile he uses water pressure from a fountain syringe held at an elevation of four feet. He makes a short attempt of only five minutes duration, and reports a very·remarkable case of a baby of nine months of age, with invagination which could be felt in the rectum, and which had been six days in existence. The child was pulseless, unconscious, in profound collapse, with great abdominal distention, and a scarcely audible heart beat could be distinguished with the stethoscope. He was afraid that rupture of the bowel would occur, but as the child's condition precluded an operation, water pressure was tried, and in a short time a large and offensive stool occurred, the condition was relieved, and the child recovered. In another case he was also successful with the same treatment. Some years ago I was called to a child who presented the symptoms of intussusception, and in a similar manner water was introduced into the rectum; the symptoms at once subsided and did not recur. In most cases, however, measures of this character have been tried and found wanting, and fortunate is it for all concerned if they have not been tried too long; hence a resort to surgical operation is the ultimate resource, without which death is almost a foregone certainty. These children of tender age are not well adapted to withstand severe surgical procedures. The abdominal incision should be made either in the middle line or over the apparent seat of the trouble. If the condition has not existed long, an effort should be made to reduce the invagination, but if it has been in existence for a sufficient length of time to produce marked stasis and œdema of the intestinal walls with beginning or actual gangrene, it will be better in many cases not to attempt the reduction of the intussusception, but to satisfy ourselves with an enterostomy, introducing a tube into the bowel and allowing the contents to escape externally, and subsequently, when the condition of the child is better, resection of the diseased parts may be done.

CASE I.—M. P., female, aged five months, admitted to University Hospital August 25, 1909, in the service of Dr. St. Clair Spruill. Temperature on admission was 105°, pulse 150, respirations 40. The child, previously healthy until the 22d inst., was taken suddenly ill on that date. Screaming with pain, the child drew up its knees and cried out as if the pain were in the abdomen; these pains came on in paroxysms. Purgatives were administered, and the following day a small amount of bloody mucus was passed in two stools; there was vomiting from the beginning at intervals. Enemata were also administered without causing a movement of the bowels, except a bloody mucus. The child became rapidly worse, and was brought to the University Hospital three days after the inception of the symptoms. At this time her condition was very serious, the respiration hurried, pulse weak and rapid, lips bluish in color, abdomen soft and somewhat distended, and there was a suspicion of a lump in the left upper quadrant of the abdomen; this, however, was not definitely made out. Leukocyte count, 21,600. Operation was performed at once, under ether anesthesia. An incision was made through the right rectus muscle. The cecum, with about three inches of the small intestine invaginated into it, was found on the left side of the abdomen in the region of the splenic flexure of the colon. There was complete collapse of the bowel below the obstruction, while above it the intestines were markedly distended. With but little effort the intussusception was reduced, there was no strangulation of the gut, and it soon recovered its normal appearance; the cecum, however, was considerably thickened from invagination. A few interrupted sutures anchored the colon into its normal position, and the operation was finished with the child in a fairly good condition. Subsequently the bowels moved twice rather freely, but convulsions soon supervened, and death terminated the scene in a few hours.

CASE II.—E. P., aged nine months, admitted to University Hospital April 24, 1909, in the service of Dr. R. Winslow. This child had had persistent vomiting for four days, with no bowel movement, the abdomen was distended, but not very rigid. Temperature on admission was 100°, pulse 120, respirations 28. The attack came on suddenly in the previously healthy child. After admission to the hospital a high enema was administered, but was ineffectual. The abdomen was opened in the middle line, and an intussusception of the ileum into the cecum was found. This was reduced without much difficulty, and the gut was found to be in a viable condition, though there was some thickening of the invaginated parts. About six inches of the ileum were invaginated through the ileocecal valve. Subsequent to the operation vomiting ceased, the bowels moved freely, and although for a while the temperature was elevated, reaching 105°, with a pulse of 160 and respirations 45, the symptoms soon subsided and the child made a good recovery.

CASE III.—M. F., aged six months, admitted to the Hebrew Hospital August 29, 1909, in the service of Dr. R. Winslow. Three days previously the child was taken sick and cried a great deal; the mother gave it a dose of castor oil but without effect. The next day a physician was called in, who administered calomel, to be followed by oil, but without beneficial effect. The next morning an enema was administered without causing a movement of the bowels, but blood was passed by the rectum. At the expiration of three days the child was brought to the hospital. It was a well-developed and nourished infant, but in an extremely serious condition, almost comatose, pulse rapid and weak, 155 to the minute, respirations 30, temperature 101°, abdomen markedly distended and tympanitic and tender on pressure. It was almost a hopeless case, but an operation was undertaken. Chloroform was administered, an incision made in the median line, and about five inches of the ileum was found invaginated into itself and then carried through the ileocecal valve and invaginated into the cecum. The intussusception was found on the left side near the splenic flexure, and not, as was supposed beforehand, in the right iliac region. The bowel was released with difficulty and showed beginning gangrene. A rubber tube was placed in the gut and drainage of the intestines established externally. The child, however, did not recover from her collapsed condition, and died three hours later.

These cases show the folly of treating acute abdominal conditions of children with purgatives and delaying to bring them to the attention of a surgeon at a period when operative procedures may be followed by success. Any case in which there is vomiting, paroxysms of pain in the abdomen, constipation, and especially when there is a discharge of blood or bloody mucus from the rectum, should cause a most careful examination to be made by the attending physician, and unless the symptoms subside almost at once, the case should be seen by a competent surgeon with a view to operating for the relief of the condition which at this time of life is almost certainly that of intussusception.

STRANGULATED HERNIA IN INFANTS.

Notwithstanding the frequency of congenital hernia, it is somewhat remarkable that strangulation takes place so seldom. It does occur, however, in a certain small proportion of cases, but I am not aware of the exact proportion between the non-strangulated and the strangulated cases. I have recently operated on one case of strangulated inguinal hernia in an infant of three weeks of age, and my former assistant, Dr. A. A. Mathews, now of Spokane, while at the University Hospital, operated on one nine days of age. These cases do not present any special peculiarities, but are attended by the ordinary symptoms of strangulated hernia, namely, vomiting, constipation, distention of the abdomen, and the presence of a painful lump in the groin. Notwithstanding the tender age of these patients, the results of operation are good, and recovery usually follows, if the operation has not been too long delayed. The question of an anesthetic in these cases is one of importance, and probably it would be better in most cases to administer chloroform rather than ether, owing to the possibly injurious effect of ether upon the respiratory passages of the child; or the operation may be done under local anesthesia, if the condition of the patient appears to demand it. The patients operated on by myself and Dr. Mathews were under the influence of a general anesthetic, chloroform in the one case and ether in the other, and made excellent recoveries from both the anesthesia and the operation. I think it is an interesting question as to the best anesthetic for administration in these early cases of surgical disease, and I should be pleased to have an expression of opinion on this point.

STRANGULATED HERNIA.

CASE I.—F. H., aged three weeks, admitted to the University Hospital March 19, 1909, in the service of Dr. R. Winslow. This child was found to have a hernia on the right side extending into the scrotum, which was irreducible and presented the ordinary signs of strangulation. It is said that its bowels had not been moved for four days, and that vomiting had been present for thirty-six hours, but we were unable to get any adequate history of the case. Operation was performed at once under ether anesthesia; the ordinary incision for inguinal hernia was made and the sac found to contain bloody fluid; the gut was markedly obstructed, but was glistening and with no evidence of gangrene, and was returned into the abdominal cavity. Vomiting ceased at once, the bowels moved promptly, and the patient was discharged well in eight days.

CASE II.—Colored male, aged nine days. Born in the out-door maternity clinic of the University of Maryland, was perfectly well until the eighth day, when he had a violent crying spell, followed by persistent vomiting. The mother noticed a swelling in the child's left groin shortly after a choking spell. A student tried to reduce the hernia, but without success, and the next day the child was admitted to the University Hospital. My former assistant, Dr. A. A. Mathews, finding the child in a serious condition, with the pulse so rapid that it could not be counted, operated at once under chloroform anesthesia. The usual incision was made, the sac opened, and the intestine found quite dark but with a glistening surface, and was returned into the abdominal cavity, the sac tied, and two or three interrupted sutures introduced closing the wound. The child began to improve at once and made an uninterrupted recovery.

APPENDICITIS IN INFANCY.

While appendicitis is very common in childhood, it occurs very seldom under twelve months of age, and I have not personally seen a case occurring under one year of age; nevertheless, it does occur at times in very young infants. The youngest cases reported, so far as I am aware, are those by Blumer and Shaw and by Fenger, the subjects being seven weeks old. I have not seen the original report of these cases, but they are mentioned in an article upon appendicitis in the fourth volume of Keen's *Surgery*, written by Dr. John B. Murphy, of Chicago. In these cases there is usually a preceding gastro-intestinal disorder; the onset is sudden and the pains violent and continuous; convulsions are common; sometimes pain is complained of in the pelvis, and a rectal examination reveals sensitiveness on the right side. Increased frequency of urination is often present, the skin over the appendiceal region is extremely sensitive, and a slight pinching of the skin causes severe pain. We must bear in mind the possibility of appendicitis occurring in young children, but before determining that such is the case a careful examination of the child's chest should be made, as it is a well-known fact that pneumonia often causes abdominal disorders, pain, tympany, vomiting, and constipation to such a degree as to lead one to suspect that a serious abdominal lesion is present. When it can be made out that appendicitis is present, of course an operation should be performed, but the results are not such as to encourage us to expect a favorable termination of the case. Kirmison and Gumbellot, in their collection of cases of appendicitis, report 9 under one year of age, all of which died, but of 26 in the second year of age, 7 recovered; some of the fatal cases were not operated on, and the 7 which recovered were operated on.

CONGENITAL HYPERTROPHIC STENOSIS OF THE PYLORUS.

About 100 cases of this affection have been reported. The symptoms show themselves in from a few days to three weeks after birth, by vomiting, loss of weight, and constipation. There is evidence of dilatation of the stomach, with waves of peristalsis from left to right, and a sausage-shape tumor may be felt in the pyloric region; the infant rapidly becomes emaciated, and unless relieved by an operation death from starvation occurs. The various surgical procedures that are applicable to similar conditions in adults may be made use of in children, but apparently gastro-enterostomy is the operation that affords the best hope of success, as of 25 cases reported, 11 recovered, and the subsequent histories of 9 of these cases are excellent. Pylorectomy is too severe a procedure for young children, but good results have followed in some cases the stretching of the pylorus, according to the method of Loreta. Some of the methods of pyloroplasty have also been done with considerable success.

CONGENITAL MALFORMATION OF THE ANUS AND RECTUM.

Congenital defects of the lower end of the alimentary canal are said to occur about once in every 10,000 births, but this is probably an underestimate, since many cases are not recorded. These malformations are found more frequently in boys than in girls, and are often associated with other defects, notably with exstrophy of the bladder and hypospadias. There are various abnormalities of the anus and rectum that are usually called imperforate anus and rectum, but which present a number of variations. To understand the method of production of these conditions, we must remember that the anus and rectum are developed separately. The rectum is formed from the primitive hind gut, and at the fourth month is in intimate association with the allantois, from which it is gradually differentiated by the growth of a septum, forming a separate canal, while the allantois subsequently forms the urinary bladder. The anus is an involution of the epiblast, which passes inward to meet the rectum. The partition between the two pouches diappears, and the rectal canal is completed. When these processes fail to occur in a normal manner, some one of the following malformations are produced, according to the classifications of Cooper, Gant, and Abbé.

A. *Imperforate anus.*

1. Congenital narrowing of the anus without complete occlusion, or without fecal fistules elsewhere.

2. Closure of anus by thin membranous tissue.

3. Entire absence of anus, the rectum ending in a blind pouch at varying distances from the perineum.

4. Imperforate anus with fecal fistula opening (*a*) into uterus or vagina, (*b*) into male bladder or urethra, (*c*) or on the surface of the body.

B. *Imperforate rectum, with anus normally placed.*

1. Membranous obstruction of the rectum.

2. Extensive obliteration or total absence of the rectum.

SYMPTOMS AND DIAGNOSIS. In some instances the anus appears normal, and it is only after the insertion of the finger that an obstruction is found to be present. Generally the anus is absent, and its normal location may be indicated by a slight depression, or there may be a perfectly smooth surface without any pit or hollow at all at the normal location of the outlet. When there is no external orifice, the condition will be speedily noticed by the physician or nurse, but when there is a normal-looking anus, it may be some while before the absence of intestinal evacuations calls the attention to the fact that something is wrong, and suggest the propriety of a rectal examination. In some cases the intestinal contents are discharged through unnatural channels, as the vagina or penis, or by means of fistulous tracts elsewhere. As has been said, most of these conditions are incompatible with life, but in a few cases life is not materially interfered with, especially when the gut opens into the vagina or vulva. The symptoms produced are those of intestinal obstruction, and they usually supervene promptly; vomiting, distention of the abdomen, obstipation, increased frequency of pulse, elevation of temperature, pain, fretfulness, crying, and, if not relieved, collapse and death in from forty-eight hours to a week. In some rare instances the child has been known to live several weeks, and in one case three months without having any fecal movement.

PROGNOSIS. The prognosis is therefore most unfavorable in the majority of cases without operation, and in the few instances in which life is preserved by means of fistulous tracts it is done at the expense of cleanliness, and with subsequent mortification and discomfort to the patient. Even with operation, both the immediate and remote results are far from favorable, and statistics of operations show about 50 per cent. of mortality.

TREATMENT. The relief of these conditions can only be secured by surgical measures. If there are fistulous or other abnormal openings, sufficiently patent for the free evacuation of the bowels, operative procedures may be postponed until the child has reached a more favorable age, but this is practically limited to those with a vulvar or vaginal outlet. In the first variety, where there is a congenital narrowing of the rectum or anus, but without complete atresia, the case should be treated as one of stricture occurring from postnatal causes, and it may be stretched by the introduction of a finger or of a bougie. In some cases, however, it may be necessary to make an incision through the anus in order to permit the introduction of dilating objects, and, of course, subsequently it would be necessary to introduce bougies from time to time to prevent contraction.

The second variety, where the imperforate anus is due to a membrane, is to be treated by incising the membrane and carefully trimming it off, after which the patency of the bowel is to be maintained by the introduction of a bougie or a finger.

In the third variety, where the anus is absent and the rectum terminates in a cul-de-sac some distance above the perineum, we have to deal with a much more serious condition than those that have just been mentioned. In this condition we may sometimes feel a bulging in the perineum caused by the pressure of the meconium when the child cries, but of course at other times this is not possible. We may facilitate this method of examination by pressing upon the abdomen of the child in order to force the intestinal contents down against the palpating finger. When this is the the case, operative procedures are undertaken, and consist in the making of an incision at the site of the anus down toward the coccyx until the rectal pouch is reached, which is then opened, the contents allowed to escape, and the lower end of the bowel brought down and fastened to the skin. When the rectum terminates at a still higher level it may be necessary to excise the coccyx and make an artificial anus at a higher point. If the rectal pouch cannot be reached from below, a left inguinal colostomy should be performed.

Fourth variety. In this condition there is imperforate anus, but the rectum terminates in a fistulous communication with the vagina, urethra, bladder, or surface of the body. The simplest of these conditions is where the rectum terminates in the vagina or vulva. In such cases the bowel empties itself freely and operation is not imperative until the child reaches a more mature age. Sooner or later, however, an operation becomes desirable. Generally a grooved director or a curved forceps may be passed through the rectovaginal opening and made to impinge upon the integument of the perineum, at which point an opening is made. The rectum may then be freed from the vaginal wall, brought down and sutured to the anal site, and the opening in the vagina may likewise be closed with sutures. This rectovaginal opening has frequently a sphincter implanted in the vaginal wall, by means of which retention of the intestinal contents is secured. Where this is the case it may be proper to enclose this sphincter with two elliptic incisions and bring this abnormally placed sphincter to its normal location in the perineum. When the fecal fistula terminates in the urethra or bladder of the male, it is an extremely difficult condition to rectify by any plastic operation, still an attempt may be made to reach the bowel and to establish an anus in the perineum; generally this will not succeed, and colostomy will have to be performed or death will usually speedily ensue. Strange to say, these cases are not always fatal; a case is reported where a man of middle age, whose rectum opened into his bladder, had continued to discharge the contents of the bowel through his urethra without discomfort or serious impairment of health. Where the fecal fistula opens upon the surface of the body it may do so by various routes, but is most likely to terminate in the scrotum or penis. Sometimes, however, the opening may be found in the gluteal, sacral, or lumbar regions. If the opening is sufficiently large to prevent obstruction of the bowels, nothing is necessary to be done until the child reaches a more favorable age for operation. When, however, the opening is small, and intestinal obstruction is threatened or has actually taken place, the fistula may be incised or dilated sufficiently to permit the free escape of the intestinal contents, or if this is impossible colostomy remains as a last resort.

Fifth variety, with a normal anus and a membranous obstruction of the rectum. This condition will not be suspected until the failure of fecal movements and symptoms of obstruction cause a digital examination of the anus to be made, when it is found that the canal is obstructed by a partition more or less dense. This may be located an inch or more above the anus. In some cases this partition or membrane may be ruptured by the insertion of the finger, but generally it will be necessary to incise it with a bistoury, and then to thoroughly stretch it by means of bougies or the finger.

Sixth variety. This is where the anus is natural as to location and appearance, but terminates in a blind extremity, while the rectum terminates at a greater or less distance above the anus, its extremity being often free in the peritoneal cavity. An attempt may be made to reach the bowel from the perineum, but when this is manifestly impossible colostomy should be performed.

IMPERFORATE ANUS.

CASE I.—Baby S. was brought to the University Hospital on February 11, 1909. He was born twenty-four hours ago; perineum is smooth, with no evidence of an anal opening; otherwise the child is normally developed. Urine mixed with meconium is discharged from the urethra, the abdomen is slightly distended, but the child's general condition is excellent. Without an anesthetic an incision was made in the perineum and an attempt to reach the rectum was made without success; a few whiffs of chloroform were therefore given and an incision made in the abdomen in the left iliac region, the muscles separated, and the sigmoid flexure sought for and brought out through the wound, a piece of gauze being placed beneath the bowel through the mesentery to prevent its retraction, and the angles of the wound sutured up to the bowel. The next day the gut was opened and a rubber drainage tube introduced into its proximal end, thus permitting the escape of the intestinal contents. Two days later the bowel was cut across and the ends sutured to the skin, establishing an artificial anus. The patient did well, the highest temperature being 100°. Was discharged in eleven days.

CASE II.—Several years ago a somewhat similar case came under my observation, in which the bowel extended as an abnormal tube along the perineum to the scrotum, forming a long fistulous track. This track was dissected out, the mucous membrane of the rectum sutured to the skin, and the child made a good recovery. I have also seen several other cases of imperforate anus in my own practice and in that of my colleagues. In one case, occurring in my own practice, the people refused to have an operation performed, and the child lived a week before a fatal termination took place.

DISCUSSION.

Dr. George W. Crile, of Cleveland.—I should like to call attention to the suture material in operating upon infants. Since the use of small round needles in bloodvessel anastomosis, I find the No. 12 needle serves admirably in the intestinal work on infants.

I have seen four cases of acute intussusception in infants under two years of age, following acute attacks of appendicitis, in which we definitely knew by histological examination and symptoms that intussusception had occurred at the start, as disclosed by operation.

Lastly, I wish to call attention to a method I have found useful in diagnosticating cases of appendititis in infants and young children. Under primary ether anesthesia, an accurate muscle spasm symptom may be elicited.

Dr. Rufus B. Hall, of Cincinnati.—First, I want to congratulate the Association upon this very complete and interesting paper of Dr. Winslow. I wish to speak of acute conditions. I will mention one case of imperforate anus.

When I was in general practice many years ago I was asked to see an infant three or four days after its birth. I did so, and found a perfectly formed anus ending in a blind pouch an inch and a half above the sphincter. With the infant crying I could feel something beyond the finger like the essayist has described. It seemed as if there might be an accumulation above. It was the child of very poor parents, and it was then under the care of a township doctor who lived nine or ten miles from my town. I was told to come there prepared to do a surgical operation. The child was *in extremis*, but I made an effort to relieve it, but I was uncertain whether I would be able to do anything or not. I did not feel like putting a knife in there before I had surgical training. But I thought I had some sense. I took a large trocar, such as we use for tapping the abdomen in cases of ascites, pushed it beyond an inch or so and pulled out the trocar, leaving the stylet, and got out material like meconium, and relieved the child. Before I was through I took a knife, made an opening, dilated it, and the child made a nice recovery and lived for six years. I lost track of the case then, as the family moved to an adjoining county. The child was perfectly well except it had attacks of constipation. When it was six and a half years of age I was again called to an adjoining county to see the same child, and while there was no money in the case I was very much interested in it. The child had complete intestinal obstruction, and I went there prepared to do an operation. When I reached the bedside of the child I examined it without an anesthetic. With my finger in the anus I found there was a firm stricture; that I could feel something that did not belong there apparently; something that was not cicatricial tissue, and by a little manipulation I felt that there was someting that was blocking up the passage. Accordingly the child was given chloroform, and when it was under the anesthetic there was very little difficulty in effecting dilatation, and a plum seed was found blocking up the passage. With forceps I removed the plum seed, dilated the stricture, and that was all the operation that was done for the relief of the intestinal obstruction. That was the only case I met in my practice in consultation that I was able to relieve.

I saw one case once in which there was no effort at formation of an anus or rectum, and I wanted to operate on that child, making a colostomy. This was many years after I saw the first case. The members of the family were ignorant and hard to persuade, and according to them the child died under the will of God, and they would not let me operate.

I wish to speak of another condition, and that is congenital stenosis of the pylorus. I have one case unreported of this condition. I operated upon an infant about six weeks of age. It was the first child of the family and weighed six and one-half pounds. Had no trouble other than that the child for about ten days began to regurgitate its food, and within two or three days all the food was regurgitated; that is, all milk. The child was carried along under the care of doctors and gradually lost flesh, and 1 was asked to see it when it was six weeks and two or three days old. As I have said, the child weighed six and one-half pounds when born. When I saw it it weighed less than four pounds. I could not feel a tumor in the region of the pylorus, but indications of obstruction were plain from the regurgitation of the food. It would take breast milk until its stomach was distended and then it would regurgitate it again. There was no movement of the bowels after the child was ten days old. Attempts had been made to feed the child by the rectum for several days preceding my visit, but rectal alimentation could not be retained. I made a posterior gastro-enterostomy, and the condition of the pylorus was that of a fibrous growth surrounding the pylorus not quite as large as the index finger of a large hand, but an inch and a quarter long, perfectly round, hard, glistening, and apparently no opening through the pylorus.

DR. F. GREGORY CONNELL, of Oshkosh, Wisconsin.—That intussusception in children is frequently overlooked cannot be doubted. It is recognized more often in England, and in Australia one meets with the remarkable record of Mr. Clubbe, who has had a personal experience of over 150 cases. In order to get better results, an early diagnosis is necessary; the sudden onset, in the midst of perfect health, with the scream of severe abdominal pain, followed by pallor, nausea, vomiting, and usually melœna, in a child that does not appear ill, with pulse and temperature often normal, is a striking clinical picture, and if Clubbe's advice—"to pay attention to the story told by the mother"—is followed, such symptoms will seldom be misinterpreted and cases overlooked.

The discovery of an abdominal mass, under ether anesthesia, will confirm the diagnosis, and should be followed by treatment. Rectal injection should be used as a preliminary step, and if the mass does not entirely disappear a laparotomy is indicated. Much harm has been done by the injudicious use of injections of water, or air, without anesthesia.

It should be remembered that intussusception may be multiple, that such a condition may recur, and that there may be a causative factor, which should be looked for.

I am familiar with one instance in which an intussusception in a youth, aged six years, was reduced after laparotomy; eight months afterward there was a recurrence of the intussusception, and at the second operation a sarcoma of the bowel was discovered. It was undoubtedly the undetected cause of the first invagination.

DR. STUART MCGUIRE, of Richmond.—I do not wish to discuss any one of the conditions described, but desire to speak briefly in regard to surgery of infants in general. I think success depends upon three factors: The first is to prevent shock by avoiding loss of time, loss of blood, and loss of heat during the operation. We must do our work quickly. What Dr. Price calls chronic surgery will kill these little patients. The loss of a large quantity of blood will produce profound and perhaps fatal shock. I believe that an infant can lose blood in proportion to its weight as well as an adult; but when we consider the weight of the infant, it is at once apparent that any material amount of blood lost would be to it a serious hemorrhage. A baby cannot stand cold, and we ought to be careful to keep it warm before, during, and after operation.

The second factor is the anesthetic. I do not propose to revive the discussion of this morning, but I will say that we get some things by heredity. I was born a Democrat, I was born an Episcopalian, and I was born an advocate of chloroform, and it is pretty hard for me to change my views on any one of these three subjects. I have never seen a death from chloroform, and I cannot conceive of a substitute which will work as satisfactory as this agent in children. I admit that many adults take chloroform badly, and there are conditions where ether or some other anesthetic might be substituted with benefit, but for the infant chloroform cannot be surpassed.

The third factor for successful work on children is a proper kit of instruments. In operating upon a baby the usual instruments are too large and clumsy. The surgeon should have what Dr. Crile calls Lilliputian instruments for work on these little patients.

Dr. JOHN C. MUNRO, of Boston.—I desire to extend Dr. Connell's remarks on intussusception. He spoke of Mr. Clubbe having had over 200 cases of intussusception, and of his success in the operative treatment. I think in his last 35 cases of intussusception he operated without a death. I asked him how he obtained such good results, and he informed me that he had trained his fellow practitioners in Sydney to recognize this condition early, although he did not think intussusception was more common in Australia than here, but the general practitioner had grasped the importance of this problem more readily than we Americans.

I would like to call attention to another point, namely, that in cases of imperforate rectum where the bulging perineum has been opened by a trocar, leaving the child with incontinence, it is a distressing condition that can be helped in a certain number of instances. I had a little girl not long ago, aged fifteen years, who had a rectum of this sort, and I found by careful dissection that I could make out a definite sphincter, and by bringing the gut down through the levator and the sphincter I gave her absolute control, so that she is all right now.

DR. I. S. STONE, of Washington, D. C.—I do not wish to discuss this subject other than to make a suggestion, namely, that twenty-five years ago Dr. Gale, of Roanoke, Virginia, recommended the use of chloroform anesthesia with the patient in the inverted position for any bowel obstruction. Dr. Gale has mentioned this time and again, and I thought it would be well to speak of it here, and I know he has relieved several cases of intestinal obstruction in this way. The transverse colon, if not the cecum, can be reached by rectal infusion or injection. I want to say, incidentally, that Dr. Gale is not here because he is ill.

DR. GEORGE BEN JOHNSTON, of Richmond.—I have seen a number of cases of imperforate anus. The first one I saw I reported at a meeting of this society which took place something like twenty years ago. It was the first operative case. I have seen several such cases in the hands of other practitioners which were surgical curiosities, but in which no operation was undertaken. In this case there was a dimple at the anal entrance, but there could be made out no opening of the bowel, and on the second day after the birth of the child an inguinal colostomy was done. This child grew to be a child of seven years of age, at which time I operated on it for a stone in the bladder, doing a suprapubic operation and removing quite a large stone from the child's bladder.

I have seen a number of other cases of imperforate anus or deformity there, and have under observation now two children under one year of age, one with the bowel opening into the vagina high up, and the other with the bowel opening into the bladder. Both of these children are thriving, and we have determined not to subject them to surgical interference until they are older.

In reference to intussusception, I think it occurs much more frequently than heretofore recognized. I believe if we could do what has been suggested by Dr. Munro, that is, educate the family doctor into the practice of diagnosticating these cases early, we would encounter a great many of them surgically that now escape our attention. I have seen two most interesting cases of intussusception, one in which there were five distinct swellings, and these cases had existed for a period of eleven days. The child was brought in with the belief that it had prolapse of the rectum. A large mass of bowel was hanging out of the anus, and on examination it was discovered that there were five distinct masses or tumors which could be felt through the abdominal wall, one of them hanging out of the anus. I opened the abdomen and reduced all five of these intussusceptions. The child made an admirable and uneventful recovery after a period of eleven days. In another infant the intussusception had existed for twenty-one days. This was likewise reduced and the child made a complete recovery.

I mention these two cases to show, first of all, that the diagnosis can be easily overlooked by reasonably good practitioners, and in the next place that all intussusceptions are not of such an acute character as to cause early death.

Referring again to the importance of educating the family doctor, and he, in turn, helping us in the matter of dealing with such conditions, a common practice, I believe, among all practitioners is that when any bowel trouble manifests itself in very young children they administer some sort of laxative, and particularly is this true if there are no symptoms which point toward dysentery being present. They try to clean out the bowels with a dose of oil or some such laxative. I look upon this as a pernicious practice. I believe it takes more courage to administer a dose of a purgative medicine in any intra-abdominal condition than to recommend a surgical operation, and I think it is our duty to preach a crusade against purgation in acute abdominal conditions, and likewise to point out to general practitioners the importance of making an early diagnosis and refering the cases to surgeons as quickly as possible.

Dr. Albert Vander Veer, of Albany, New York.— With reference to the remarks made by Dr. Johnston, I will say that in my district the general practitioner now reaches these cases promptly and, without giving them too much medication, calls in a surgeon.

I have had a chance to observe a number of cases of imperforate rectum. One of my early operations, done over twenty-five years ago, was in a case like that reported by Dr. Hall, in which I made use of the trocar. Take a case in which we have the rectum formed below, in which we can introduce the finger an inch and a half into the lower portion of the rectum, with an entire diaphragm across the rectum shutting off the upper portion of it; those cases are favorable for treatment. In the patient upon whom I operated twenty-five years ago I succeeded after the method spoken of by Dr. Hall. By gradual dilatation she went along very well. Her mother learned to introduce the finger into the rectum to assist in dilating the canal. When this patient was much older I was called to see her in consultation, and found she was then suffering from chronic Bright's disease, from which she died. She had the most interesting case of contracted kidneys I have ever seen. I have had three cases where the length of time was quite remarkable.

Another case came to the hospital on the twenty-third day with obstruction of the bowel. The patient, a girl, had been given a certain amount of nourishment. Her abdomen measured thirty-six inches. It was greatly distended. We succeeded in treating the case with the trocar, and withdrew an enormous amount of fluid. She made a good recovery. The cases which have disturbed me are the ones where the obstruction is situated high up, along the upper portion of the rectum. I had a case three years ago in a child who was otherwise healthy, in which obstruction had existed for forty-eight hours. I endeavored to reach the seat of obstruction from below, but did not succeed, and finally resorted to a colostomy. The child lived and did well, and at the end of its second year I opened up from above, made an opening and introduced a good-sized rubber tube down through the perineum, establishing an opening in that way. It did very well for a few months, but the canal insisted on closing. There was no continuity of the intestine, and, as a matter of course, it healed and contracted after a time, but we managed to keep it open by the use of bougies, but it was difficult to do so. At the end of the third year I opened above, dissected a portion of the intestine free, made a good canal, and brought down the intestine, but the operation was possibly too severe, and as a consequence the child died at the end of forty-eight hours.

I remember seeing one case in which the intestine opened down by a continuous sinus on the under surface of the penis. This one I saw when the child was six months old. A discharge had taken place. I made an opening through the perineum, getting into the caliber of the bowel above and establishing good bowel connection in that way. Then I dissected out the sinus below on the under surface of the penis, and had the good fortune to have it unite by stitches, thereby establishing a very good rectum. I saw that boy when he was ten years of age, and he was in good condition.

Dr. John C. Wysor, of Clifton Forge, Virginia.—I want to report a case I had in which there was no sign of an anus or any bulging of the perineum. I operated on this patient, a child, aged two days, doing a left inguinal colostony. This relieved pain and suffering, and the child did very well for about five days, when, during a fit of crying, the stitches gave way and the child died.

I cannot refrain from saying a word or two about chloroform, inasmuch as Dr. McGuire has mentioned it. I attended the New York Polyclinic some years ago. I knew Dr. Wyeth's prejudice in regard to chloroform. Those of you who have read the first edition of his book on surgery will remember what he says of the use of chloroform. He says that a child under the age of six years should be given chloroform in preference to ether, and gives some ten or twenty conditions in which it should be given instead of ether. Some years afterward I was in New York and went to Dr. Wyeth's clinic. It was about a year after a prominent politician died following the administration of ether, and I was surprised to see five or six patients upon whom Dr. Wyeth operated at this chinic were given chloroform. Some of you doubtless remember the controversy between the late Dr. Hunter McGuire and Dr. Wyeth in *Gaillard's Medical Journal* on the relative merits of chloroform and ether. When I asked Dr. Wyeth at his clinic if he had not changed his views recently, he patted me on the shoulder and said, "Yes, doctor, I am ashamed of my narrowness."

GASTROMESENTERIC ILEUS FOLLOWING GASTRO-ENTEROSTOMY.

BY THOMAS *C*. WITHERSPOON, *M.D.*,
Butte, Montana.

IN March of this present year I had an experience with gastromesenteric ileus, so called, which I believe will prove interesting to relate, and I therefore present the details in this paper.

I shall not attempt in any wise to cover the literature upon this important subject nor enter into a polemic discussion. The fact that I performed a gastro-enterostomy, and later, on the ninth day, reopened the abdomen and ascertained fully the existing conditions, makes the case an instructive one, and I believe one which throws a certain shade of light on the question of causation of this important lesion.

The best way to get directly to my subject is to relate the history of this patient. A man, aged forty-nine years, having been a resident of Montana for twenty-eight years, leading an out-door, active life, such as is characteristic of our western sheriff, had been suffering for some while from gastric symptoms which were diagnosticated as resulting from ulcer of the stomach.

On March 25, I made a median incision in the epigastric region and found the ulcer. The portion of the stomach involved was the usual ulcer-bearing area near the pylorus. The stomach was not apparently dilated. The ulcer did not involve the pyloric orifice, but was situated about an inch to the left along the lesser curvature.

The induration was fairly marked. An examination of the neighboring lymph nodes showed no epithelial invasion, so we took it for granted that the lesion was non-malignant.

A short posterior loop gastro-enterostomy was made. The opening, when finished, would easily allow two fingers to invaginate a portion of the wall of the jejunum through the opening into the stomach. Care was taken to stitch the transverse mesocolon to the line of the gastro-enterostomy by interrupted catgut stitches.

Before closing the abdominal opening, the appendix was examined by touch and found to be adherent and slightly thickened. A criss-cross incision was made at the usual site and this organ removed.

The gall bladder was apparently normal and no other lesion could be found. The abdominal wall was closed by catgut in layers; two deep silkworm-gut stitches were introduced for tension and the skin closed with a continuous fine silkworm gut.

There was nothing unusual in the progress of the case for eight full days. The temperature and pulse reached their greatest elevation on the day following the operation, both being at that time 100. He was fed by rectum for four days, then given small quantities of broth by mouth. Later, orangeade with albumin in small sips and beef juice were allowed, and six days after the operation oatmeal gruel was added to the diet list. This diet was adhered to for the remainder of the eight days following the operation. On the morning of the ninth day the temperature was 98°; respirations, 20; pulse, 72. At nine o'clock that morning he began to complain of pain in the region just left of the wound over the costal border and extending round to the back. His temperature and pulse were normal at the time.

The dressings were changed, thinking I might find some reason for the pain. Upon snipping the stitches in several places, I discovered the skin union had not progressed well; in fact, it showed a slight tendency to open. There was, however, no redness nor inflammatory swelling about the wound. He was given a grain of codeine and $\frac{1}{100}$ of atropine about twelve o'clock, at which time he complained of being nauseated and likewise of an increase of pain. There was still no evidence of a dilated stomach.

About 1 P. M. he was resting quietly from the injection. His temperature had fallen at two o'clock to 97.6°, his respirations were 26, but his pulse had gone to 110. Bowel movements were urged by glycerin and afterward by alum injections. I found his pulse at 4.30 had dropped to 96, and at ten o'clock that night to 85.

The patient continued, however, to suffer from the nausea; vomiting became more and more frequent. The vomited matter was at first yellow, later dark. An examination revealed at this time a largely distended stomach; the greater curvature was found below the umbilicus. He refused absolutely to have his stomach washed. At twelve o'clock (midnight) the pulse showed a decided loss in volume, though it had not increased in rate, and as the patient continued to vomit, I decided to reopen the abdominal wound. This was done under ether narcosis. I found no union in the wound, and as the outer silkworm gut and the inner catgut stitches were cut, the walls fell apart. There was a sero-bloody fluid here and there throughout the wound.

The stomach was immensely dilated; in fact, it reached well down to the pelvis. I experienced considerable difficulty in bringing the organ up through the abdominal wound, which was fully five inches long. So great was this difficulty that I increased the size of the wound. I was much impressed with the fact that a dilated stomach was like a great heavy bag, hard to handle and return to its normal position.

The walls were somewhat thinned, but there was nowhere any sign of peritonitis. After bringing the stomach out of the wound in order to allow an exploration of the former field of gastro-enterostomy, I found the union complete in every particular. The transverse mesocolon was firmly united to the line of suture, though the symptoms had led me to fear a hernia at this site. The opening between the jejunum and stomach was just as it was at the end of the operation, that is, it admitted two fingers.

The bowels were flat, contained little or no gas or fecal matter. The portion of the jejunum proximal to the anastomosis was not dilated, nor did it show any pathological change to the eye or touch. The duodenum was not dilated. The pylorus was patulous and the distention was wholly limited to the stomach. Finding this state of affairs, and no evidence of inflammatory or other lesion save an absolute paralytic stomach wall, the question arose, What could I do to relieve the patient? Under the circumstances I decided there was but one course to follow, that was gastrostomy.

A portion of the stomach was brought through an opening to the left of the original incision, between the outer fibers of the rectus muscle. This was opened and drained by means of a large rubber tube. The large incision was closed with through-and-through figure-of-eight silkworm gut stitches. It might be well, in passing, to state that the portion of the stomach wall which was opened and drained was that immediately anterior to the base of the omentum on the anterior floor of the organ. This was sutured in the rectus, split high up, just under the costal arch. Fixing the lower portion of the stomach in this way to the abdominal wall I thought would prevent a return of the viscus toward the pelvis. The fluid in the stomach did not flow through the tube, but had to be pumped out in order to diminish the size of the organ and relieve the pressure upon the surrounding structures.

The tube was connected with a bottle at the side of the bed. Vomiting immediately ceased, and after a primary rise of pulse and temperature to a moderate degree, they returned to normal by the end of thirty-six hours.

The drainage from the tube was not free for several days, indicating a flaccid condition of the organ. It was eight days after the operation when the drainage tube was removed, because the stomach was apparently not able to take care of itself earlier. The mucous membrane of the stomach evaginated into the opening upon removing the tube, and for five days very little drainage took place out of the wound. During this time the patient drank freely of buttermilk, broth albuminades, beef juice, and gruels. The bowels moved freely; stools appeared to be normal.

All pain subsided after this second operation and recovery was uneventful save for the difficulty experienced in causing the gastric fistula to close. This difficulty might seem to be due to a possible obstruction to onward flow from the stomach. Had I not examined the gastro-enterostomy carefully when reopening the abdomen I might have thought so, but this I at least proved to my own satisfaction did not exist. The only explanation of a prolonged recovery from the fistula was the low position of the gastric opening itself, being at the bottom of the viscus. The patient I have lost track of for several months, and do not know his present condition.

The salient features to which I desire to direct attention are these:

1. There existed an ulceration with a catarrhal stomach.

2. A gastro-enterostomy was performed, making a good opening between the stomach and bowel.

3. Following the operation there was absolutely no evidence of stomach or bowel dilatation until the ninth day, and that within twelve hours or thereabouts after that time, the stomach dilatation was so great that its greater curvature reached the pelvic cavity.

4. The stomach at the second operation resembled a large inert bag full of fluid, and after this organ was opened the fluid still remained within its wall and had to be pumped out through a tube.

5. It required about eight days for the stomach to regain its tone so that it could perform its function of propelling its contents onward.

6. There was no attempt at union in the abdominal wound.

7. The reopened wound, which did not heal between the first and second operations, healed quickly and fully without inflammation after the second operation.

The conclusions to which I am led are these:

The gastromesenteric ileus in this case was not due to obstruction. The second operation proved that the opening between the stomach and bowel was still patulous. The pylorous was not at all contracted, nor was the duodenum dilated.

The stomach itself was absolutely paralyzed and incapable of contracting, even after pumping out its fluid contents, and this paralysis lasted fully a week after the gastrostomy.

The lack of union in the abdominal wall, which portion of the wall is supplied by the same spinal segment as that which innervates the stomach, was caused by some trophic changes in the spinal cord.

The only explanation of this apparent lesion of the cord which seems tangible is the one of chemic intoxication, as the question of simple shock from operative procedure was certainly excluded by the lapse of eight full days without symptoms.

The source of this intoxication would seem to be from the alimentary canal itself.

During the eight days of convalescence the patient was allowed some albuminous foods, which possibly constituted the chemic base for such an intoxication.

The lesson, if a lesson might be taught by a single case, is:

1. The uselessness of gastro-enterostomy as a means of drain for a paralyzed stomach.

2. The need of early stomach washing before marked paralysis and dilatation can be detected to relieve tension and possibly to diminish intoxication.

3. If after several washings the stomach continues to dilate, the necessity of making free drain by means of gastrostomy.

4. The necessity of keeping the stomach and bowel as free from alimentary material during the first week or ten days after operative procedures on the alimentary canal as the patient's general condition will allow. I believe the nitrogenous foods are the most harmful.

Having seen a reasonable number of these cases, and believing the majority of gastromesenteric ileus attacks are due to a similar cause, this case throws light on the entire class. I believe it is reasonably apparent that the attack resulted from a trophic change in the spinal segment which has to do with innervating the stomach. The probability is that injury, operative shock, psychic shock, over-feeding, and other causes which upset normal alimentary function or lead to intoxication might bring about this condition. I have for a long time considered the term gastromesenteric ileus misleading, and prefer to look upon the condition as a paralysis of the stomach from a central condition.

Among the many instructive findings which might refer to central lesion are:

The marked quantity of fluid due to secretory activity and the large amount of gas formed in a paralyzed bowel.

A discussion of these, however, would take us beyond the limit of such a paper, and I conclude with the suggestion that every case of gastromesenteric ileus which resists stomach washing should be drained by means of a gastrostomy, and that such a drain be maintained until the stomach wall has regained its tone.

DISCUSSION.

DR. F. GREGORY CONNELL, of Oshkosh, Wisconsin.—The case reported by Dr. Witherspoon is most interesting and instructive, but it would seem as though more benefit would be derived from its study had the condition been called paralysis or dilatation of the stomach, or some equivalent term, instead of gastromesenteric ileus. The condition called gastromesenteric ileus is generally accepted to apply to an obstruction of the duodenum between the vertebra and the root of the mesentery and the superior mesenteric vessels. This is but one of many possible causes of dilatation of the stomach, and was positively absent in the case reported by the essayist, which was undoubtedly of nervous origin. Hence the necessity, in order to avoid confusion, of differentiating between these types of dilatation of the stomach.

DR. WALTER C. G. KIRCHNER, of St. Louis.—Some years ago a great deal of attention was paid to this class of cases, and a number of such conditions were reported under the name of acute dilatation of the stomach. Certain explanations were given for this cause, and one that seemed plausible was traction upon the mesentery, closing off the pyloric orifice, and in this way obstructing the stomach. This traction was supposed to be due to the patient being in Fowler's position, in which position many of these patients were placed. My own opinion is that these conditions are probably of nervous origin, just as Dr. Witherspoon's case would seem to be. In one instance I did a Wertheim operation for cancer. A few days following the operation an acute dilatation of the stomach resulted. The patient's condition became so critical and the pulse so rapid and almost imperceptible that I was afraid to remove the patient from the bed, and so under local anesthesia a gastrotomy was performed, and the patient's condition immediately relieved. A great deal of gas and fluid were drained from the stomach, but from that time on, however, convalescence was uninterrupted. The condition in that case was similar to the one described by Dr. Witherspoon, only in my case the stomach was not quite down to the pelvis. I was led, therefore, to the conclusion, and this is emphasized by the conclusion reached in Dr. Witherspoon's case, that gastro-enterostomy is of little service in these cases. I think the nervous element is the chief feature in this condition.

DR. WITHERSPOON (closing).—I dislike to take up any more of the time of the Association, but I cannot refrain from mentioning one or two points: First, with reference to Dr. Connell's advice in segregating these cases. I would like to know how it is done. Symptomatically, clinically, and surgically they all look alike. As a matter of fact, I have for a long time doubted whether pulling upon the mesentery, thus closing off the duodenum, has anything to do with the condition. I have never seen it demonstrated. The history of these cases is so nearly alike that it seems to me the question of segmental disturbances naturally comes to one's mind, particularly when backed up by clinical history of this kind. One case I am going to report at the meeting of the Western Surgical and Gynecological Association was very much in the same line in which there was obstruction of the bowel. The obstruction was potential and brought about by old and well-marked adhesions. I made an incision in the right rectus, severing its fibers, extending the incision into the territory supplied by the eleventh and twelfth dorsal nerves. The patient recovered, but not until after some days, during which time he suffered from a distended bowel and from a condition which caused us no little degree of mental uneasiness The area supplied by the eleventh and twelfth nerves healed .primarily. The area supplied by the tenth, which area is al so supplied by the same segment of the cord which supplies the bowel, which was involved chiefly about its middle or lower third, did not heal, but opened up, and at the end of twelve days, when the stitches were snipped, the upper wound gaped while the lower part of the wound closed nicely. The upper part of the wound showed the same condition that this case presented. These two cases made me think seriously as to the possibility of this trouble being largely segmental, and the only explanation for such segmental disturbance, it seems to me, not having any other light, is that it is due to a trophic chemical auto-intoxication from the cord itself.

EXTRA-PERITONEAL DRAINAGE AFTER URETERAL ANASTOMOSIS.

By John Egerton Cannaday, *M.D.*,
Charleston, West Virginia.

WHILE the subject of ureteral anastomosis has been most carefully worked out experimentally and otherwise, I do not believe the matter of devising drainage to guard against a possible leakage of urine has received all the attention the subject merits.

It is a well-known surgical fact that wounds of the ureter when made extra-peritoneally and drained, heal readily and give but little trouble; in fact, Van Hook showed experimentally that wounds involving over half the diameter of the ureter unite readily and do not interfere with the normal outflow of urine onward to the bladder. When there is plenty of ureter to spare the invagination method as described by Van Hook is perhaps the simplest and easiest. In suturing the cut ends I have been forcibly reminded of the description given of the ureter by the demonstrator of anatomy in my student days, when he said the diameter of the ureter was about that of a goose quill plucked from a crow's wing; however, it is a little larger than that.

I had felt for some time that if cases of ureteral anastomosis could be treated as extra-peritoneal wounds and drained, the results would be bettered. I append an illustrative case.

Thelma W., a robust young demimondaine about twenty-five years of age, had been suffering for two years or more with chronic salpingitis following an acute attack. There had been a most active adhesive process, and the left ureter had been drawn up for at least one and one-half inches from its normal bed, an apparent adhesion band across an inflammatory mass. The condition of the uterus and adnexæ were such that a hysterectomy was done. The incision was carried low down so that only a small portion of the cervix was left. One inch of the ureter was removed. The cut ends of the ureter were recognized, and since they were not long enough for lateral anastomosis, an end-to-end anastomosis was decided on. For the purpose of making certain that the structure was ureter, a probe was passed upward toward the kidney, then downward into the bladder. The cut ends of the ureter were easily held in position for suturing by the small hemostats devised by Crile for bloodvessel anastomosis. A small probe passed into either cut end of the ureter helped materially in placing the fine sutures of anastomosis at the proper points. The ends were easily approximated and united with eight No. 00 catgut sutures. A stab wound was made just mesial to the anterior superior spine of the ilium. In the left lateral portion of the pelvis the removal of the remains of an adherent cystic ovary and a badly adherent distorted tube had left a considerable raw surface. Above, however, a fair-sized apron of parietal peritoneum was preserved.

After a good-sized, split-rubber drainage tube with a gauze wick had been carried through the stab wound and extra-peritoneally down to a point near the point of union of the ureter, I began to cover the abdominal end of the drainage tube and the ureteral anastomosis by suturing closely a portion of the lower sigmoid to the flap of parietal peritoneum with fine catgut. This was continued until the ureteral wound and the drain were rendered entirely extra-peritoneal. The first layer of suture was reënforced by a second row. All denuded areas were carefully covered with peritoneum and the clean abdominal wound was closed without drainage.

For fear of possible urinary extravasation and infection

the patient was kept in a sitting position for forty-eight hours. There was evidently a slight leakage of urine, for the patient's temperature rose to 103° F., and fluctuated for three or four days. The rubber-tube drain was removed in thirty hours and a small gauze strip inserted in its place. In twenty-four hours this was removed. The drainage stopped almost immediately after this and the patient made an uneventful recovery. She left the hospital against orders the seventh day. The tenth day there was a rise of temperature one degree above the normal, and the patient had a severe cramping pain localized in the line of the ureter. Morphine hypodermically was required to relieve the pain. From that time to the present, four months, the patient has been in perfect health.

In case of suture of the right ureter, rectum and parietal peritoneum could easily be made use of to bury the ureter. When one can drain the vicinity of the anastomosis, the dangers of leakage from imperfect coaptation and of secondary leakage from sloughing are largely obviated.

DISCUSSION.

DR. HOWARD A. KELLY, of Baltimore.—I do not think we ought ever to close up a wound with the ureter sutured without drainage of some sort, as there is apt to be a little leakage at some time—temporarily at least. I think when the ureter is divided and is to be anastomosed, the best method of anastomosing it is to take the lower end and slit it. If this represents the lower end (illustrating on the blackboard) of the ureter, slit it down and then run a suture through the upper end, so that when you tie the suture you close it. You can run a grooved director through the lower end, take a needle threaded with the suture, then pass it through the upper end and bring it well down the ureter. That enables you to pull the ureter down into the divided lower end. You can suture this round and round to the ureter, which is invaginated into it, and the slit opening prevents any constriction. I think that is the simplest and most rapid way of reuniting it, but I fully agree with the author of the paper that if we drain we ought to do so extraperitoneally.

DR. RUFUS B. HALL, of Cincinnati.—I want to emphasize what the last speaker (Dr. Kelly) has said with reference to drainage. Dr. Cannady's patient evidently, from her temperature, had a little leakage into the peritoneal cavity, and abdominal drainage plus the other for a few hours would undoubtedly have obviated this rise of temperature. If he had not done such good surgery he probably would have lost his patient without the abdominal drainage.

DR. J. WESLEY BOVEE, of Washington D. C.—The first ureteral anastomosis I did was done without drainage, and there was no trouble from it. The woman had no symptoms referable to the anastomosis. The operation was done fourteen years ago.

In the other operations I have done I have drained, but I have not had any leakage, and it seems to me we can suture the duct without any drainage. Of course, a good deal depends upon the character of the urine, and I believe many times we can safely drain intraperitoneally. We may have a pus case, or one with adhesions, when we think of draining intraperitoneally, and under such circumstances we can safely trust to the intraperitoneal drainage instead of establishing drainage extraperitoneally in addition.

I am not in favor of trying to suture through the lower portion of the ureter to draw the segment of duct inward. I believe that an end-to-end anastomosis does very well, it answers quite satisfactorily, and probably is applicable in a larger number of cases than any other form of anastomosis. We find so many cases in which so much continuity of structure has been removed accidentally that it is with difficulty we can draw one into the other. It is advisable in such cases to draw it in a trifle on account of tension, and this is the class of cases in which drainage is advisable. There is an additional difficulty in drainage, and that is, we are apt to put drainage against the wound in the ureter, and that is inadvisable. If we put in drainage we should have it lay loosely, close to the ureter, but not against it.

DR. J. SHELTON HORSLEY, of Richmond.—There is one point I wish to call attention to—the danger of extraperitoneal drainage after ureteral anastomosis. This was emphasized by a case reported by a surgeon of the Mt. Sinai

Hospital, New York. He operated and removed a stone from each ureter and drained extraperitoneally with a tube, and in each case a terrific hemorrhage followed within a few days from ulceration into the iliac artery. The iliac artery was ligated on both sides, and the patient fortunately recovered. There is, therefore, considerable danger attending extraperitoneal drainage with a rubber tube in these cases.

DR. CANNADY (closing).—In this particular case there was not sufficient ureteral tissue to do an anastomosis by the invagination method. If that was the case I should have done it in that way, because it is the easiest way to do an anastomosis. I do not believe it to be the best way, because in doing an end-to-end anastomosis we get approximation of like anatomical structures.

The reason for not draining in this case intraperitoneally was because it was a clean case and there was no reason for that method of drainage.

SKIN STERILIZATION BY TINCTURE OF IODINE.

By I. S. Stone, M.D.,
Washington, D. C.

During the past decade we have been using the tincture of iodine as an antiseptic with constantly increasing satisfaction. Its penetrating quality and efficiency, with almost entirely non-toxic action, renders it free from many of the objections raised against the antiseptics in general use. In the work in the gynecological department of Columbia Hospital the surgeons long since abandoned the disagreeable iodoform, and it is absolutely certain that one never needs this drug in gynecological practice. Since Claudius exploited his method of sterilizing catgut, we have had the greatest satisfaction in relying upon iodine for every possible use instead of all other so-called antiseptics, especially in the various conditions requiring sterilization of the interior of the uterus and vagina, including all vaginal operations, and we have never had cause to regret the practice. Our attention was called to the use of iodine for sterilizing the skin by a paper written by Antonio Grossich, of Fiume, published in the *Centralblatt für Chirurgie*, October 31, 1908, No. 44, p. 1289.

The essential facts in this paper are as follows: Grossich had been using iodine in emergency surgery for a year before he commenced its use in all kinds of surgical work. He found that soap and water cleansing of injured fingers and hands was followed by redness and infection, even when the usual antiseptics were applied, and that those treated by iodine applications healed without these complications, or, in other words, by primary union. He then began to use the method in all classes of cases with dry shaving, but without further preparation, before applying the tincture of iodine, and always had perfect healing. He then made careful microscopic examinations, in order to ascertain the cause of this difference in results. He alludes to the development of the superficial layers of the skin and their elevation and separation from the basal layers. The spaces between these layers are occupied by the various forms of bacteria, fat, sweat, etc. The inter- and intracellular capillary and lymph spaces all communicate with these layers of epithelium, and it is conclusively shown that iodine penetrates into all of these various clefts and openings of the skin. The alcohol of the tincture dissolves the fat which is always found in the capillary spaces, while iodine has a special penetrative quality of its own, and forms a chemical combination with the fatty acids of the skin, which combination is quickly absorbed. The soap and water cleansing is wrong in principle, or at least the skin thus prepared is harder to disinfect, because, first, the loose epidermic scales are made to close the spaces which contain bacteria, and secondly, these spaces are filled with the soap solution, which prevents the entrance of the antiseptic solution. The particles of soap cannot easily be washed away with water, and actually form a protective coating for the germs which are hidden beneath. Grossich gives his house patients a bath the day before operation, dresses them in fresh linen, and applies the iodine just before operation. He is convinced that iodine gives the best skin sterilization and absolutely prevents infection from the side of the patient. He gives a final application of iodine after closing the wound, just before placing the usual dry gauze dressings. On the seventh day he removes the sutures, and the patient generally leaves the hospital on the day following. In our hospital work we follow the above plan, and have seen no unpleasant results save some blisters from the use of a strong tincture of iodine. We certainly have seen no case of wound infection in a clean, non-infected case.

Since the paper by Grossich the subject has been taken up by many surgeons, and we have yet to hear of any unfavorable or undesirable results. The most elaborate study of the effect of iodine upon the skin and its complex elements, together with the resident bacteria, has been undertaken by Walther, of Paris (see *Bull. et Mém. de la Soc. de Chirurg.*, March 16, 1909, p. 345, etc.). Walther has contributed a most valuable paper, which has apparently withstood the criticism of the surgical society of Paris without yielding an inch from the main position announced by Grossich. He has not only found the claims made to be correct in clinical work, but also in a histological and bacteriological way. Sections of skin were cut after treatment with iodine, which was subjected to precipitation by means of a solution of nitrate of silver. This precipitation he has used to show in microphotographs how far the iodine penetration extends. His beautifully illustrated article must carry conviction to those who may read the interesting lines.

The experiments of Walther show that the bacteria usually found in the skin require several minutes for complete sterilization. He obtained growths in culture media after five minutes, but never after eight minutes of preliminary treatment of the skin by the tincture of iodine. He therefore advises waiting ten minutes before making the incision. Walther finds it absolutely safe to waive preliminary skin washing with soap and water, alcohol, etc., but finds the use of ether advisable, since the skin is penetrated deeper by iodine after it has been washed with ether. He has used the skin of patients and that of guinea-pigs to test the penetrative power of iodine, and he summarizes his results as follows: The skin is painted with iodine and sections made which are placed in a solution of nitrate of silver to precipitate the iodide of silver in the tissues. The application of iodine alone without previous use of soap and water affords a thorough disinfection, as shown by the microscopic and bacterial examination. Every available space and cleft is reached. The granulations of iodide of silver are abundant in the epidermis, and especially in the germinative clefts (couches germinatives), the hair follicles, even those most deeply situated in the thickness of the dermis, are strongly impregnated by the iodide of silver. On the contrary, the sections having been cut from the skin which had been previously soaped, while in most respects satisfactory as to superficial layers, although more irregular, do not show the iodide of silver granulations in the deep capillary follicles, and hence the sterilization is not so complete as with the previous method.

Tincture of iodine is made by adding 70 grams iodine and 50 grams iodide potassium to 1000 c.c. of alcohol, 95 per cent. (or rather add gradually until the whole amount equals 1000 c.c.). The exact strength of the solution used by different surgeons varies greatly. In our work we are satisfied as yet to use 25 per cent. of the tincture for ordinary skin sterilization, but have a weak solution—3j of tincture to Oj water—for ordinary uses, such as vaginal cleansing preliminary to plastic operations.

The advantages of this method of sterilization are apparent to everyone who desires a safe, sure, and speedy method of skin sterilization, as in emergency surgery. It is quite possible that thirty seconds is long enough for ordinary plastic work, and the sterilization is as effective as that by the use of mercuric bichloride, 1 to 1000 solution, applied for a much longer time. There are many good reasons for the use of a better method of skin sterilization, the chief of which are as follows:

1. To save time. The patient is ready for operation immediately after sleep is induced by the anesthetic. No

time is spent in washing, etc., which to be effective requires at least ten minutes.

2. The patient may be kept warm and dry during the entire seance, including the time of anesthesia and operation.

3. If the incision must be extended, or one made in another place, this quick method is most desirable.

4. The operator's hands may be sterilized with iodine, as the stain can be removed by a weak solution of aqua ammoniæ.

LITERATURE. The use of iodine for skin sterilization is well described in the two papers mentioned below, and we hesitate to mention many others, notably by American authors, however confirmatory their character, because we could only prolong our contribution. Grossich, Antonio (Fiume), *Zent. f. Chirurg.*, 1908, October 31, No. 44, p, 1289; Walthar (Paris), *Bull. et Mém. de la Soc. Chir.*, March 16, 1909, p. 345 *et seq.*

DISCUSSION.

DR. HOWARD A. KELLY, of Baltimore.—If, as Dr. Stone has said, the other method of sterilization of the skin commonly used succeeds in 99 per cent. of the cases, with only one failure, why not continue the commonly used method in the 99 per cent. and use the method of iodine sterilization of the skin in the 1 per cent. that remains?

DR. J. WESLEY BOVEE, of Washington, D. C.—Since I came back from my summer vacation I have been using iodine for sterilizing the field of operation exclusively in my work. The method I have employed was suggested by Porter, a British army surgeon, and based upon Grossich's plan. When you have a field that needs shaving, shave it a sufficient time before operation for the water that you use in the process to completely dry out of the skin before you use the iodine. In abdominal operations I have followed this plan: The patient is shaved in the afternoon on the day previous to the operation. When the patient comes to the anesthetizing table she gets the first painting of tincture of iodine, and when I am ready to make the incision she gets the second coating. There is no scrubbing or any other preparation whatever. From the time of the shaving to the time of the first application there is no protection to the surface any more than on the face after shaving. I have prevented blistering, I think, thus far by using alcohol when the wound is closed to take up the iodine. In the first place, you will find the iodine fades away along the line of incision. When the fluids are brought in contact with the skin about the incision, the solution will dilute the iodine at the line of incision, and there is not so much danger of injury. As soon as I finish the operation I take alcohol on a piece of gauze and soak the surfaces farther away from the line of incision, and, in my judgment, that lessens the tendency toward injury by the strong iodine. This is applicable in so many ways that I have been impressed with its usefulness. In the first place, there is less time required in the preparation of patients. One night, in a case of ectopic pregnancy, in which the abdomen contained the largest amount of blood I have ever seen in any condition whatever, and in which there was only 10 per cent. hemoglobin and 1,130,000 red corpuscles, with an immensely distended abdomen, I went to the hospital as soon as I could, examined the woman, had her taken to the operating room, and after sterilizing the skin with iodine I operated with a gratifying result. We used salt solution in the vein. I have been much pleased with this method of preparation, and I expect I shall use it exclusively unless something comes up which makes me believe it is not an advantage over former methods of preparation which I have employed.

DR. HALL.—Do you use full strength?

DR. BOVEE.—Yes—of the official tincture.

DR. THOMAS C. WITHERSPOON, of Butte, Montana.—I feel that it would not be wise to let what has been said in this paper go absolutely unchallenged, because I have had experience which makes me feel that iodine is not as trustworthy as we have thought it to be in the past.

About two years ago I adopted the rule of sterilizing the catgut with the well-known 1 per cent. iodine solution, and I used also as an adjunct the sterilization method proposed by Dr. Willard Bartlett, of sterilizing it in hot vaseline or oil. I had my catgut arranged in little jars. On one Thursday night I had to operate for general peritonitis in a young woman who had brought on infection by criminal abortion. She suffered from streptococcic peritonitis. While I was operating I called for a dressing forceps to insert a rubber tube as a suprapubic drain into the lower part of the pelvis, and the nurse, who was most efficient and careful in that sort of thing, handed me the forceps to introduce this tube, which became infected. She had not noticed the slight smear on the forceps when I put them down. The following Monday I was called upon to do three operations, in which I used No. 2 catgut, one of the cases being a simple appendectomy. The case progressed nicely for thirty-six hours and then developed evidences of general peritonitis. On making a suprapubic opening for the purpose of draining, on examining the pus I found streptococcic infection. I operated on two other cases, one a case of appendectomy, in which drainage was resorted to, and the other a case of ununited fracture, where I cut down on the fracture and united it, using No. 2 catgut to sew up the connective tissue about the bone. In each case I had infection. I then made a painstaking and careful examination, and found that in jar No. 2, from which this nurse had removed a piece of catgut, I had infection of most of the strands of catgut in that jar, and the bacteria grew actively on agar-agar and gelatin culture-media. That case was operated on Thursday night for streptococcic general peritonitis. This nurse removed a loop of gut with forceps from the jar, and I did not see that she had used the infected forceps, and the next time I saw the jar was on Monday. In the meantime the catgut had remained in a 1 per cent. solution over Friday, Saturday, and Sunday, and certainly if iodine had been an efficient sterilizing agent with this infection it would have removed the possibility of such an occurrence. I had infection in the three cases, and that the source of my infection was the catgut was proved by culture experiments.

Dr. Stone (closing).—As to what Dr. Witherspoon has said about the catgut, I should simply say we do not know whether the catgut was the cause of the infection he speaks of or not. I should be inclined to think, however, that one case like the one he mentioned does not prove that iodine in the proper strength fails as a sterilizing agent to inhibit bacterial growth. Additional evidence is necessary to establish that fact. In regard to the matter of cleansing, Dr. Bovée has emphasized what I said in my paper, namely, that iodine sterilization of the skin has an advantage over the former method of scrubbing. We know that scrubbing causes maceration of the skin and fills the pores with soap and epithelium, so that it is impossible for antiseptics to enter. That is the reason why, as a groundwork, sterilization of the skin by iodine is superior, because it does enter and penetrate deeper into the skin than any other known chemical agent.

A LARGE CYSTIC TUMOR DEVELOPING FROM THE ILIOPSOAS BURSA, CONTAINING LARGE FREE CARTILAGINOUS MASSES, AND COMMUNICATING WITH THE HIP-JOINT.

By Thomas S. Cullen,
Baltimore, Maryland.

In November, 1908, I was asked by Dr. A. H. A. Mayer to examine a man, aged forty-six years, who had what appeared to be a very unusual pelvic tumor. About ten years before, the patient had begun to limp, and a year later consulted a physician, who told him that he had a tumor of the left hip. The condition gradually had become worse. For about a year the man had noticed that every time he put his weight on his left leg "something slipped in his hip."

The patient was a tall, rather anemic-looking man. The chest sounds were normal. The left leg was stiff and when walking he held the left hip-joint as immobile as possible. Occupying the left iliac fossa and extending beyond the median line was a firm oval mass, 8 by 10 cm. This was continuous with a smaller mass which passed below Poupart's ligament and extended to the left of the hip-joint anteriorly. The large mass seemed to fill the left half of the pelvis. In some places it appeared to consist of bone, but at other points felt cystic. It seemed to be intimately connected with the pelvic bone. The glands in both groins were palpable.

The left leg was three-quarters of an inch shorter than the right. On flexion of the leg the pelvic mass receded somewhat, but on extension the tumor again became prominent. Flexion, extension, adduction, and abduction were accompanied by a dull crepitation in or near the hip-joint. On carefully questioning the patient, it was learned that the swelling had been first noticed just below Poupart's ligament.

OPERATION. An incision was made just above and parallel with Poupart's ligament and the extraperitoneal tumor exposed. After displacing the anterior crural nerve, which was markedly stretched over the tumor, and splitting the muscle which lay over it, it was found necessary to sever Poupart's ligament, as a portion of the tumor lay beneath it. The pelvic portion of the mass was loosened up easily on its anterior and posterior aspects, but on the outer side was firmly attached to the ilium, and below seemed intimately related to the anterior portion of the hip-joint. After being walled off with gauze it was opened and there was an escape of clear viscid fluid, yellowish in color. Lying free in the cavity were five irregularly lobulated, hard, cartilaginous masses (Figs. 1 and 3). After these had been removed a sixth was found fastened down beneath Poupart's ligament. When this nodule had been taken out, a finger carried downward and forward passed directly into the hip-joint anterior to the head of the femur. The bones of the joint were perfectly smooth.

The pelvic sac was gradually dissected free at a point considerably below Poupart's ligament. It was then cut away and the remaining portion which formed the margin of the entrance into the joint was trimmed, turned in on itself, and snugly brought together with catgut sutures, thus securely closing the hip-joint. A small drain was laid in the upper angle of the wound far removed from the joint and the incision closed.

For a few days the patient did remarkably well, but then became delirious and talked incoherently. It was learned that on a previous occasion he had shown similar cerebral disturbances, and that it had been necessary to confine him for a time in a sanitarium. Dr. Henry J. Berkley, who saw him in consultation, felt that his mental condition had nothing to do with the operation. The wound, after draining for a few days, closed completely, and the patient left the hospital in excellent physical and mental condition five and one-half weeks afterward. He was able to walk without much difficulty.

December 6, 1909, Dr. Mayer informed me that the patient occasionally has some discomfort in his leg, but no pain in the hip-joint. He still uses a cane.

DESCRIPTION OF SPECIMEN. The walls of the sac were composed of fibrous tissue, and scattered throughout them were plaques of cartilage and definite bony masses (Figs. 1 and 2). Some of these fragments of bone were very small; others reached 3 cm. or more in diameter. The inner surface of the sac presented a trabeculated appearance (Fig. 2), evidently due to the unequal and gradual distention of the cystic tumor. Notwithstanding the uneven appearance, the inner surface was everywhere covered by a smooth membrane. The fluid contents were clear, yellowish in color, and rather sticky.

The six irregular, white, cartilaginous masses filling the cavity are shown in their natural size in Fig. 3. They were lying perfectly free, and five of them popped out as soon as the sac was opened. The sixth could not escape, as it was firmly held down by Poupart's ligament, and its lower end entered the hip-joint.[1]

ORIGIN OF THESE CYSTIC TUMORS. One of the largest, if not the largest, bursa in the body is that situated beneath

[1] The specimens were demonstrated to the class and then drawn. During my absence in Europe they were unfortunately mislaid, and have not yet been located; consequently, have thus far been unable to make a careful histological examination to determine definitely whether the central portion of the cartilaginous masses contained bone or not.

the tendon of the iliopsoas muscle. This complex muscle arises from the body of the twelve dorsal vertebra, from the bodies of all the lumbar vertebræ, from the transverse processes of all the lumbar vertebræ, and from the iliac fossa. The combined tendon is inserted in the trochanter minor. In order to reach this the iliopsoas muscle must curve around the crest of the ilium. It is beneath the muscle where it curves over the bone that the bursa is found. It lies beneath Poupart's ligament below and lateral to the iliopectineal eminence. According to some authors, it may attain the size of a hen's egg.

According to Joessel,[1] the iliopsoas bursa or the bursa mucosa subiliaca lies between the partly tendinous portion of the iliac muscle and the front of the iliopectineal eminence. Anteriorly it is firmly attached to the iliopsoas muscle, posteriorly to the iliopectineal eminence, and likewise to the thin portion of the capsule of the hip-joint. This thin spot is well seen in Fig. 232 of Cunningham's *Anatomy*, 1909, page 296. It is bounded on the outer side by the iliofemoral ligament, below by the pubofemoral ligament, and on the inner side by the cotyloid ligament.

Joessel further finds that occasionally the fibrous capsule at the thin point of the joint is wanting and then nothing but the synovial membrane separates the joint from the bursa. Occasionally the synovial membrane is lacking at the thin point, and in these cases there is a direct communication between the hip-joint and the bursa. This opening explains how purulent accumulations of the joint may extend to the iliopsoas bursa and then appear under the iliopsoas muscle, and also how psoas abscesses may travel down the muscle and eventually cause involvement of the hip-joint. An extended consideration of the subject would necessitate a discussion of practically all diseases of the hip, and would naturally lead us too far afield. I

[1] Topographisch-Chirurgische Anatomie, Band i, S. 169.

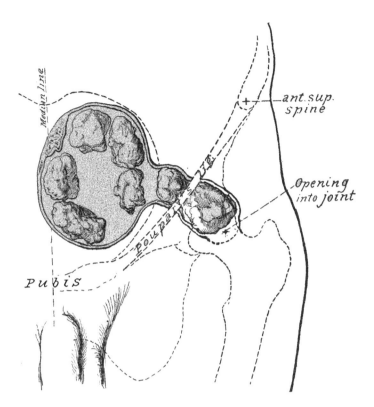

FIG. 1.—A cystic tumor developing from the left iliopsoas bursa containing large free cartilaginous masses and communicating with the hip-joint. Occupying the left half of the pelvis is a cystic tumor which on its outer side was firmly attached to the pelvic wall. The cyst walls were composed chiefly of fibrous tissue. The thickening in certain areas noted in the walls is due to deposits of bone. The cyst cavity was distended with clear, yellowish, tenacious fluid, and also contained five free and irregular cartilaginous masses. A narrow prolongation of the cyst passed downward and forward beneath Poupart's ligament and opened directly into the hip-joint. Filling this portion of the cyst was a large free cartilaginous mass. All the cartilaginous masses are shown in their natural size in Fig. 3.

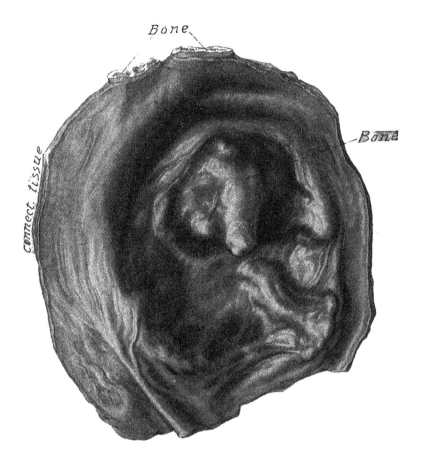

Fig. 2.—Part of the sac of a cystic tumor developing from the iliopsoas bursa. The picture represents the inner surface of the cyst. The walls vary from 1 to 2 mm. in thickness, and in them are seen cross sections of plaques of bone. In other portions of the walls cartilage was noted. The inner surface presented a distinctly trabeculated appearance evidently due to the uneven stretching of the sac. Projecting into the cavity is an irregular bony mass fully 3 cm. in diameter. The sac was lined with a smooth glistening membrane; it contained clear, yellow tenacious fluid and the six cartilaginous masses depicted in Fig. 3.

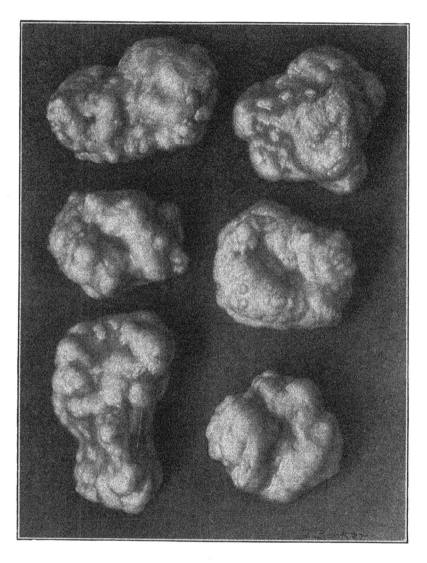

FIG. 3.—Cartilaginous masses lying free in a cystic tumor developing from the iliopsoas bursa (natural size). These masses were pearly white, very irregular, but perfectly smooth. They were rather lighter in weight than bone. Their general arrangement in the cyst is shown in Fig. 1.

shall consequently limit my remarks chiefly to those cases in which cystic tumors similar to this have been noted, and in which little or no evidence of inflammation has existed.

When consulting the literature I found a most instructive and painstaking article on "Diseases of the Bursæ of the Hip," by R. Zuelzer.[1] I have examined in the original the references given by this author, and have found them in the main so well epitomized that I shall draw largely on his descriptions and conclusions.

It has been noted that the bursæ that are regularly found are usually developed during fetal life, while the less constant ones appear at a later date. Virchow and Schuchardt found that the small subcutaneous bursæ developed out of a connective-tissue network resembling cavernous tissue. Eventually a cavity was formed, in which, as a result of the continuous movements and rubbing, the connective tissue gradually atrophied. The walls of these bursæ consist of dense connective tissue, and contain very little elastic tissue. The inner surface is lined with one layer of so-called endothelium, and the contents of the bursa resemble those of the joint. They are slightly tenacious, thick, and usually just enough in amount to keep the walls of the sac smooth.[2]

Cases of Cystic Development of the Iliopsoas Bursa as Collected by Zuelzer.

Hoffa. The patient, a workman, was struck on the right foot and the left arm. He walked home at once, a distance of about two miles, remained without treatment for fourteen days, and again went to work. A year later he com-

---

[1] *Deutsche Zeitschrift f. Chirurgie*, Band 1, 1899.

[2] Those interested in the development of bursæ should not fail to read the excellent paper on Luetic Bursopathy of Verneuil, by Dr. John W. Churchman, resident surgeon in the Johns Hopkins Hospital (The American Journal of the *Medical* Sciences, September, 1909).

plained of pain in the region of the right hip. On examination the leg was found slightly flexed, abducted, and rotated outward. At the hip was a painful tumor which was clearly visible and palpable; it lay under Poupart's ligament between the psoas and the pectineus muscles, and was of the consistence of bone. On flexion of the leg, however, fluctuation could be detected. The trochanter was in its normal position, and movements of the hip-joint were easily made. Abduction, flexion, and rotation inward were, however, somewhat limited. The pain extended down to the knee. The corresponding leg was somewhat thinner than the other. This case was diagnosed by a colleague as an impacted fracture of the neck of the femur, and the tumor was thought to be a callus formation which was pressing on the crural nerve and causing pain. There was no shortening of the leg.

Ehrle. A cooper, aged thirty-three years, for thirteen years had suffered with pain in the leg and down its inner side. Four months before coming under observation he noticed a tumor situated slightly below Poupart's ligament. This was ovoid in shape and lay under the large vessels. On extension of the leg the tumor became hard. On flexion fluid could be detected. Extension and rotation outward produced pain. By flexion it was clearly seen that the psoas muscle was lifted up. The hip-joint was free.

Herdtmann. The patient had been squeezed between two cars, the chief pressure coming on the left hip. The patient was carefully watched, as he was supposed to be a malingerer. On examination, however, a painful swelling of the bursa beneath the tendon of the iliopsoas muscle was found. Flexion of the leg or rotation inward caused much pain in the joint.

Mommsen. This surgeon saw a patient who had an elevated, clearly fluctuating, painless tumor which projected from the region of the iliopsoas muscle and passed out beneath Poupart's ligament. It lifted up the femoral artery. On pressure the tumor diminished in size.

Mommsen. The same author reported a case of a man, fifty years old, who without apparent trauma complained of difficulty in walking on account of a gradually increasing swelling in the right inguinal region. The tumor was as large as two fists and was situated deep in the right iliac fossa. It was firm in consistency and only slightly movable. It was thought to be a sarcoma of the fascia of the hip. At operation its lower pole was found firmly attached to the capsule of the joint. The cyst walls varied from 3 to 5 mm. in thickness and the failure to detect fluctuation was due to overdistention of the cyst.

Schäfer. The patient, a man coming to Volkmann's clinic, complained of a tumor the size of a child's head situated at the flexion of the thigh and lying under Poupart's ligament. The man had fallen and injured his hip a year and a half before. The tumor projected only slightly above the normal skin surface. It was buried deeply in the muscle of the thigh, was elongate oval, and followed the long axis of the psoas muscle. The thigh was markedly flexed. When the leg was extended the tissue was of stony hardness. With extensive flexion some fluctuation could be detected. A second tumor, the size of an apple, was present at the edge of the gluteus maximus. This tumor also on extension was tense, but on flexion of the hip it became softer. Its contents could be made to disappear, and, as a result, the anterior tumor became more distended. The cystic tumors communicated with one another. The movement of the hip-joint was free. The pain radiated from the hip to the knee.

Fricke. This author described a case of a carter who, without apparent cause, had a tumor in the hip region. It lay over the right trochanter and passed inward under Poupart's ligament and extended downward over the upper third of the thigh. It really formed three tumors. The outer portion was as large as a child's head and markedly distended. The second lay on the inner side of the thigh, and the third, the smallest, lay between them. All three fluctuated, and the fluid could be pressed from one tumor into the other. The position of the thigh was normal, but movement of the hip was impossible on account of the severe pain which was caused, especially by flexion and rotation. The tumor itself was not painful on pressure, but pain was reflected down to the knee.

Heineke observed a case in the Greifswald clinic in which, after a rheumatic inflammation of the hip-joint, a very prominent and distinctly fluctuating tumor developed. This followed the direction of the iliopsoas muscle from Poupart's ligament downward and raised up the femoral artery. On pressure the tumor diminished, but on removal of the pressure the tumor again became prominent. Passive motion of the hip-joint was free and painless. In this case there was accumulation of fluid in the iliac bursa, and this communicated with the hip-joint, which also contained an excess of fluid.

Wood[1] reported a case in a thin man, twenty-eight years old, who two years previously, while convalescing from typhoid fever, had sprained his left hip. Walking was associated with severe pain. Six weeks later he noticed a swelling in this region. There was swelling both in front of and behind the hip, and fluctuation was definite. A diagnosis of gluteal abscess was made. The patient, on account of well-marked contraction of the iliopsoas muscle, was unable to extend the leg. The tumor ruptured, and there was a spontaneous expulsion of particles of bone as large as beans. The hip-joint was freely movable and not painful. This is one of the very few cases in which the bursa contained foreign bodies.

[1] This is the only case of Zuelzer's that I could not confirm, as the reference is incorrect, and consequently I have not been able to obtain Wood's original article. I was unable to trace the case either in the Index Medicus or the Index Catalogue of the Surgeon-General's Library.

Couteaud. This patient was a man, aged thirty-one, who was very strong and who had done heavy work. Six years previously he had had syphilis In the left inguinal region and on the inner side of the thigh was a prominent tumor the size of an egg. This was smooth, rounded, painless, and could not be made to disappear. The skin over it was freely movable. On examination fluid could be detected in the pelvis, and this fluctuation communicated with the tumor. The hip-joint was normal. The tumor was punctured, and clear, citron-yellow, slightly tenacious fluid came away. In this case the chief pain was in the region of the knee.

Since Zuelzer's paper several cases have been recorded. The most interesting one is that of Delbet.[1] This surgeon gives a very short account of a case in which he diagnosticated a cystic tumor of the iliopsoas bursa (a hygroma) before operation. On opening the sac he found three foreign bodies, each of which was the size of a large nut.

DIAGNOSIS. In summing up his article, Zuelzer points out that these tumors may be of various sizes, and that the swelling indicates primarily the anatomic position of the subiliac bursa. As the tumor increases it may extend far below Poupart's ligament, sometimes reaching to the middle of the thigh. It may consist of one tumor or be made up of several. It may spread out on either side of the iliopsoas muscle or extend in various directions, and may communicate with the joint. When more than one tumor exists it is often possible to press the fluid from one tumor into another. On releasing the pressure the fluid at once comes back. The tumor may extend forward beneath Poupart's ligament and then backward along the course of the iliopsoas muscle, as in our case.

In some cases fluctuation can be detected, but in others

[1] Corps étranger contenu dans un hygroma de la bourse du psoas, Bull. et. Mém. de la Soc. de Chir. de *Paris*, N. S., t. xxviii, 1902, p. 1264.

the tension is so marked, or the cyst walls so thick, that the tumor is supposed to be solid.

The skin is, as a rule, freely movable over these tumors, provided inflammatory conditions are absent. Many of the tumors are painless, but when one remembers that the growth develops beneath the crural nerve and puts it on marked tension, as in the case reported, it is but natural that any excessive movement of the hip-joint should be accompanied not only by local pain, but also by pain referred to the knee.

Zuelzer found that the typical position of the leg in these cases is in abduction, outer rotation, and slight flexion of the hip. In this position there is naturally a minimum tension on the crural nerve and on the iliopsoas muscle. In these cases the hip-joint is, as a rule, perfectly normal, the great trochanter bears its normal relation, and there is no shortening of the leg. In this way it is possible to exclude completely fracture of the neck of the femur, luxation and diseases of the hip. In my case there was three-quarters of an inch shortening. The joint itself was perfectly normal.

ETIOLOGY. The majority of these cases have followed some injury, although syphilis and rheumatism are also supposed to be contributing factors. In my case the connective-tissue walls of the cyst contained bone. This should occasion no surprise, as this fibrous tissue is similar to and continuous with that forming the joint. The presence of large free foreign bodies in the sac is most unusual, but when we remember that small, free cartilaginous bodies are not infrequently found in the knee-joint, it should not appear strange that a sac communicating with the hip-joint might contain similar products. The foreign bodies, in the case reported, however, were exceptionally large.

TREATMENT. In times past local applications were sometimes made; at a later date some of the tumors were aspirated, but the fluid tended to return. In cases similar to mine complete removal of the sac is the only satisfactory solution of the problem. Here it was necessary not only to get rid of the secreting surface, but also to remove the large free foreign bodies. Under no circumstances should irritants be injected into the sac, as was formerly done. The surgeon cannot, as a rule, determine definitely before operation whether these bursæ communicate with the joint or not. The results from operative treatment should be most satisfactory.

Monroe's beautiful atlas containing a description of all the "Bursæ Mucosæ" of the human body, published in Edinburgh in 1788, should be read by every surgeon. It will undoubtedly stimulate increased study of this subject and materially help to clear up many imperfectly understood conditions originating in the bursæ in various parts of the body.

DISCUSSION.

Dr. John C. Munro, of Boston.—I have been very much interested in Dr. Cullen's paper, and wish to say that Dr. Lund has had three cases similar to his in the last year or so, but whether he found cartilaginous or solid bodies I do not know.

Dr. Cullen (closing).—I think that since the attention of the profession has now been drawn to this subject more cases will be found and reported.

A SIMPLE METHOD OF EXCISING VARICOSE VEINS.

By William S. Goldsmith, *M.D.*,
Atlanta, Georgia.

THE function and location of the superficial veins of the lower extremity expose them to varying degrees of dilatation not usually existing in the deeper group and rarely seen elsewhere except in the veins of the scrotum and rectum. The relationship of the scrotum and testes and the influence of the sphincter ani and portal circulation explain in part the etiology of varicocele and hemorrhoids.

But the varicosities of the saphena, for instance, are not dependent upon the vacillating changes of the digestive system or any deviation from a normal sexual apparatus.

As etiological factors it is difficult to fasten upon any one or more clearly defined causes. The matter of age, sex, occupation, or remote physical conditions develop curious inconsistencies.

No one so clearly points out these perplexing facts as Reichel in Von Bergmann's *Surgery;* to wit: "Mechanical factors preventing the return of venous blood certainly play an important part; regarded as such are certain valvular insufficiencies of the heart, abdominal tumors, especially pregnancy, the wearing of tight garters, tumors at a higher level—in view of the height of the blood column thus pressing upon the venous valves, and hard work combined with long periods of standing. But these facts alone are not a sufficient explanation; there is no doubt that pregnancy greatly favors the production of varicosities, but that the gravid uterus is not always the essential cause in preventing the return of venous blood is proved by many cases in which the varicosities developed to a considerable size in the first months of pregnancy when there could be no question of pressure of the uterus upon the abdominal veins or of any considerably increased intra-abdominal pressure. On the contrary, large abdominal tumors attended by marked intra-abdominal tension are not infrequently unaccompanied by varicose veins. These mechanical factors, therefore, can be only accorded a coöperative significance; the actual causes leading to atrophy of the walls or of the valves of the veins and to dilatation are unknown. It is certainly not the atrophy of old age, as the disease usually develops between the twentieth and fortieth years, often soon after puberty, and only in a few cases after middle life. In the etiology a certain significance is attached to inherited and racial peculiarities."

The last sentence quoted is of peculiar interest since this condition has never been observed by me in the black negro, and only in a mild degree in those of mixed blood. Occasionally a severe type of the disease is seen in a light-colored negro, but careful examination will develop a cause other than a primary thinning of the wall of the veins or of defective valves. Negroes are also singularly immune from varicocele, and an exceedingly small percentage develop hemorrhoids.

The so-called varicose ulcer, so prevalent among the negroes, is largely syphilitic or tuberculous in origin and aggravated by the filthy neglect and superstitious habits of the race.

The majority of my cases have been in white males from twenty to forty-five years of age. The inherited tendency has not been observed. Occupation has been in nearly every case a prime factor. Men in active life, pursuing vocations necessitating long standing positions, were the subjects of operations.

The numerous ingenious operations for the relief of this distressing condition will not be discussed here, as the treatment of varicose veins by surgical means is ofttimes attended by the difficulty of selection of a method, and not infrequently the question of expediency hastens the decision.

The ease and dispatch of multiple ligation, without the stress of general anesthesia, encouraged the performance of many operations which were incomplete, not wholly curative, and making directly impossible the complete obliteration of a functionless vessel. The exception, of course, occurs with cases in which, for justifiable reason, it is essential that local anesthesia be employed, or that some dangerous local infections limit the scope of the excision.

About two years ago the necessity of devising some means which would shorten the time involved in the excision of the saphena, and limit the trauma incident to such an exposure, led me to the practice of using scissors in making the dissection instead of the knife. The undoubted advantages gained by correcting these details resulted in superior wound repair, and practically excluded wound infection.

Ordinarily, the removal of a long section of a vein is tedious, bloody, and mutilating. These objectional features are largely overcome after exposing and ligating the main trunk by lightly outlining with a sharp knife the course along the vessel. The tissues overlying the vein are next incised with scissors, the lower blade having a blunt point and the instrument resembling a bandage or dressing scissors. As there are no branches given off from the exposed or external surface of the main vessel, the bleeding is slight and in nowise obscures the skin guide or soils the gaping wound developing behind.

It is pleasing to note how quickly the large vessel is exposed, lifted from its bed, laterals clamped and cut, leaving a comparatively dry wound.

Below the knee the veins are more superficial, and there

is such a limited space between the vessel and skin that the scissors dissection must be attended with a greater degree of delicate manipulation.

The large wound is closed with interrupted silkworm-gut sutures threaded on long straight needles, a dozen or more being provided, and this step adds much to the economy of time necessary in the operation.

PLASTIC INDURATION OF THE CORPUS CAVERNOSUM.

By Horace J. Whitacre, B.S., M.D.,
Cincinnati, Ohio.

Plastic induration is a progressive, painless, connective tissue thickening in the fibrous tissue sheath of the corpus cavernosum, which appears in men over fifty years of age, and is not the result of local disease in the penis.

Fibrous tissue changes in the penis, which result in a serious disturbance in the sexual and urinary functions of this organ, have been described in the literature since 1743, when La Peyronie first wrote on the subject. A dissertation by Herman Neumark on plastic induration, published in 1906, gives a bibliographic list of eighty-nine articles, and many articles have appeared since this time. This abundant literature on the subject has been so fully summarized by Neuwark, by Stopezanski (*Wiener klin. Woch.*, 1909, xxi, No. 10, 318), and by others that it is unnecessary for me to enter extensively into the subject.

Two cases of this sort have presented themselves to me within the past year and my failure to contribute greatly to their relief has led me to seek further information in our society. The literature on the subject furnishes little hope for such cases, and I feel it a duty to report upon an unsolved question in surgery.

Symptoms. The disease occurs between the ages of fifty and sixty-five. The patient may notice the appearance of nodules or a hardening of the penis, but does not often present himself for medical advice until there is a bending of the penis in erection or an incomplete erection. When the penis is flaccid it presents an entirely normal appearance, the skin and subcutaneous tissue are entirely normal, there is no difficulty in urination, and there is no pain. On palpation, hard nodules, plates, or cords are found on the upper surface of the corpora cavernosa, and particularly in the septum. The most typical site is in the septum near the symphysis. From here an elongated definitely circumscribed tumor may extend forward for one to two inches, or detached, more or less separate, nodules may extend as far forward as the glans penis. These nodules are very hard, have a smooth surface, are somewhat elastic, and appear to be fairly well circumscribed. They are not sensitive to the touch. Spreading out over the upper surface of the corpora cavernosa there may be plates of this same tissue. These plates may be in saddle form or confined to one side. Such plates are likewise, as a rule, well circumscribed, have a smooth surface, and are quite hard. They may exceptionally extend completely around the penis to give a ring like construction, or they may take the form of lateral longitudinal bands. The nodules in the septum may be the size of a pea or a bean, and the elongated tumors may attain the diameter of a lead pencil. These nodules develop painlessly, as has been stated, and grow progressively until they reach a certain size, when they remain stationary. They show no tendency to diminish in size or to disappear.

The most important symptoms are presented in erection. The tumors or plates lead to a bending of the penis, when erect, at the site of the induration. When the induration is mainly in the septum, the penis will bend upward toward or actually against the abdomen. When on one side, the curve will be toward this side. A great variety of shapes are possible. Depending upon the nature and degree of disturbance with the circulation, the distal portion of the penis will be much smaller when erect than the proximal portion, or it may be less hard, or it may be entirely flaccid. Such deviation or such incomplete erection will make coitus impossible. Erection may furthermore be attended with pain, or pain may be experienced only at the time of emission, because of a kinking in the urethra. The nervous symptoms attendant upon such a disturbance of function are usually quite marked, and suicide may result. When a patient attempts to straighten the curve forcibly a fracture of the corpus cavernosum may occur and the symptoms of this condition will be added.

PATHOLOGICAL ANATOMY. There has been some confusion in the classification of indurations of the penis because of a failure to accurately define the pathological process. Ricord, in 1847, gave the following most excellent classification, which has not been followed by all writers on this subject: (1) Traumatic indurations; (2) inflammatory indurations; (3) syphilitic indurations; and (4) plastic indurations.

Not a great many microscopic examinations have been made in the plastic type of induration, but the examinations reported are uniform in the findings. The structure is essentially a dense connective tissue with a predominance of fibers, few cells, and few bloodvessels. The connective tissue fibers are for the most part arranged in bundles or whorls. Some observers have described an occasional embryonic cartilage cell. The cells often show fatty or other degenerative changes, but no evidence of inflammation. There are few elastic fibers in the centre of such a nodule, more in the circumference. The bloodvessels adjacent to the nodules show evidence of an endarteritis.

No cause is known for the development of this lesion. Trauma, inflammation, and syphilis are not etiological factors. Gout, rheumatism, diabetes, leukemia, smallpox, typhoid, typhus, cellulitis, and a great variety of other general diseases have been suggested, but the connection is certainly not clear. It has been noted that some of these patients likewise suffer from Dupuytren's finger contraction, as does one of my patients. The microscopic findings are practically the same in the two conditions.

DIAGNOSIS. The differential diagnosis concerns itself with the exclusion of traumatic, inflammatory, syphilitic, and malignant tumor lesion.

PROGNOSIS. As regards recovery, it is extremely unfavorable.

TREATMENT. Therapeutic medication has given no results. Treatment by iodine has been extensively used, and is advised by many writers as the only medication likely to improve the condition. Massage, hot and cold applications, mercury preparations, rubbed on and injected, plasters and salves have likewise been used without result. Waelsch obtained complete healing after the injection of fibrolysin, but the same agent used by other authors has given no results. Operation has not given good results because of the deformity which is likely to result from scar tissue formation. The operative treatment would seem to be the only one which is likely to give results, however, and my only contribution to this subject will be the description of an operation which it seems to me will be less likely to cause scar tissue deformity. I have not seen a description of this operation in the literature.

CASE I.—H. T., aged sixty-three years, merchant, married. No member of family has suffered from similar trouble, from Dupuytren's finger, nor from keloid. Neither gout nor rheumatism is a family characteristic. Patient has enjoyed fair health except for rheumatism during past few years. This has been mainly in form of rheumatism pains. Had gonorrhea in youth, which was well in a week. Has never had chancroid, abscess, or other inflammation of the penis. Never had syphillis. Has not had Dupuytren's finger contraction.

In June, 1908, first noticed tendency of penis to bend upward against abdomen when in a state of erection. This has slowly grown more marked. There has been no interference with urination, intercourse is still possible, and no pain is experienced at the time of emission. There is no pain except when an attempt is made to straighten the penis when erect.

PHYSICAL EXAMINATION. The penis is of medium size, and normal in appearance when flaccid. Three hard nodules can be felt—one in the septum, at the base of the penis, which is about one inch long and one-fourth inch broad; a second, also located in the septum, three-quarters of an inch long and beginning one-half inch behind the corona; a third nodule or plate of firm tissue is found on the right side of the penis and separate from the other nodules.

At the first examination there was a question of malignancy, and a fragment of tissue was removed from the largest nodule at the base of the penis for microscopic examination. The naked eye appearance spoke so strongly for a benign condition that a large part of this nodule was removed at this time under cocaine anesthesia. Microscopic examination showed a fibrous tissue structure.

Under urgent solicitation a second operation was performed a few weeks later, by a technique which I have not seen described, and which seems to me worthy of report. The danger of deforming cicatrices and of adhesions between the skin and corpus cavernosum has been urged by many writers as a reason for refraining from operation on the body of the penis, and I had been convinced by experience that this danger exists. I believed that a semilunar incision in the pubic skin just above the base of the penis would give access to the greater part of the corpus cavernosum, and that it would avoid all adhesions. An incision two and one-half inches long was accordingly made in this way. Excellent exposure of the mass at the base of the penis was obtained, and there was no difficulty at all in pulling out the entire length of the body of the penis in a sort of loop through this incision. All fibrous tissue was then dissected away as fully as possible down to the vascular part of the corpus cavernosum. A large amount of firm connective tissue was removed. An effort was made to remove tissue symmetrically and to stop just short of opening up the sinuses of the corpus cavernosum. This was not always possible. When as much had been removed as seemed wise, there was still a great amount of connective tissue visible which it seemed might readily act as a basis for rapid regeneration.

Healing was rapid after operation, and there was not the slightest adhesion between the skin and deeper tissue, and there was no apparent development of a deforming cicatrix at the site of the wound. There was marked induration in the line of dissection on the dorsum of the penis, however, which lasted for a few weeks. This softened greatly in time, but there is today a well-defined indurated fibrous mass in the septum and on the right side. The induration is very much less in amount and the penis feels more normal on palpation, yet the symptoms are not relieved. The patient states that the penis still bends upward and that erection is not quite as firm as before operation, but coitus is still possible.

CASE II.—C. B., aged fifty-three years, bartender. This patient gives a history of no such trouble in any other member of the family, neither have any members of his family suffered from keloid or Dupuytren's finger contraction. Patient has never suffered from rheumatism, gout, or diabetes. He has twice suffered from gonorrhea, the last time in 1886. He recovered promptly from the gonorrhea each time, and had none of the usual complications. He has never had syphilis and has never suffered from abscess or ulcer on the penis. In October, 1908, he first began to notice that his penis became markedly bent to the right side at a point one inch back of the corona when in a state of erection. This slowly became more marked until coitus became impossible. He states that the penis beyond the point of bending does not become as rigid as the proximal portion.

He has noticed no pain at the time of intercourse and there is no obstruction to the flow of urine.

Physical Examination. A robust, well-developed man, who looks the picture of health. Except for Dupuytren's finger contraction of slight degree in both hands, the physical examination is negative except for penis. In the penis there is a plate induration about one inch in length along the right side of the corpus cavernosum and about one inch from the corona. There is some induration in the septum, but there are no distinct nodules. The proximal portion of the penis seems to be soft and normal.

On January 18, 1909, a longitudinal incision was made on the side of the penis over the site of the induration, and the more or less circumscribed connective tissue mass was dissected away from the corpus cavernosum. Care was taken to suture the divided structure in layers and to obtain primary healing, but postoperative erections could not be prevented; some stitches were pulled out and there was an adhesion of the skin to the corpus cavernosum.

An attempt was made later to liberate the skin from the scar without a satisfactory result. This experience led to the development of the operation described in Case I. On July 28 the pubic incision was made; a much more extensive incision of indurated tissue was made not only on the right side, but likewise in the septum. The old scar adhesion was also liberated. The wound healed primarily. The penis maintained full erectile property after operations, and the scar adhesion was relieved, but the penis still bends to the right when in a state of erection.

In both of these operations the results have not been satisfactory as regards the cure of the deformity, yet two valuable points have been developed: (1) The operation can be done by the method described without serious danger of increasing the deformity by operative scars; and (2) the corpus cavernosum will stand a very extensive dissection of its fibrous tissue sheath without losing its erectile power.

I have been so strongly impressed by the danger of destroying the erectile power of the corpus cavernosum in both of these operations that I feel certain that I did not make my dissection sufficiently radical. I now believe that a more radical removal would not be dangerous and might bring better results.

EXOPHTHALMIC GOITRE.

By John B. Deaver, M.D., LL.D.,
Philadelphia, Pennsylvania.

So much has been written upon this subject within the last two years that it seems almost like trespassing upon the time of this Association to discuss any aspect of exophthalmic goitre. Still we are not in full accord in all our own views, and even in those matters on which there is agreement simple reiteration is of value in leavening the medical lump. "Line upon line, precept upon precept," is needed to convince and overcome professional inertia.

At the present time the central fact which has been established both by clinical observation and by surgical and experimental evidence as to the cause of the symptom complex of exophthalmic goitre is its dependence upon an overacting hyperplastic and usually hypertrophied thyroid which produces its chief effect through excessive discharge into the circulation of some substance possessing a powerful toxic action.

Whether the enlargement and heightened activity of the gland be primary or in response to a reflex, toxic, or physiological call, or whether the substance elaborated be normal or altered in its composition, and whether the symptoms be due to poisoning by excess of a physiological product or by the harmful action of a pathological substance, we are not yet prepared to state.

The meagreness of our knowledge concerning the cause of this serious condition naturally prevents our founding a system of treatment based upon the solid foundation of its ultimate mode of origin. Let us admit at once, therefore, that the profession does not possess anything like a specific for the disease. In such a case it is our duty to assert the likelihood of spontaneous recovery from the affection. Then, by the use of such methods as empiricism and our limited knowledge of the essential characters of the disease may commend, to counteract or palliate its effects. Often we find that palliation is truly curative, since it affords opportunity for Nature to assert herself and reëstablish the normal state.

There is probably no disease with a wider range of symptomatology. The cardinal features, exophthalmos, tachycardia, tremor, and goitre, have been so emphasized that their absence is given a negative value that is not deserved. As long ago as 1860 Trousseau insisted upon this point, and adduced cases in point, calling them "formes frustes," a term which is still occasionally encountered. He pointed out, and the observation has been verified many times since then, that any one or more of the cardinal symptoms may be missing.

In addition to these masked or incomplete forms, there are rudimentary forms in which the thyroid derangement is but slight and perhaps temporary. Exophthalmos is often lacking. It is easy to overlook a moderate enlargement of the thyroid. Indeed, I have at times had difficulty in satisfying myself in regard to this when the operation subsequently showed the gland to be twice its normal size, or even larger. The tachycardia, tremor, and other nervous symptoms in such cases are thus easily consigned to one of the neurological scrap baskets, such as neurasthenia or hysteria. Many of these patients undergo spontaneous cure, and doubtless others would be cured or prevented from developing the full distressing syndrome if early and appropriate palliative treatment should be adopted. Such cases are the exclusive property of the internist. Upon them he may direct his full armamentarium of rest, bal-neotherapy, dieting, x-rays and electrotherapy, serum treatment, milk from thyroidectomized animals, thymus tablets, sodium phosphate, and symptomatic medication. In any event nine-tenths of the benefit derived will be due to rest; physical and mental quiet.

So many remedies have been proposed that it is too ardu-ous even to mention them. I have been impressed, how-ever, with the fact that in many cases where the patients could be taken into a hospital, controlled and kept at rest during the trial of any method of treatment, it was noted that nervousness abated and usually some gain in weight followed. These favorable features were often heralded as the result of the unimportant factor in treatment, while rest was deprived of its due tribute.

In a percentage of cases there will be a return to normal or to a state of comfort under measures purely medical. Every patient, therefore, is entitled to a trial of medical treatment. From one-fourth to one-third of all patients will be so relieved as to obviate any surgical measures.

What of the remaining two-thirds under medical or expectant treatment? A few, probably 3 to 4 per cent., will speedily perish of toxemia. A larger number will live for a number of years before the toxic degener-ations of the organs become incompatible with life. The largest number will be carried along in a miserable condi-tion of body and mind to become the prey of intercurrent infections, or if, after a number of years, partial recovery should take place, it is only to find that the physical powers are depleted and the individual's life ruined.

Hyperthyroidism may be succeeded by hypothyroidism, and myxedema arise to close the unhappy picture. It is seldom that there is a return to normal health after a pro-tracted period of severe thyrotoxicosis. I have seen cases of so-called medical cure in which the last state of the patient was at least as bad as the first. Lethargy, hopelessness, and a profound change in disposition almost made me question the use of such a cure. The mortality of the medical treatment of exophthalmic goitre is not small, but the question is not all one of mortality. The pursuit of health is as much a primary right as is that of existence. Men risk their lives daily in the pursuit of pleasure, sport, or livelihood. How much more will a man risk for his health and the joy of living? Moreover, it can no longer be contradicted that in the group of cases which surgery claims, the mortality is less than under purely medical treatment. The operative mortality has steadily diminished until today it is under 5 per cent. in competent hands, while the great master of this procedure, Kocher, can point to a mortality of 1.5 per cent. in his last 153 cases. The results of surgical treatment are swift, brilliant in 80 per cent. of the cases, satisfactory in 90 per cent., and unsatisfactory in only about 10 per cent. The results of medical treatment are slow, seldom completely satisfactory, more often disappointing, and show a large mortality, partially concealed by its being spread out over a period of years and often brought about indirectly by intercurrent disease to which the weakened state of the patient lays him liable.

This is the outlook under the general methods of medical treatment. The special methods of non-operative treatment for which more was claimed seem to afford no better prognosis.

It is now evident that the *x*-rays have no specific action in controlling the disease.

The serum question is not so well settled. Certainly it has failed to sustain the high hopes it aroused in the beginning. Until it has more signally demonstrated its rights to consideration, it cannot be a legitimate excuse for not employing any method which has been demonstrated to be of value.

It appears to be far more rational to remove a superfluous portion of the gland than to attempt to allay an activity of whose causes, conditions, and regulating influences we are ignorant. Surgical intervention is indicated when it becomes evident that cure is not resulting after Nature is given a reasonable opportunity to restore the balance, and assisted in her attempts by palliative methods shown to be of value. Occasionally this is apparent in a very few weeks. Sometimes in cases with remissions and relapses it may take some months, but it is never necessary to wait until the heart is greatly weakened and dilated, the nervous system shattered, and emaciation marked, before coming to such a conclusion. A determined effort must be made to secure from the internist, as soon as possible, every case which is not yielding to non-operative treatment. Such a desirable state of affairs would largely do away with the necessity of selection of cases. As it is, we find a few patients who, while they would undoubtedly be benefited by the loss of a large part of the gland, would undoubtedly render up their lives in the attempt.

The selection of the cases appropriate for operative treatment and the choice of the best moment for operation are questions of the first importance. Generally speaking, the more severe and the longer the duration of the toxic symptoms the greater the risk.

The heart is the chief index of operability. Dilatation with high pulse rate during recumbency, especially if associated with arrhythmia, are unfavorable, and indicate postponement with all the aids of hygiene and palliative treatment, until subsidence or slight remission gives a more favorable moment for attack. A light, nourishing semiliquid diet, daily sponge baths, fresh air, and prohibition of muscular exertion are essential. X-rays and sera have not seemed to me to have any specific effect. Drugs are often of use for symptoms. The bromides and opium are of service in restlessness, excitement, and tachycardia. With a weakened, dilated heart, especially if there be arrhythmia, digitalis is of service. If there be much capillary dilatation, as often is the case, the use of nitroglycerin is unnecessary. If the countenance be pale, however, and the heart laboring, I do give nitroglycerin, and have seen some remarkably brilliant results from this combination. An ice bag over the precardium also is useful. For excessive sweating belladonna or atropine may be used, but I hesitate to employ it because of its well-known physiological action in paralyzing the cardiac inhibitory fibers of the vagus. Under such treatment usually we may count upon a certain degree of improvement, but in some cases nothing seems to be able to allay the tachycardia. We must then be content to abandon operation altogether or to do simply a ligation of one or both superior thyroid arteries. Reduction of the blood supply may cause marked improvement and give opportunity later for excision of gland substance. Sympathectomy has proved a failure. I have done a number of sympathectomies, and in the majority of cases the disease was but little influenced. In one case my patient, after making a good operative recovery, suddenly fell dead as she was walking about the ward. I cannot but feel that the removal of the important cervical sympathetic may have caused this fatality, and in any case I believe this operation to be totally valueless.

If an enlarged thymus can be demonstrated or reasonably suspected, it is wiser not to operate. Capelle remarks that "a large Basedow thymus is, so to speak, pathognomonic of a weak Basedow heart, incapable of standing the stress of an operation." He points out that in 66 autopsy reports an unusual size of the thymus is recorded in 79 per cent., and reports 4 cases in which sudden death after operation was associated with large thymus. In view of the dangers of lymphatism in other conditions, it seems quite probable that we have here a contra-indication of importance. The possibility of thymic death must be considered and excluded as far as possible by investigation of the thymus before operation is decided upon. Enlargement may be demonstrated by percussion over the manubrium sterni, occasionally by palpation during inspiration, by Röntgenoscopy and by signs of status lymphaticus elsewhere, such as enlarged, pale red tonsils, enlarged spleen, or follicular hyperplasia of the lymphoid tissue anywhere in the body.

The blood picture also, as Kocher has pointed out, is important in respect to prognosis. There is a moderate leucopenia due to deficiency of the polymorphonuclear neutrophiles. At the same time, the monuclear cells are relatively or at times absolutely increased. In general, the lymphocytic increase is proportional to the severity of the disease, but is sometimes absent in severe cases. In these the prognosis is serious. This is comparable to what we know of the polymorphonuclear leukocytosis in acute infections.

Riedel, having had six postoperative deaths from bronchopneumonia, lays particular stress upon the condition of the bronchi. The choice and administration of an anesthetic, always of importance, is especially so here. In spite of the authority of Kocher and some other surgeons, I can see no advantage in local anesthesia. These patients are particularly liable to be restless and clamorous. Fear and emotional storms are important factors in the outcome, as emphasized by Crile, and under local anesthesia both are at their height. The surgeon is hampered, the duration of the operation is increased, and the danger of infection of the wound is greater. I have not found ether, carefully given, to be more harmful than the stress of an operation under local anesthesia. I do not think chloroform is advisable. The care of the anesthetist has much to do with the successful outcome. The patient should be kept just beyond the point of struggle or nausea, but never deeply anesthetized. The open gauze method of administration I believe to be the best, and in these cases I vary my usual rule of no morphine, and give $\frac{1}{6}$ grain of morphine and $\frac{1}{100}$ grain of atropine as a preliminary to the anesthesia. The morphine has a beneficial sedative action and the atropine diminishes secretions of the mouth and bronchi. I have had no experience with spinal anesthesia in operations upon the neck. If it can be given safely in this location it will be indeed a boon. My experience with spinal anesthesia in the lower region of the cord, while I have had no fatalities, has not been such as to give me sufficient courage to employ it in the cervical region.

In the usual type of diffuse hyperplastic enlargement of the thyroid most frequently associated with this condition I confine my operative intervention practically to two procedures. I have already spoken of ligation of the superior thyroid arteries. This I do in the extremely severe cases, and at times in the extremely mild ones, in the former cases thinking to diminish the severity sufficiently to permit more radical operation, in the very mild cases with the idea that perhaps the more serious operation may be avoided.

When reduction in the thyroid tissue is the object, I practically always remove the larger of the two lobes, which is most commonly the right. The usual collar incision is made and the flap reflected upward. Splitting the ribbon muscles vertically almost always gives enough space without their division. In enucleating the thyroid the successive fascial coverings should be divided until one is beneath the true capsule. The superior pole is first freed, and the artery ligated immediately after it penetrates the substance of the gland. Then working from above downward, still leaving the capsule undisturbed posteriorly, after ligating the inferior thyroid artery, the lobe is freed, except for a small portion of the gland which lies above the sulcus between the trachea and esophagus. This is tied off just as one would treat a pedicle, and the remainder of the lobe cut away. By this method the recurrent laryngeal is never seen, and runs no risk of injury unless crushing forceps are too recklessly used. The cut surface is touched with pure carbolic acid and alcohol for their coagulating action, to guard against too rapid absorption of toxic material from the stump.

Injury to the parathyroids is averted by keeping within the capsule and by ligating the thyroid arteries just within the substance of the gland. While it may be true, as some observers have reported, that the parathyroids may lie within the capsule, it is generally agreed that this is exceptional. Charles Mayo has called attention to the fact that they may lie within a split in the capsule, hence the necessity of leaving the entire posterior capsule.

Their blood supply comes from small terminal arteries derived from the inferior thyroid artery or from an anastomotic branch between the superior and inferior thyroid arteries. Halsted has shown that in certain instances the origin of these arteries is so close to the thyroid gland that a ligature outside will certainly include the parathyroid branch. Since ligation of this nutrient artery entails death of the gland, I avoid this in the manner stated, by tying the thyroid artery within the first bits of thyroid tissue penetrated after the artery has pierced the capsule. This is substantially the same method as I employed before the importance of the parathyroids became known. I never had a case of tetany then, nor have I since. I have never made an attempt to transplant a parathyroid, though I think it quite proper and advisable to do so where one is found to have been removed with the goitre.

To close the operation it is necessary simply to place a few sutures to draw together the split muscles. Occasionally it will seem well to partially obliterate the bed of the excised lobe with a few stitches. A rubber tube is laid down to the stump of the thyroid tissue and brought out through a puncture in the flap, which is completely closed. Free drainage to the stump of the gland is important.

In all these steps iodized catgut is the only ligature material used, and I have seen no contra-indications to its use, while the advantages of absorbable material are too well known to be commented upon. The wound is closed with linen thread.

In the less frequent cases of hyperthyroidism due to adenomatous growth or to hyperplastic changes in persisting simple goitre, it is necessary to vary the procedure. Encapsulated adenomas are usually best removed by intraglandular enucleation.

In large diffuse goitrous enlargements it may be necessary to excise a part of each lobe. If possible, the most normal appearing position of the gland is selected for preservation, and an amount left which is about equal to the volume of the normal gland.

In working upon both lobes it is necessary to observe especial care to avoid removing or destroying the blood supply of the parathyroids. After-treatment also must be symptomatic, as is the preliminary treatment. Saline by rectum is a valuable aid, and bromides may be administered in it. Morphine, digitalis, sometimes nitroglycerin, and always efficient nursing are needed to tide the patient over the first twenty-four or forty-eight hours during which the danger is of death from acute hyperthyroidism. Those who pass safely through this period usually make an uninterrupted recovery.

Now, as to results, I have already stated that approximately 90 per cent. will prove satisfactory.

Where the desired benefit is not obtained, it is often due to the inroads made by the disease upon the general health. As Charles Mayo aptly remarks, "Such cases should be compared to the removal of a bullet with the expectation of obtaining relief from all injury caused by its passage." The majority of these patients, however, are among the most grateful which the surgeon has, which speaks volumes for the benefit derived.

In conclusion, I would summarize the factors which are most important for successful surgery upon exophthalmic goitre as follows:

Selection of the cases and choice of time for operation.

Careful anesthesia, my personal preference being for ether in the absence of definite contra-indications.

Avoidance of mental excitement.

Suiting the operation to the case, *i. e.*, not to do an excision upon a patient who can only endure a ligation.

Quick, skilful operation.

The avoidance of injury to the recurrent laryngeal nerve and to the parathyroid glands by preservation of the posterior capsule and of the parathyroid arteries.

Adequate drainage of the wound.

PERFORATION AND RUPTURE OF THE GALL-BLADDER.

By *F. T. Meriwether, M.D.,*
Asheville, North Carolina.

From the literature of the diseases of the gall-bladder, one would think that perforation and rupture were uncommon, but in looking over a series of cases of prominent operators, in 2135 operations for gall-bladder disease, I find no less than 87 cases of perforation and 31 cases of rupture.

A large number of the cases of perforation are those in which the perforation occurs and no infection following, the stone or stones being walled off or encysted, but about one-third were acute perforations with infection, necessitating immediate or at least early operations. The mortality of these acute cases was 24 per cent., a large percentage in these days of accurate diagnosis and clean operations.

The mortality of the cases of rupture, non-traumatic, was 37 per cent. Nearly all of these cases of rupture were due to distention of a gall-bladder with pus and with a stone blocking the cystic duct.

The necessity for operations upon all gallstone cases when diagnosticated independent of the relief from pain and the other symptoms, is shown by these few cases, for undoubtedly if all cases of rupture or perforation could be gotten together there would probably be a mortality of about 1 per cent. of all gallstone cases from these causes alone, and possibly even more.

This is analogous to the condition found in appendiceal attacks when we operate not altogether for the relief of symptoms, but to prevent gangrene perforation and the consequent sequela of local and general peritonitis.

It is necessary to educate the physicians to make a correct diagnosis before the condition of one is grave, for it is astonishing how slow some are in diagnosticating gallstones, waiting for jaundice, intense pain, and fever, really symptoms and conditions due to complications or sequelæ. The more I see of gall-bladder work, the more I see the urgency of advising an operation when the diagnosis can be made. Even in my limited experience I have seen two cases of spontaneous rupture in gall-bladders not gangrenous, and perforation three times, both cases of rupture not having been diagnosticated, though there must have been tumors large for quite a time, and the cases of perforation presented symptoms that should have led to correct diagnosis, but in none of them were they diagnosticated until just before operation, which was done in two of the cases of perforation, and in the other case not until just before death.

In the latter case a diagnosis was made of probable impacted stone in the common duct, but the operation was refused. The stone perforated Sunday afternoon, and the patient died Monday night from acute peritonitis, postmortem showing a perforation in the common duct.

In one case of rupture I had made a diagnosis of gall-bladder disease some months before, but the patient doubted the diagnosis, and passed into the hands of other physicians; and when I was called a second time the bladder was enormously distended, and was evidently leaking enough to cause peritonitis. She refused operation again, and twelve hours later, when seen, she was dying, and the gall-bladder tumor then had disappeared. A limited postmortem showed free pus in the abdominal cavity.

Mrs. R., Birmingham, Alabama, aged sixty-two years, with history of attacks of what had been diagnosticated as appendiceal colic, having had these attacks for several years at intervals of two or three months.

Otherwise her health was fairly good. Had never noticed any jaundice, though the urine during these attacks became dark. Was seized with pain Thursday afternoon, nausea, some vomiting, slight rise of temperature, pulse 80 to 96.

Dr. Lucius B. Morse, of Chimney Rock, N. C., made a probable diagnosis of gallstone, and put her upon appropriate treatment.

She developed a low grade of peritonitis, ran a temperature of from 100° morning to 102° evening, the pulse increasing daily until on Sunday night when I saw her it was 120 and quite weak.

Marked tenderness over the gall-bladder, increasing tympany, loss of liver dulness, grass-green vomiting, a chill Sunday morning, a leaking skin, urine scant, leading to a diagnosis by Dr. Morse of a perforation with a commencing peritonitis.

He called me over long distance phone, and with Dr. Elias drove twenty-six miles.

We operated by the light of kerosene lamps.

There was no attempt by nature to wall off.

The bladder was about three times its normal size, and had a clean-cut perforation in its posterior wall half way between the fundus and the commencement of the cystic duct. There were several ounces of a turbid fluid in the abdominal cavity, a few flakes of exudate, and I picked out several small stones, seven in number, loose in the cavity, the gall-bladder being empty. The ducts were patulous.

The patient's condition being bad, I walled off the gall-bladder with gauze, and carried a rubber tube into the perforation.

Dr. Morse reported that in about five weeks the fistula had closed. Evidently, the stones had been pocketed in a small pouch of the bladder and by erosion had caused gangrene of the wall there and perforated. In no other way could it be explained how so few stones could bring about this condition.

Very probably I left one or more small stones in the abdominal cavity. The innocuous character of the bile in this case was remarkable, for the patient's condition commenced to improve immediately after the operation.

Another case, Mr. W., had a history of frequent attacks of colic with jaundice. The patient was aged eighty-three years, and at the time I saw him had evidently had peritonitis for five days. He was intensely yellow, and at the umbilicus the color was walnut. Temperature, 99.5°; pulse, 140. A rapid operation showed the upper wall of the bladder perforated, the opening the size of a half dollar, with slight attempts at walling off. There was probably seven or eight ounces of free bile in the abdominal cavity, and the liver seemed to be literally studded with small stones, looking as if the gall-bladder had exploded and blown the stones into it. Possibly there had been adhesions between the bladder and the liver which had given way.

The gall-bladder still contained a large number of stones, and a large stone was tight in the common duct. Several free stones were found in the abdominal cavity.

Gauze and tube drainage was used, but the patient died after four days, from exhaustion.

Free bile in the abdominal cavity is not very irritating, and if nothing but bile is discharged only a local peritonitis supervenes and the perforation is sealed by adhesions, and the stones if any are encysted.

The perforations are very apt to be clear cut, like a typhoid perforation. If pus or infectious organisms are present in the bladder, a violent peritonitis is set up, with consequent early death. But if only bile or clear mucus is present, the peritonitis is of a low grade, and the patient may survive several days.

In the two cases I operated upon for perforation the umbilicus was distinctively yellow, and showed more marked jaundice than the rest of the abdomen, a symptom pointed out by Ransohoff, of Cincinnati.

This is no doubt due to the absorbtion of the free bile in the cavity by the abdominal wall, and the umbilicus being the thinest part of the wall, it showed more marked there.

Of course, operation is the only treatment.

Whether or not to do cholecystectomy or cholecystotomy depends upon the condition of the patient and the dexterity and the experience of the operator.

Undoubtedly cystectomy is the ideal operation, but if the patient's condition is such as to indicate that a prolonged or severe operation would cause death, cystotomy is the thing to do.

In my two cases to have removed the gall-bladder would have resulted in death, for neither patient would have stood the more severe operation. Still we must realize that, with increasing experiences, a cystectomy is but little more dangerous than cystotomy, and we get rid of the danger of fistula and possible reinfection and formation of stone.

Personally, I believe an incomplete operation with a living though crippled patient, is better than an ideal operation with a dead one; but we all have our limitations, and undoubtedly one more dextrous and experienced can undertake the complete removal with as much or more safety than some of us can do a simple incision and drainage.

But when drained, after the patient gets stronger, we can then remove the gall-bladder at a time of election.

Virtually all of the cases are in bad shape, and I believe the operation in most surgeons' hands should be incision, wiping out the cavity, and drainage. Irrigation is bad, for it merely scatters the pus and infectious material, and I doubt if any more can be removed than by judiciously wiping out with gauze, using the finger to carry it into the pockets of the abdomen, particular up and behind the liver, where in my experience pus both from the gall-bladder and appendix is likely to have gone, and which gives rise to the peritonitis and deaths following so many cases of disease of these organs.

THE PRINCIPLE OF THE TEALE FLAP APPLIED TO AMPUTATION OF THE PENIS.

By William M. Mastin, M.D.,

Mobile, Alabama.

In a case of carcinoma of the glans penis where amputation was performed, some ten years ago, the hemorrhagic oozing from the corpora cavernosa was so persistent and troublesome—despite the use of numerous ligatures together with the application of the cautery, and finally only yielding to inversion and firm suture of the sheaths of the cavernous bodies—that I sought some modification of the usual operative technique by which this complication might be avoided or controlled.

It then occurred to me that this could be accomplished by the application of the principle of the Teale method of amputation of the extremities, that is, by incising the cavernous structures horizontally, forming a long lower or posterior flap, and bending this upward on itself, to be snugly sutured to the upper transversely divided end. It seemed probable that this would secure the necessary pressure hemostasis, and, at the same time, produce a symmetrically fashioned stump.

With this idea in view, the following technical steps were evolved, and the completed operation has resulted so admirably in several instances that I venture to offer it as a very satisfactory method of performing partial amputation.

First Step. With a constricting band encircling the base of the penis, the integumentary flap is formed either

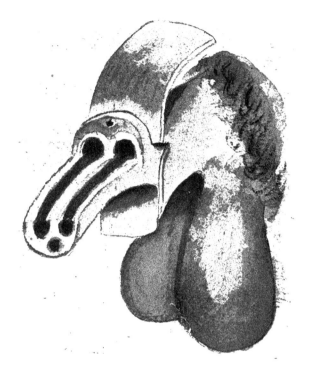

FIG. 1.—Showing the cutaneous and cavernous flaps formed.

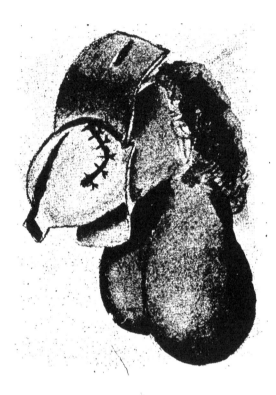

Fig. 2.—Showing the urethra dissected loose and split dorsally, and the cavernous flaps stitched in place.

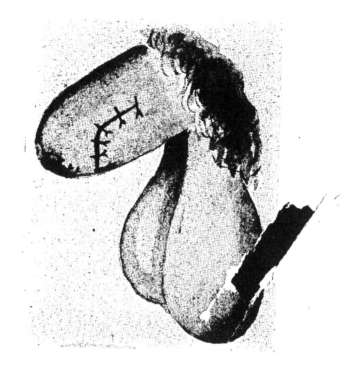

Fig. 3.—Showing the skin flaps sutured and
the operation completed.

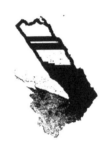

by a long anterior and short posterior oval flap, or by the anteroposterior rectangular Teale flaps—the anterior long flap corresponding in length approximately to one-half the circumference of the organ, and the short posterior flap to one-fourth of this length. This character of flap is preferred to the circular cuff method, since the cutaneous scar is placed underneath and behind the urethral outlet. The skin flaps are then freed and retracted.

SECOND STEP. The two cavernous bodies are now transfixed laterally by a narrow knife, somewhat in advance of the base of the skin flaps, and split down to the extent of giving the proper length to the proposed flap, at which point the edge of the knife is turned downward and the lower segment, containing the corpus spongiosum, cut through. The upper segment is next divided transversely on a level with the point of the original entrance of the knife, thereby severing the remaining attachments of the diseased portion to be removed.

THIRD STEP. The spongy body, enclosing the urethra, is next dissected from its bed to the required distance, the vessels ligated with fine chromicized catgut, and the cavernous flap turned upward and sutured to the superior half of the corpora cavernosa. One or two lateral sutures give both additional support and greater security against bleeding.

FOURTH STEP. Finally, the urethra is divided at an angle obliquely downward, then split either laterally or on its dorsal surface, and stitched, in the ordinary manner, to a button-hole opening made in the anterior skin flap. The cutaneous flaps are approximated with interrupted sutures of horsehair or fine silkworm gut.

The hemostasis is complete, and a shapely, well-rounded stump is formed. The line of skin union is posterior to and away from the urinary meatus. In addition, the urethra and cutaneous flaps are not in contact with the usually transversely divided cavernous stump, and, therefore, the urethral meatus has less tendency to become strictured and deeply depressed, or of an infundibular form, produced by the contracting cicatrix, as frequently occurs after the usual circular amputation.

Another advantage, and which is possibly the most important feature of the operation, is that a more radical removal of diseased tissue, with a minimum of shortening of the organ, can be effected by this method. Observation has definitely shown that epitheliomatous disease of the penis oftener originates superficially about the corona glandis and the mucus surface of the prepuce than elsewhere on the organ, and that the route of extension is by way of the main lymphatic trunks occupying the dorsum. The lymphatic radicles of the anterior extremity of the penis largely converge to these large dorsal channels, which pass backward in the subcutaneous tissue, on both sides of the dorsal bloodvessels, to empty into the lymph nodes of the groins and pelvis. Consequently, by dividing the corpora cavernosa laterally and cutting away the upper halves—as far back as the pubis if necessary—the lymphatic ducts coming from the diseased area are in greater part removed; and the lower halves composing the flap, which are less rich in lymphatics, are utilized to give increased length to the stump. Furthermore, the bilateral skin incisions can be prolonged on either side into the inguinal regions, the upper skin flap reflected upward on to the pubis, and the dissection extended so as to include the groin glands, as in the operation practised by Nicolls, of Glasgow (see *Annals of Surgery*, February, 1909, p. 240, *et seq.*). Again, on account of the lymphatic distribution to the dorsum of the penis, and the consequent greater danger of the cutaneous lymphatics in this locality being infected, the integumentary flaps can be reversed—that is, taking the long flap from the under surface and the short flap from the dorsal aspect of the organ.

This procedure is, necessarily, restricted to the early stages

of the disease where the neoplasm is limited to the glands
or prepuce, and before infiltration of the spongy and cavernous bodies occurs—the dense fibrous sheaths of the latter
resisting carcinomatous invasion until late in the progress
of the disease—allowing sufficient sound tissue for safe
utilization in the formation of the flaps.

The accompanying drawings indicate the several stages
of the operation.

TUMORS OF THE KIDNEY. WHEN OPERABLE?

By Henry O. Marcy, M.D.,
Boston, Massachusetts

Operations for large tumors of the kidney are sufficiently rare to prove interesting for study.

Case I.—A man, aged about sixty years, had been ill for a long time, was greatly emaciated and anemic. The urine gave no evidence of renal lesion. A tumor had slowly developed, distending the abdominal cavity; was movable, rather tense, symmetrical, fluctuating. Diagnosis not determined; probable cyst of the left kidney. Section in the left of the median line. After a careful dissection of the posterior peritoneum a thick-wall cyst was easily enucleated almost without hemorrhage. Its attachment to the kidney was separated, removing a portion of the cortical tissue, leaving the cyst unbroken, which weighed about eight pounds. The wound in the kidney was sutured with kangaroo tendon, the capsule introflected and closed with a light continuous suture. Another layer closed the posterior peritoneum. The abdominal wound was united in lines of buried sutures without drainage. The patient made an easy and uneventful recovery.

Case II.—A sea captain, in middle life, of temperate habits, just returned from a long voyage to Africa, for some months had suffered from pain in the left side with a slowly increasing swelling. On admission to the hospital a rather firm non-fluctuating tumor distended the abdomen. It was more pronounced upon the left side, extending under the floating ribs. At times blood and pus in the urine. A very great sufferer for some weeks, and had been under the observation of Dr. Joseph Lockhart, of Cambridge.

An oblique incision was made extending from the floating ribs well within the crest of the ilium. It was the intention not to open the peritoneal cavity, but this was accidentally incised for perhaps two inches, and was closed by continuous suture. The enormous tumor was everywhere adherent and most extraordinarily vascular. The hemorrhage for a few moments imperilled life, until the vessels of the kidney were seized and clamped. Notwithstanding care, the tumor was considerably broken in abstraction. After the removal of the mass the hemorrhage was comparatively easily controlled and most of the great pocket coapted by lines of buried tendon suture. Drainage was used. There was a local infection, probably from the tumor contents. The patient made a slow and painful recovery, and died the following year from a recurrent disease of the liver.

Diagnosis, primary cancer of the kidney.

CASE III.—J. K., aged fifty-two years, admitted to hospital November, 1906. First seen two years ago; pain in right side, then in bed for some weeks, passing bloody urine with clots. Is anemic. Prior to this good general health. Tumor of the right kidney about double fist size; advised operation; thought malignant. Has gradually grown worse, until at present a large solid nodular tumor of the right side extending quite over to the left of the middle line, with a rather sharp, well-defined border. The lower edge is quite below the umbilicus. An ill-defined depression between the tumor and the liver. Is slightly movable and not painful on pressure. From the ensiform cartilage, in a line with the left crest of the ilium, to the base of the tumor measures ten inches; the same in the middle line; to the right crest, eleven inches. Urine light colored, acid; heavy line of albumin; specific gravity, 1010; pus, uric acid crystals, no casts. Operation advised as the only hope of recovery, especially since the duration of the disease indicates a non-malignant growth. Clamped the renal vessels without especial difficulty, and removed by enucleation. Much hemorrhage; oozing from the abraded surfaces. The entire pocket was closed with buried sutures, leaving room for a gauze drain. This controlled the hemorrhage. Rallied satisfactorily from the operation, and without warning became pulseless, and death occurred at eleven o'clock, evening of the operation, probably from embolism. Dr. Councilman examined the tumor; hydronephrosis; many of the large veins filled with clots. The weight of the tumor was *ten* pounds.

CASE IV.—Mr. F., aged sixty-one years, captain of the coast guard; good habits; well until about a year ago. Some months ago noticed swelling on the right side, with bloody urine, much pain, loss of flesh and strength, anemic. Tumor has rapidly increased in size until at admission it extends from beneath the liver to the crest of the ilium. Not tender on pressure, slightly movable. Probably sarcoma. Operation permissible. Undertaken reluctantly. Tumor everywhere adherent, and extraordinarily vascular. Clamped and sutured the great vessels. The bloody oozing was controlled with extreme difficulty, and that only by firm packing. Intravenous injection of two pints of salt solution. Death occurred about twelve hours after the operation, probably from loss of blood. The abdominal cavity was not opened, the operation being postperitoneal. The tumor was an immense sarcoma, the central portion friable, easily breaking down under pressure. The extraordinary advance of the disease proved that the operation was ill advised.

CASE V.—Mrs. M., aged fifty-nine years; well until six months ago, during which time she has lost forty pounds in weight; occasionally there has been blood in the urine. Has consulted a number of distinguished surgeons, with much variation of opinion. Admitted to hospital February

22, 1908. Large movable tumor in right side extending from the base of the liver quite to the umbilicus. Urine normal; doubtful if there is any secretion from the right kidney. Postperitoneal incision extending quite within the crest of the pelvis. The tumor was enucleated without any special difficulty, and the renal vessels clamped. The renal artery was ligated separately, and the tissues carefully sutured over the vascular stump. The entire pocket was closed with lines of buried tendon sutures, then the abdominal wall, and a subcutaneous suture closed the wound, eleven inches in length, which was sealed with iodoform collodion, without drainage. Rallied well from operation; convalescence rapid, without incident. Primary union. Discharged. Tumor was about the size of a cocoanut. Cancer had invaded the renal structure, only a small portion of which was unchanged. A firm recent clot absolutely plugged the ureter, probably due to an examination made by a New York surgeon just previous to admittance. The growth was entirely within the capsule, owing to which a favorable prognosis was given. Patient seen in October, 1909. Is in excellent general health; of normal weight and strength; has no discomfort. The urinary secretion quite normal.

CASE VI.—Mrs. L., aged forty-eight years; well until a year since. Normal weight, 125 pounds; now 80 pounds. For the last months has suffered from nausea, vomiting, and pain, especially upon the right side. Has been under the care of a number of rather eminent physicians. Diagnosis had been made as probably cancer of stomach. Physical examination shows a well-defined movable tumor in the region of the right kidney about the size of a double fist, not especially painful on pressure; undoubtedly a tumor of the right kidney. Postperitoneal operation not especially difficult. Closed the entire wound with lines of buried tendon sutures and sealed with iodoform collodion. Union primary; convalescence easy and rapid, followed by a marked increase of flesh and strength. The tumor was a hydronephrosis of the kidney caused by an enormous calculus, which distended the pelvis, with a prolongation running down into the ureter.

The object of the report of these cases is especially to show that tumors of the kidney should be favorably considered from an operative standpoint. That by a careful physical examination they may be detected, and in a measure be differentiated.

The profession in general should be instructed to carefully determine such conditions and advise an early operation, since it is now generally accepted that removal of the kidney under favorable conditions is not especially dangerous.

It is rare that diseased conditions involving a considerable hypertrophy of the organ are self-eliminative, but, on the contrary, steadily go on to a probably fatal termination.

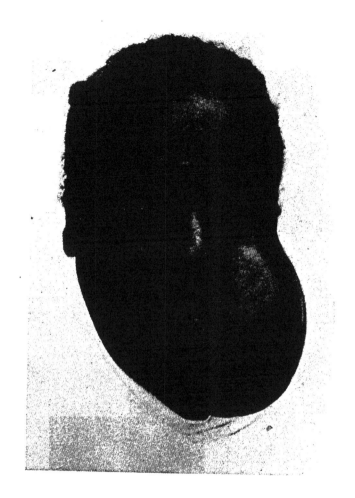

Basal-celled epithelioma of lower jaw.

BASAL-CELLED EPITHELIOMA OF LOWER JAW.

BY EDWARD A. BALLOCH, *M.D.*,
Washington, D. C.

THE patient was a colored woman, aged fifty-five years, who entered Freedmen's Hospital March 25, 1909. Owing to her limited mental capacity the history was not very satisfactory. Family history negative. In 1892 the left lower wisdom tooth was extracted with difficulty. Soon after this it was noticed that the lower jaw on the left side was enlarging, and it has grown in size steadily since that time. Two years ago she was struck on the affected side of the jaw by a door, which was slammed in her face. Since that time the tumor has increased in size very rapidly, and there have been pain and hemorrhage, which were not present before.

Externally the tumor presented the appearance shown in the accompanying photograph. Upon inspecting the mouth there was found an ulcerating, fungating mass, which nearly filled the oral cavity and which pushed the tongue to the right side of the hard palate. No demonstrable enlargement of cervical glands. The oral portion of the tumor bled readily. Clinical diagnosis, malignant degeneration of a cystic tumor of left side of lower jaw. A small portion of the mass was removed and submitted to the pathologist of the hospital and by him pronounced to be a basal-celled carcinoma.

Operation, March 29, 1909. Removal of left half of lower jaw, a portion of the right half, and extirpation of cervical glands on both sides. At the operation the growth was found to extend beyond the symphysis and to involve the medulla on the right side. The section of the jaw was made about an inch to the right of the median line. The bone was disarticulated at the left temporomaxillary articulation. The glands of the neck were not enlarged, but were removed on both sides. The floor of the mouth was reconstructed and the wound closed without drainage. Recovery was uneventful and she left the hospital April 17, 1909, in good condition. She has not been heard from since.

Inspection of the specimen showed it to consist of a series of bone cysts, containing a colloid substance. Springing from the alveolar process was the ulcerating fungous mass, already alluded to.

The specimen was sent to the Army Medical Museum and the following report, made by Dr. J. S. Neate, gives a full account of the microscopic pathology of the tumor:

In sections of this tissue taken from the buccal surface prior to operation, which I was enabled to see through the courtesy of Dr. H. W. Lawson, it was found that the columns of cells or ingrowths, composed of epithelial cells with their inner layers consisting of a more flattened or fusiform type, had invaded the tissue from the mucous surface and constituted the essential tumor growth. These processes of deeply staining cells, in the arrangement of their outer layers, always exhibited the palisade type of the basal cell layer of the skin and a tendency to form irregular acini or incomplete cysts, roughly simulating a cystadenoma. The supporting stroma consisted of a connective tissue in various stages of development and sometimes quite fibrillar, and contained well-formed and numerous bloodvessels. Mucoid change and degeneration was present and leukocytes were found infiltrating the degenerated area. A few patches of epithelial cells were seen which had reached further development than the predominating basal cell, but there is no evidence of pearl formation or the characteristic prickle cell. For these reasons the tumor was diagnosticated as a basal-celled epithelioma or a benign epithelioma, as it is sometimes called.

On receipt of the tumor at the Army Medical Museum the growth was found to contain several large cysts with flakes of bone in their walls and evidently developed in connection with the jaw bone, while others possessed fibrous walls and with many of microscopic size were situated remote from the bony area. The large cysts contained vestiges of hemorrhagic debris, and some were lined with columnar epithelium. Sections taken from the interior of the neoplasm differ from those first examined only in the fact that there is relatively more degeneration, and areas are to be found where the epithelial cells are somewhat more varied in type than the parental basal cell.

The presence of these bone cysts suggests as the point of primary origin some defect in or injury to some undeveloped enamel organ or rudimentary tooth follicle. The tumor may be classed by some, therefore, as an adamantinoma, which, after all, is a basal celled epithelioma, differing only in its point of origin rather than in cellular structure.

When the enamel germs differentiate into enamel organs they consist of an outer layer of columnar epithelial cells which are to be regarded as a direct continuation of the basal cells from the epithelium of the oral mucous membrane, or, still better, the enamel ridge. The epithelium of the interior of the organs is also derived from the stratum Malpighii. These, however, undergo changes in shape and later become stellate. The development of the enamel organ from the dentinal ridge is, in effect, basocellular downgrowths enclosing areas of cells of the branched types, with more or less orderly arrangement. Add to these conditions an exuberant disorderly growth, cyst formation, and possibly enamel cells and dentine, and we have the epithelioma adamantinosum.

A differential diagnosis between this subtype and the commoner basal-celled epithelioma is more a matter of academic interest than of practical import. Briefly considered, it will depend upon the situation of the tumor, the period of formation, and the resemblances which the structure affords to that of the various phases shown in the evolution of the enamel organ. Unfortunately in this tumor the demonstration of branched cells, enamel cells or dentine is very uncertain. We do have, however, the presence of bone cysts and a clinical history not incompatible with a theory of dentinal origin.

On the other hand, we have a distinct picture of ingrowths from the oral mucosa. The conclusion is therefore admissible that like many other epitheliomatous growths there was more than one point of origin and that the basal cells of the oral mucosa later participated in the newgrowth.

SOME CASES OF SURGICAL SHOCK, WITH REMARKS.

By J. G. Earnest, *M.D.*,
Atlanta, Georgia.

WHAT is known to surgeons as shock pure and simple is generally conceded to be a reflex impression upon the nerve centres, caused by irritation of sensitive nerves, from wounds accidentally received, or as a part of necessary surgical operations resulting in paralysis of the vasomotor system. Mansell-Moulin tersely expressed the belief generally held when he said shock is an example of reflex paralysis in the strictest and narrowest sense of the term, a reflex inhibition affecting all the functions of the nervous system.

Recently this view has been questioned by gentlemen of acknowledged ability in the profession, notably by Dr. Eugene Boise, of Grand Rapids, who says: "When we regard surgical shock from the standpoint of the clinician, and when we reason from physiological facts which are beyond dispute as to the conditions which we see in shock, we are forced to the conclusion that the true pathology of uncomplicated shock is a hyperirritation (a spasm) of the entire sympathetic system."

As a matter of fact, when surgeons speak of shock as a result or complication of an operation, we are dealing with a condition where it is often difficult to say which plays the major part, the reflex influence transmitted through the nerves, the effect of the anesthetic on the nerve centres, or the loss of blood. The resulting condition, no doubt, in most cases being the outcome of the combination.

S Surg   33

I wish to cite a few cases illustrating some phases of this condition. The first seems a very marked case of shock from what would seem a most insignificant cause. A married woman, aged · thirty-five years, mother of three children, general health good, somewhat inclined to obesity, had a very small rectovaginal fistula.

It was just inside the sphincter, and as the vagina was relaxed there was no difficulty in bringing it into easy reach by simply introducing the finger into the rectum and bringing it to the mouth of the vulva. I proposed to divide the tissue between the membranes and surround it with a purse string suture, after Tate's method, which I explained to her would take only a few minutes. She preferred to stand the operation without any anesthetic or sedative. When I had been operating two or three minutes the nurse said to me, "She is not breathing." I asked about the pulse. She replied, "She has none." I at once abandoned the operation, found the pupils widely dilated, and no pulse or breathing that I could detect. Her head was immediately lowered, her hips elevated, and artificial respiration commenced. After four or five minutes she began to breathe, but very slowly and irregularly. The pulse was barely perceptible. One-sixth of a grain of morphine, with $\frac{1}{150}$ of atropine, was given hypodermically, while the nurse injected hot water into the rectum. In about thirty minutes the pupils began to respond slightly and the patient regained consciousness. The breathing and pulse were still bad, but improving slowly at the end of the first hour. It was more than two hours before I felt safe to leave her in the care of a nurse. On the following morning I found her up and dressed, with normal respiration and pulse. The fistule was closed, under ether, some months later, when she experienced nothing unusual. This seems to me an uncomplicated case of shock in which the patient would likely have died if she had not had prompt assistance, notwithstanding the apparently trivial nature of the exciting cause.

April 19, 1895, Mrs. H., aged twenty-seven years, had a section at the Grady Hospital for pyosalpinx, with cystic ovary of the left side. The appendages of the opposite side were normal. Her heart and kidneys were normal. The adhesions were not troublesome, and in ten minutes after opening the abdomen I was tying off the tube and ovary, when the anesthetist said to me, "She has no pulse." While the assistants were lowering the head and elevating the foot of the table I cut away the mass and, observing that she was not breathing, had artificial respiration immediately begun and a strong secondary current from an electric battery applied to the spine and over the heart. In the meantime I hurriedly closed the small opening in the abdomen with a few through and through stitches. This was at 2.30 P.M. From that time until 11 P.M. she breathed only by artificial respiration and her heart beat only when under the stimulus of electricity. She had hypodermic injections of strychnine and atropine. The rectum was injected with saline solution, I believe we got some benefit from the inhalation of oxygen gas. I used no saline infusions, for the reason that the hemorrhage seemed so insignificant it was of minor importance. Her life was so unquestionably saved mainly by the persistent use of artificial respiration and electricity for a period of eight hours and a half. At eleven o'clock she suddenly sighed, like a child after a crying spell, and then began slowly to breathe and her heart to act. In ten minutes after that she had a fairly good pulse and nearly normal respiration. Just how much the anesthetic had to do with this condition it is difficult to say, but from the length of time it lasted I am inclined to believe it was due almost entirely to shock, and the anesthetic probably played an insignificant part only. One thing this case impressed upon me was that a suitable battery should be a part of the furniture of every operating room, and it should always be ready for immediate use. This case certainly could not have been saved without the battery. The fact that in the first case recited the pupils were widely dilated and failed to respond in the slightest degree to the influence of light, and there had been no anesthetic or drug of any kind used, seems a strong point in favor of reflex paralysis rather than reflex spasm. As to the treatment, I believe that morphine is the most important remedy at the beginning, whether we believe in the theory of spasm or paralysis, as it is within proper limits a powerful stimulant to the heart and at the same time relieves the excessive nerve conductility, which probably plays an important part in these cases. The patient should be placed in Trendelenburg position and artificial respiration begun at once; at the same time a moderately strong faradic current of electricity should be turned on, applying one electrode (of not less than two inches in diameter) over the spine opposite the lowest point of the shoulder blades, while the other electrode is applied directly over the heart. The strength of the current and length of time necessary to keep up the application, of course, must be determined for each individual case. Saline infusion is indicated in nearly all cases, and, if there has been serious hemorrhage, is of paramount importance as soon as there is sufficient circulation to insure its absorption. Atropine and strychnine are valuable aids.

We hear occasionally of cases of delayed shock, and before closing the subject I will relate a case that possibly belongs to that class. I at least have been disposed to so class it, mainly on account of the fact that I could never account for it on any other theory. The patient, a married woman, aged thirty-three years, one child, six years old. On October 19, 1904, I made an abdominal section at the Halcyon Sanitarium for the removal of a cyst of the left ovary, two inches in diameter. The operation was simple, no complications. The patient rallied promptly and had a good night. At nine o'clock next morning I was called, and the nurse informed me that the patient had suddenly developed symptoms of internal hemorrhage. I found her temperature subnormal; skin cold and clammy; pulse, 140. My first impulse was to open the abdomen at once. After a little reflection, I could not believe that there could be any hemorrhage from so small a pedicle tied with the utmost care. So I decided to wait. After free use of strychnine and other stimulants for several hours, with no improvement but growing rather worse, I opened the abdomen and found the ligatutes intact and no bleeding. There was no improvement for twenty-four hours. She then began gradually to pull up, and made a good recovery. If this was a case of delayed shock, it was the only one I have ever seen. I have suspected that cases reported as shock coming on several hours after operation are generally cases of internal hemorrhage.

AN UNUSUAL TYPE OF BLADDER TUMOR.

By Robert C. Bryan, M.D.,
Richmond, Virginia.

The case which the writer wishes to record briefly is that of a cavernous angioma of the bladder. Angiomata of the mucous membranes, except in the larynx, rectum, and tongue, are markedly uncommon, but few instances having been noted.

In the indexed catalogue and case reports at the United States Army Medical Museum, Washington, no such condition has been reported, nor has the writer been able to find any reference to vesical angiomata other than that of Albarran, "Tumeurs de la vessie," Paris, 1891; Langhans, Virchow's *Archiv*, 1879, lxxv, 291.

Tumors of the bladder constitute less than 1 per cent. of all neoplasms. By far the larger majority are epithelial in origin, which, starting as papilloma, or, as it is called by Virchow, "papillary fibroma," may later undergo malignant change. As is known, men are much more frequently attacked by tumors of the bladder than are women, which are in 40 per cent. (Hurry Fenwick) of all cases multiple. And further, vesical growths are more frequently found about the base and ureteral outlets than in other parts of the bladder. Senn, in his *Pathology and Treatment of Tumors*, says: "Cavernous angiomas are found essentially in the deep connective tissue of the bones, liver, spleen, and kidney, and are composed of a tissue almost identical with that of the corpus cavernosum penis, that is, of irregular blood spaces connecting freely with one another and separated by fibrous septa of variable thicknesses."

This is of great developmental interest; the proximity of the bladder to the corpora cavernosa suggests an embryological misplacement which may be worthy of consideration as an etiological factor of the unusual location of the tumor in this instance.

Mr. O. B. S., aged thirty-five years, single, contractor, presented himself on July 13, 1909, for an intermittent hematuria. The patient denies absolutely, and shows no evidence of, a venereal infection. He is a big, muscular, healthy-looking man, who now appears somewhat run down and anemic. Other than an attack of typhoid fever sixteen years ago, he has never had an illness of any consequence, and has always enjoyed the very best of health. The heart, liver, and lungs are normal, nor can any abnormality be found.

Four years ago he had a severe attack of pain in the right side, which radiated toward the right knee and testicle. There was vomiting and considerable prostration at the time. A physician who was called in pronounced it appendicitis, and advised operation. The condition, however, cleared up in a few days, and aside from a little soreness about the neck of the bladder, the patient considered himself quite well, until one year later, when there was another such attack of colicky pain in the right side. On this occasion a small dark brown stone the size of a grain of wheat was voided; no blood, however, was noticed in the urine, and again in a few days he enjoyed his usual good health. Five months later he had another seizure of pain in the same place. No stone was passed, nor was there any passage of blood. The patient was confined to the house only for a day on this occasion, but was influenced to try a water-cure treatment at a sanatorium. Here he was much benefited, gaining in weight and spirits. During the last two years he has had no severe attack of pain, but feels constantly a soreness in the right side, which is uninfluenced by exercise, posture, or excesses. For the last twelve months, at varying, irregular, and unsuspected intervals, he has noticed blood in the urine, which is usually mixed in with the urine, of a dark-brown coffee color, and absolutely painless on passage.

From July 9 to 13 it has been constantly present. From July 13 to 17 the urine would be clear in the morning, only to cloud up during the day, at times becoming a dark or tarry red. It was now that he was referred to the writer by Dr. E. C. Fisher, of Richmond, Va., under whose care he has been for only a short while.

Examination. Urinalyses were repeatedly made. Nothing suggestive was ever found, blood constituted the bulk of the sediment. In the absence of significant epithelia no definite opinion could be ventured. The prostate was normal. A stone searcher was carefully used, with a negative result. An *x*-ray picture of the right pelvis and ureter and of the bladder showed nothing. The right kidney was palpable to the second degree, but not enlarged or painful. The left kidney could not be palpated. Deep pressure over the region of the appendix was uncomfortable, though not painful. The urethra was normal and of a medium caliber. The bladder held twenty ounces. The cystoscope showed the right ureteral mouth rather small and somewhat congested, the *right bladder field* normal and the mucosa healthy. The left ureteral mouth larger than the right, and somewhat pouting. The *left bladder field* showed a broad sessile tumor of a dark red color, situated well up in the fundus, upon the posterior wall and a little to the left of the mesial line. It appeared to be about the size of the thumb nail and projected into the cavity of the bladder to a slight degree. The left ureter was catheterized; the specimen, however, failed to show any significant cellular elements. The tumor was supposed to be a papilloma.

On July 22, by suprapubic cystostomy, the tumor was located with difficulty, owing to the collapsed condition of the bladder. With serrated scissors it was carefully dissected out of the mucosa, the base was thoroughly seared with the

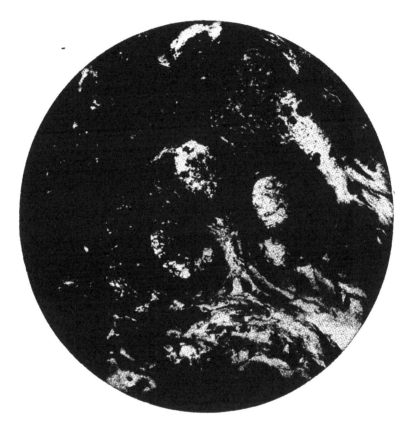

FIG. 1.—A cavernous angioma of bladder tumor.

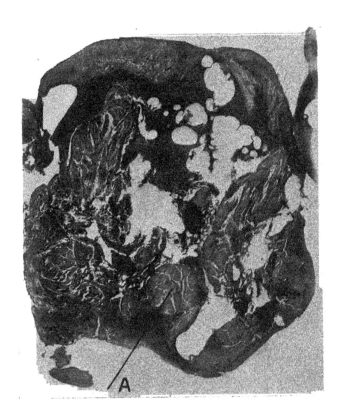

FIG. 2.—A cavernous angioma of bladder tumor.

Paquelin cautery, the free edges of the mucous membrane were now stitched together with catgut, the bladder sewed to the abdominal wall, and drainage established. There was little hemorrhage, the patient reacted well, and made a good recovery.

The tumor measured about three-eighths of an inch in diameter, and was pronounced by Dr. E. G. Hopkins, Pathologist of the Virginia Hospital, to be a cavernous angioma.

A review of the history would lead us to believe that this patient had two coincident lesions. The passage of the stone along the ureter, possibly to where that tube crosses the iliac artery, was responsible for the first attack of pain, the so-called appendicitis; the excursion into the bladder and its expulsion one year later explain the second. The third seizure of pain in the right iliac fossa, which was unaccompanied by either stone or hematuria, may be considered as an attack of appendicitis or as a ureteral diverticulitis.

The hemorrhage in the last two years has been caused by the angioma, which, doubtless of congenital origin, would have lain dormant and given rise to no hematuria had not the stone excited the walls of the bladder to violent and unusual muscular effort.

THE CANCER PROBLEM

By Roswell Park, M.D.,
Buffalo, New York.

I HAVE always had a feeling of pride in being a member of this Association, and that feeling is very much enhanced today in enjoying the privilege of participating in your work.

I regret very much that Dr. Coley is not here to consider the subject which was assigned to him, because what I shall say to you with reference to cancer will be said practically impromptu; but it is such a very important subject that I hope that what is said may provoke some discussion.

This problem of cancer is the most important one before the medical as well as the surgical profession today. Cancer is certainly on the increase, not only as a disease of modern life, but from other and mysterious causes, and I believe the statistics collected from all over the world establish this fact. In New York State we lose about thirteen thousand people from tuberculosis every year. When I began to especially study this disease there were some fourteen thousand deaths each year from tuberculosis, and about five thousand deaths from cancer. From tuberculosis the mortality has now been reduced to about eleven or twelve thousand per year, while the mortality from cancer has risen to nearly eight thousand. This is not attributable to faulty methods of diagnosis alone.

Our studies have also established the fact that cancer is prevalent in certain localities and in certain houses. A few years ago we made a map of the city of Buffalo, the like of which has been attempted in only one or two other places in the world, in which all houses where the disease had occurred within ten years were marked, and we established the fact that there were certain places where cancer was far more prevalent than in others, and we noted a considerable number of houses in which several deaths from cancer had taken place.

With regard to the matter of heredity, I think it can be stated as a fact that the disease *itself* is not transmitted by inheritance, but I am quite sure that there is a possibility of transmission of predisposition. This is a very important question, not only for the laity but for physicians. For instance, a woman suffering from cancer will come to you and ask if her daughter is likely to have it. And again the daughter, whose mother has had cancer, will come to you and ask if she is likely to have it because her mother had it. Let us suppose the case of a mother who bears a daughter at the age of twenty-five. When the mother is fifty years old and has cancer of the breast is there any reason for the daughter to fear that she is likely to have that disease? I think perhaps there is, *but simply because of the liability of the transmission of a predisposition.* It is not possible to inherit disease which was not present when the individual was born.

With regard to the infectious nature of cancer, when I began to teach the doctrine in this country, some twenty years ago, I was smiled at everywhere, and found very few friends of that theory either here or abroad. Yet now the infectivity of cancer is quite generally established. Last year at the meeting of the International Society of Surgeons, held in Brussels, this question was under discussion for three days, and of some three hundred surgeons present out of a membership of six hundred, I found a large majority in attendance there believed in the infectivity of cancer, although there are naturally still some doubters. By that theory it is just as easy to explain all the phenomena of

cancer as it is by any other. It is proved every day by
clinical evidence. What stronger evidence can there be
than the numerous instances of cancer following the use
of the knife or trocar? Numerous instances have occurred
in tapping for ascites due to intra-abdominal cancer, and
it has been subsequently found that a track or streak of
cancerous tissue follows the path of the trocar. What
other inference can one draw except that of infectious character of the fluid which leaks out or oozes along the path
of the instrument? That has been noted by numerous
observers and many times in my own experience. It is
known to follow the knife as well, and we have more and
more frequently noted instances of rapid dissemination
of cancer after the removal of a small piece of tissue for
microscopic examination. I think it can be shown that
this is a dangerous procedure unless the microscopic
examination is completed within a few moments after the
removal of the section and the operation made practically
continuous with the examination. How else can you explain
contact infection? And such contact infection can be
seen in almost every case of intra-abdominal cancer, as
well as intrathoracic cancer. How else can it be explained
except as an autoinoculation? How else can you explain
cases of malignant ovarian cysts, papillomata or dermoids,
with infection of every bit of peritoneal surface which has
come in contact with the disease, the infection leading to
adhesions or to the development of papillomatous or carcinomatous outgrowths at thousands of points on the interior
of the peritoneum? How else are you to explain the rapid
dissemination of cancer after incomplete operations, as
every one of you has seen? How else explain the phenomenon of metastasis? Is there any other disease, known
to pathologists anywhere, characterized by metastasis as
is cancer, in which you are not profoundly impressed by
the very fact that metastasis furnishes the most indisputable
proof of the infectiousness of the disease? The very fact

that metastases occur during cancer is the best demonstration of its infectivity, and for me every instance of metastasis in a given case is an expression of a reinfection from the original source. If that does not mean that it is an infectious disease, what does it mean? You cannot explain it on any cell theory except the distribution of the *contagium vivum,* or whatever you would like to call it, from the original source and its distribution all over the body. How else can you explain the horrible phenomena of malignancy, such as the general dissemination of medullary carcinomata or sarcomata as you may witness in serious cases?

What shall be said about the influence of trauma in connection with the theory of the infectivity of cancer? It may be that there is a predisposing cause; or it may be that it opens up pathways or ports of entry for infection just as it does in tuberculosis. I think whatever we may say with regard to the relation between trauma and tuberculous disease, we may say as to relations between trauma and carcinoma.

What about the results of inoculation? Well, they are extremely successful, particularly in certain animals, but we have found so far scarcely any exception to this fact that the transmission must be between animals of the same species. Here has been the great excuse for those men who do not wish to believe in the contagiousness of cancer. In our laboratory in Buffalo thousands and thousands of instances in small animals have been furnished, and recently in fish we are seeing these same evidences, and they have been reinforced by many thousands of instances in the other laboratories of the world. The great trouble is that, cancer being transmissible only between animals of the same species, we are not at liberty to make experimentation in our own race. But that which we are not at liberty to do intentionally is done for us constantly in operations where knife or contact infection follows. It is done by accident. It is done by the ordinary process of disease.

It is done many times unintentionally, and we see the same results. Nobody makes experiments deliberately, nor publishes his work showing that cancer can be transmitted from animals to man, nor from man to man, and here is where I make a plea for the scientific use of criminals for the purpose of legitimate investigation. There are a certain number of individuals who are worthless, who are useless, who are antagonistic to society, who have no proper purpose in this life, but who might be made useful under proper rulings of the courts. Under suitable precaution if they could be made available for purpose of investigation, I feel confident that experiments on individuals of this class would be followed by startling revelations, and it is the only way by which I can see that some of these criminals can ever be made in the slightest degree useful to mankind.

The contagiousness of cancer is no longer uncertain. We have far more proof for its contagiousness than we have for that of leprosy, or some of the other diseases that are considered more or less contagious. But this is certainly true of leprosy. There is not one one-hundredth part the danger attending leprosy that attends cancer. But we are met with the statement that the infectious organism of cancer is not yet known. That is true. But neither is it in rabies, neither is it in scarlatina, nor many other diseases whose contagious or infectious nature we do not hesitate to accept. It is no argument to say that it is not yet identified. We know it by its results, although we do not yet recognize it face to face.

Now the problem of attack upon cancer from the practical side, as it were, is, of course, of scarcely lesser importance than its pathology. But in order to make the attack effective we must make an early diagnoses. What shall be said about the early diagnosis of cancer? It is most difficult, undoubtedly, in many instances impossible. Under every means of investigation and exploration the diagnosis is sometimes impossible. Why is that true? Is it our fault?

Here is a question the laity put to us very often; they say, "Why are you unable to recognize this disease?" The answer is found in this, and it is surprising that it has not been more generally recognized, for so far as I know, except in my own work, there is scarcely any allusion to it in English literature; yet it is a fact, namely, that *cancer as such has no distinct symptomatology.* That is not our fault. It is our misfortune that it has not a distinct symptomatology of its own. When you can *feel* it you may recognize it, but there is not one *symptom* produced by cancer, either early or late, which may not be produced by some other disease. Therein we find our excuse for failure to recognize it early, and therein we find our difficulty in coping with it. The more you think of this statement the more it will impress itself upon you, and the more anxious you will become to get nearer some early symptomatology. Possibly Dr. Crile has come as near to it as any one yet with his studies of hemolyses, yet these are not absolutely reliable nor available, because such work requires technique and skill of the highest order.

There are a few words I would like to say in regard to the possibility of cure of carcinoma or cancer in general. As yet the knife is the only remedy in the hands of the profession generally which offers any certainty, and not even that unless we get at these cases relatively very early.

Here is a general thesis which I think you will accept: *If* cancer could be early diagnosticated or recognized, *if* it were accessible to our present means of attack, and *if* it were thoroughly removed, it could be cured; but there are *"ifs"* standing out in tremendous proportion and they are now apparently insuperable. We often cannot recognize it early; it is not always in an assailable position, nor is it possible to make a radical removal, which should be made in order to cure it; and yet when these conditions can be fulfilled then the disease is curable, but it will require that we get at the disease much earlier than we do at present.

Delay in operating on these cases is partly the fault of the patient and partly the fault of the profession. It is a horrible reproach to our profession that some of its members make excuses for putting off operations on these cases when early operative interference would do much for many of them. Some members of our profession rather encourage delay for the purpose of an alleged study which is futile. They encourage delay at a time when action is most desirable. What we need to do is to ourselves practise, and then preach by precept and example the earliest possible attack upon cancer. A well-founded suspicion of internal cancer justifies the earliest possible exploration for its recognition, while such exploration should be followed by radical operation if it be possible to make it. It is a sad mistake to take a case of suspected cancer of the stomach and test it for weeks, and treat it for months, until all hope of doing good has passed. We should impress the desirability of an early exploratory operation, and no man should be trusted to do this unless he is both prepared and competent to go on with the work and make a radical removal at the same time if indicated or permissible. In other words, in every case in which there is a suspicion of cancer an exploration should be made at once, and no time should be lost or wasted in the use of drugs. I think it may be generally stated at an early date whether an operation should be done or not. That certainly is true of cases of uterine cancer, of cancer of the tongue or the rectum, and of many other organs, and in fact this statement should be broad and general enough to cover every instance. If doubt arise as to what one ought to do it is practically too late to do anything, except to make a palliative operation. That may be worth while, but it is mighty late and it is usually too late to offer a prospect or promise of cure.

What can be done with non-operative measures, such as are held out by quacks and charlatans, and undoubtedly by a few honest men? I do not know whether there really is much or anything in the so-called Alexander treatment, or in methods of that kind, but we read of selected and occasional instances in which apparently good has been done. I believe there is such a thing as the spontaneous retrocession of malignant growths. They cure themselves, but I do not think that this occurs once in several hundred cases. It is barely possible that in the administration of some non-operative remedy, spontaneous relief in a way may follow, but x-rays, for example, rarely cure in those cases where operation ought to be thought of first. Just as a practical hint in connection with the use of the cathode rays, I will say that their efficacy can be enhanced by the use of the thyroid extract. In other words, we get better effects by giving the thyroid extract internally while using the cathode rays than by the latter alone.

I know that what I have said without time for preparation has formed a desultory presentation of this most important subject, but I simply wanted to put before you a few thoughts in reference to cancer, and am very much obliged to you all for the marked attention with which you have listened to me.

EXSTROPHY OF BLADDER: MAYDL OPERATION.

By HORACE J. WHITACRE, B.S., *M.D.*,
Cincinnati, Ohio.

EXSTROPHY of the bladder is a distressing congenital deformity, which occurs infrequently and must be treated surgically.

I wish to report the case of a young woman, aged twenty-one years, who was operated upon successfully one year and seven months ago by the method devised by Maydl, and who has remained well up to the present time.

Case Report. C. T., female, aged twenty-one years, single. Was admitted to Christ Hospital May, 1908.

The family history of this patient was entirely negative. There has been no congenital defects in any other member of the family. Patient has suffered from the ordinary diseases of childhood. Had diphtheria at the age of five, otherwise has always been strong and healthy. She began to menstruate at the age of thirteen, and this function has always been normal and regular. The present deformity has existed since her birth.

Physical examination reveals an unusually healthy, robust-looking girl five feet seven inches tall and well developed, a rather handsome girl. There is no abnormality except in region of the bladder. The pelvis is broad and the symphysis pubis is separated for an interval of at least four inches. In this interval between the pubic bones the urethra is completely cleft and appears as a groove lined with mucosa. This groove is continued upward into a globular mucous membrane tumor about three inches in diameter. This tumor projects at least two inches above the surface of the abdomen and is covered by mucous membrane, which represents the posterior wall of the bladder. At the base of the tumor the mucous membrane is fused into the skin of the abdomen along a rather sharp line. In the lower portion of this tumor the ureteral openings are plainly seen and constantly discharged clear urine. The mucous membrane covering the bulging mass is much reddened, secretes mucus abundantly, and bleeds easily. The clitoris is entirely absent and the labia are rudimentary. The vaginal outlet appears as a puckered, contracted aperture just below the urethral groove, and seems directed more forward than downward. The perineum and anus are normal, and vaginal examination reveals a normal vagina, cervix, uterus, tubes, and ovaries. When the patient is in the dorsal or in the Trendelenburg position the bulging tumor mass is reduced and remains inside the abdominal cavity, leaving a corresponding cleft or aperture between the recti muscles. Rectal examination reveals no abnormalities.

Operation, May 21, 1908. Nitrous oxide ether anesthesia. Time of operation, one hour and forty-five minutes. Nine ounces of ether used. The surface of bladder was very thoroughly cleansed, particularly at the ureteral openings, and a ureteral catheter was passed into each ureter. The bladder was then dissected away from the underlying tissue down to the trigone, where an area of mucous membrane about one and one-half inches square, or perhaps more nearly in the shape of an ellipse, was left intact. This area included both ureteral openings. This segment of the base of the bladder was then dissected up from below and the ureters sufficiently exposed to give the necessary mobility. The abdominal cavity was then opened low down and the sigmoid flexure brought into the wound. The gut was grasped in a gastro-enterostomy clamp and thoroughly protected by gauze sponges. The ureter bearing segment of the bladder was then placed alongside the sigmoid and a preliminary continuous silk suture used to unite the outer connective tissue portion of the wall of the bladder to the peritoneum of the gut. A sufficient incision was then made in the gut and a continuous chromic gut suture was passed through all coats of the gut and of the bladder in a manner entirely analagous to that used in making a lateral anastomosis of the hollow viscera. This row of sutures was continued entirely around the fragment of the bladder and the opening into the bowel, so that the mucous surfaces of the bladder bearing the ureters become continuous with the lining mucosa of the sigmoid. The ureteral catheters which had up to this time kept the field clear from urine were removed just before the mucous membrane was turned in. The preliminary reinforcing suture of silk was now continued anteriorly around the first line of suture. The peritoneal cavity was then closed down to the point of anastomosis and the defect in the abdominal muscles closed over as completely as possible. An opening below, the size of a fifty cent piece, was left and packed with gauze. A rubber tube was inserted into the rectum and allowed to remain for the purpose of carrying off urine and gases.

The patient endured the operation well and reacted promptly. The amount of urine secreted appeared to be normal. The rectum was washed out daily with normal salt solution. On the eighth day the rectal tube was removed. The urine gave very little or no irritation and was passed about every six hours. The stools were usually soft and fluid. The patient left the hospital twenty-three days after operation with the wound entirely healed, and there was no tendency to hernia. On December 1, 1909, I communicated with this young woman, who states that she has been and now is in good health. She has some pain in the back, which is associated with menstrual irregularity, but never has fever. There is no irritation of the rectum by the urine. The urine has been discharged every two or three hours lately, but I would judge from her letter that this frequency is exceptional. There is sometimes an escape of urine involuntarily.

The best result that can be obtained by plastic operations in the treatment of exstrophy of the bladder is to construct a cavity which will at the best hold 100 c.c. of urine. It is impossible to get retention in such a cavity, however, and all such operations have been abandoned.

The only operations which may be considered are those which divert the urine into the bowel and utilize the sphincter ani for retention.

Simon, in 1851, first directed the urine into the rectum, basing the operation upon the facts that in many animals there is a cloaca, that the ureters are sometimes found at birth opening into the rectum, and that those patients who have developed fistulæ between the bladder and rectum learn in time to control more or less perfectly the discharge of urine from the anus.

Thiersch, in 1881, established a permanent connection between the bladder and rectum.

It was observed, however, that the implantation of the divided ureters into the rectum was promptly followed by infection of the kidneys, and Maydl conceived the idea of avoiding ascending infection by preserving the normal vesical opening of the ureter. After previous experimentation upon animals he first performed his operation on man in 1892.

Enderlen has calculated a mortality of 25 per cent. in 110 cases. These deaths have been due to shock, peritonitis, chloroform, and pyelonephritis. The largest percentage of deaths have been from pyelonephritis.

This operation gives a satisfactory cure for the distressing symptoms of constant dribbling of urine, the rectum is practically always tolerant, and the sphincter ani is usually efficient in retaining the accumulated urine for three to eight hours. The operation would be quite satisfactory were it not for the dangers of the operation and the danger of ascending infection of the kidney.   The dangers of operation are (1) the anesthetic, (2) peritonitis, (3) shock, (4) persistent urinary and fecal fistula.

The question of anesthesia need not be discussed.   The dangers of peritonitis arising from the opening of the peritoneal cavity have been very greatly reduced with the perfection of the operation.   The important features of this development have been more careful preparation of patients, improved asepsis, the omission of drainage, the dropping back of the spot of suture, and closing up fully except perhaps for a gauze wick.   Maydl gives the warning to cut widely in removing the piece of bladder wall in order to preserve its nutrition.   The danger of a urinary and fecal fistula has been greatly reduced by attention to this point and by the omission of packing.   The dangers from shock can be greatly reduced by performing the operation in two stages.   The transplantation can be done at one operation and the excision of the bladder mucosa and other plastic work at a later date.

The operation of Maydl was suggested as a means of avoiding the ascending infection which is almost certain to follow the implantation of the divided ureters.   It has certainly succeeded in reducing greatly this danger, but the danger still remains.

Ewald[1] in discussing the postoperative dangers of kidney infection, states that we should not lose sight of the facts (1) that many patients die from such infection without operation, (2) that many patients probably have had a beginning infection at the time of operation, and (3) that older individuals because of the exposed state of the mucosa suffer from ulceration and scar formation in the region of the ureteral openings, which cause an interference with the closure of the opening.

Lendon, of Adelaide Hospital, Australia, first performed, in 1899, an extraperitoneal operation in which both ureters

[1] Wiener med. Woch., 1909, No. 2.

were transplanted into the rectum. Peters, of Toronto, two months later, did practically the same operation on a boy aged five and one-half years.

In this operation a button or rosette of mucosa immediately surrounding each ureteral opening is outlined and the ureter dissected out for a short distance. An extraperitoneal blunt dissection is then made backward to the region of the rectum, a blunt instrument is forced through the rectal wall from the rectum on each side, and the mucous button is seized by this forceps and drawn into the bowel. This much simplified operation bids fair to replace the Maydl operation, but the danger of pyelonephritis still remains. Time limitations do not permit of a discussion of the relative merits of these operations.

The general conclusion of the author, as based upon personal experience and an incomplete review of the literature on exstrophy of the bladder, would be that the operative treatment is fully justified, notwithstanding the danger of kidney infection, that either the Maydl or the Lendon-Peters operation should be performed, and that functional results are excellent.

THE INCREASE OF CANCER.

By WILLIAM B. COLEY, M.D.,
New York.

IT is a remarkable fact that a disease so widely prevalent as cancer and one that has from time immemorial held first place in the amount of suffering that it inflicts upon its victims, and is now approaching front rank in the number of those victims, should have received such meagre attention from both local and national boards of health. Antituberculosis leagues have become universal, government boards of health and scientific medical bodies all over the world have long since instituted a well-organized campaign against the white plague, with results that even now justify the hope of speedy control with the possibility of ultimate conquest. While much has been written upon the question of the increase of cancer, many of the papers have been attempts to explain away the figures of the vital statistics, which in every civilized land during the last half century have shown a steady increase in the number of deaths from cancer.

The purpose of the present paper is to go over the evidence at present at our command, in the hope of arriving at some conclusion as to whether cancer is increasing or not.

Roger Williams, in his recent book on the *Natural History of Cancer,* states that the disease has doubled in frequency in periods ranging from twenty to thirty years, the annual increase averaging from 3 to 5 per cent.

Williams refers to the unique statistical study of cancer made by Ekblom (*Hygeia,* January, 1902) for the small Swedish town of Fellingsbro. Taking the average for the first and last decennial periods of the century, he showed that the cancer death rate increased from 2.1 per 100,000 living in the former period, to 118 living in the latter.

The only statistics in Great Britain which compare with these statistics as regards the period of observation, are those of the Scottish Widows' Life Insurance Fund (Edinburgh, 1902). The records of this Fund show the proportion of deaths due to cancer to the total mortality among males since 1815:

	Per cent.
1815 to 1844	0.93
1845 to 1858	1.79
1859 to 1866	3.00
1867 to 1873	4.56
1874 to 1880	4.93
1881 to 1887	5.44
1888 to 1894	6.88

PERCENTUM RATIO OF DEATHS FROM CANCER TO TOTAL DEATHS.
EXPERIENCE OF ÆTNA LIFE INSURANCE COMPANY OF
HARTFORD FROM 1870 TO 1906.
(For which I am greatly indebted to Dr. E. I. McKnight
and Dr. E. A. Wells, of Hartford, Conn.).

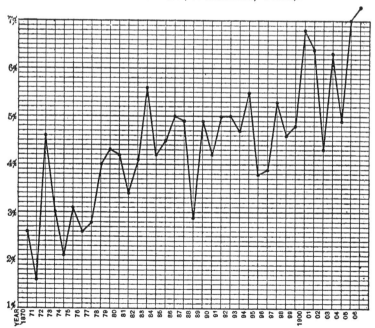

Year.	Total deaths.	Deaths from cancer.	Per cent.
1870	426	11	2.6
1871	432	7	1.6
1872	486	8	4.6
1873	579	18	3.1
1874	474	10	2.1
1875	527	16	3.0
1876	536	14	2.6
1877	544	15	2.8
1878	502	20	4.0
1879	532	23	4.3
1880	542	23	4.2
1881	593	20	3.4
1882	565	23	4.1
1883	656	37	5.6
1884	645	27	4.2
1885	667	30	4.5
1886	715	36	5.0
1887	719	34	4.9
1888	783	23	2.9
1889	761	37	4.9
1890	817	34	4.2
1891	897	45	5.0
1892	1019	51	5.0
1893	1013	48	4.7
1894	956	53	5.5
1895	1052	40	3.8
1896	1029	40	3.9
1897	1044	55	5.3
1898	1051	48	4.6
1899	1114	54	4.8
1900	1215	83	6.8
1901	1303	84	6.4
1902	1267	55	4.3
1903	1386	87	6.3
1904	1432	70	4.9
1905	1388	97	7.0
1906	1514	111	7.3

The records of the German Life Insurance Company strikingly confirm the foregoing figures. The cancer mortality among males from 1885 to 1889 amounted to 3.7 per cent. of the total deaths, and among females to 11.4 per cent.; from 1889 to 1895, however, the ratio was 11.4 for men and 12.9 for women.

In England and Wales the later statistics have separated the rural population from the urban. The cancer rate in the rural districts seems to have suffered much less than in the urban. Considerable difficulty, however, results from the fact that a number of rural cases of cancer go to the city for

operation, thus adding to the mortality of the urban population by at least the number of such cancer patients as die

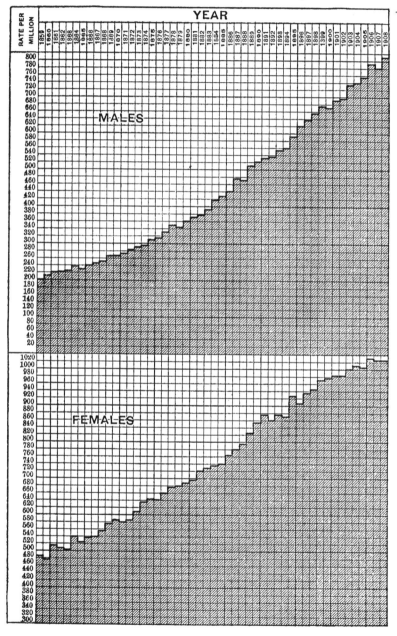

Increase of cancer in England and Wales.   Report of Registrar-
General, 1908.

from operation. It is probable that the majority of patients who come to the city for operation and recover return to their respective homes, where they remain until death.

During the last six years, in England and Wales, 176,019 persons died of cancer. Of these, 104,418 were females and 71,601 males. Of 10,000 males dying of cancer, 2172 had cancer of the stomach; of 10,000 females, 2259 had cancer of the uterus. Of the males who died of cancer in this period, 43,092 died of cancer of the intestinal tract: Stomach, 15,553; intestine, 5439; rectum, 7277; esophagus, 4505; liver and gall bladder, 9328.

London, per 100,000: 1851 to 1860, 42; 1861 to 1870, 48; 1871 to 1880, 55; 1881 to 1890, 68; 1891 to 1900, 85; 1901 to 1904, 92.

Berlin, cancer and tumors: 1881 to 1885, 55; 1886 to 1890, 65; 1891 to 1895, 75; 1896 to 1900, 85.

Average for Ten Years, 1896 to 1905 per 1000 Living.

Switzerland	1.29
Netherlands	0.95
Norway	0.90
England, Wales	0.83
Scotland	0.81
German Empire	0.74
Victoria	0.72
Austria	0.70
New Zealand	0.63
Ireland	0.63
South Australia	0.61
Prussia	0.61
New South Wales	0.59
Tasmania	0.50
Italy	0.53
Queensland	0.50
Japan (average five years)	0.49
Spain (average six years)	0.44
Western Australia	0.38
Hungary (average seven years)	0.35
Servia	0.09
Ceylon	0.06

French statistics show that the increase has been general, and not an increase of obscure internal or abdominal cases that could be accounted for by increased accuracy in diagnosis.

France, Denmark, Sweden, and Bulgaria, causes of death tabulated for towns only.

CANCER DEATH RATES.

Among the places showing the lowest death rate from cancer in the State of New York are: Hudson, 36.8 per 100,000; Little Falls, 17.5 · per 100,000; Ithaca, 156 per 100,000; Johnstown, 115 per 100,000.

In New York City in 1908 the rate was 75.4 per 100,000.

The difference in the different boroughs of New York is noteworthy:

In the borough of the Bronx the rate is highest, being 95.8; it is lowest in Queens, namely, 68 per 100,000.

The mortality of the white and colored population, under the same conditions, in New York City is practically the same, viz., 75.4 white; and 71.8 colored.

The death rate of the colored population shows most extraordinary differences in the different boroughs: In Manhattan borough it is 57.5 per 100.000; in Bronx, 244; in Richmond, 150.

It is very difficult to explain these differences, especially as the general cancer death rate throughout the South is distinctly lower in the colored race than in the white. It is also lower in New York City in general.

The marked, constant, and general increase in the death rate from malignant growths in the twenty-eight principal cities of the United States from 1883 to 1907 is clearly shown in a paper by Roy F. Edwards.[1] These 28 cities, in 1883, with a total population of 6,097,585, showed 2960 deaths, or a rate of 48.5 per 100,000 living. In 1895 the population of

[1] *Medical Record*, December 18, 1909.

these cities was 9,157,682, with 5377 deaths from cancer, or a rate of 58.7 per 100,000 population. In 1907, with a population of 12,524,695, there were 9686 deaths from cancer, or a rate of 77.3 per 100,000. Thus, in a period of twenty-four years the death rate increased from 48.5 to 77.3 per 100,000.

These figures were taken entirely from local bureaus of vital statistics. Actually, the death rate from cancer is far greater than the rate shown by the vital statistics, for the reason that there is prevalent among the laity a strong prejudice against the name cancer, the result being that in many cases of death from cancer, especially metastatic cancer with internal complications, the family physician, out of respect for this feeling on the part of the family, will assign some of the secondary causes in place of the actual primary cause of malignant disease.

The great extent to which this is true has recently been shown by Guilliot, of Reims, France, who made a careful comparative study of the number of cases certified to have died of cancer, and the actual number known to have died of cancer in a given locality in a given period of years, and found that the number who had actually died of cancer was exactly double the number certified to have so died.

American Average per 100,000 *Population.*

Cancer.	1900 to 1904.	1901.	1902.	1903.	1904.	1905.	1906.	1907.
Registration area . .	66.5	64.5	68.3	68.6	70.6	72.1		
Boston	89.6	88.2	87.5	93.2	95.7	105.6	100.1	104.6
Massachusetts . . .	83.0	82.0	86.7	85.0	86.3	92.9	90.3	93.5
San Francisco . . .	124.0	115.2	128.3	125.3	134.3	125.0		
Indiana	47.0	44.0	47.0	49.0	50.0	55.0	53.7	57.1
Vermont	81.0	70.0	69.0	93.7	87.0	84.2	85.3	99.0
New York City . .	68.5	69.0	66.0	69.5	71.4	72.0	74.0	76.8
New Haven . . .	..	..	..	79.4	71.9	92.4	83.3	100.5
Providence, R. I. . .	..	..	..	80.8	96.9	97.2	93.5	108.7

Registration area, 1900 36,846,981
Registration area, 1907 41,758,037
Estimated population, 1907. 85,532,761

Lowest Rates of Cities in the United States.

Louisville, Ky.	50.1
Paterson, N. J.	56.1
Detroit, Mich.	65.0

Highest Cities.

San Francisco	125.0
Boston	104.0
Providence	108.7
Lowest rates, Indiana, average 1901 to 1905 . .	49.5
Highest rates, Maine, average 1901 to 1905 . .	86.7

Deaths from cancer registration area in the United States for 1907 was 30,514, or 1494 more than in 1906, and a rate of 73.1 in 1907, compared with 70.8 in 1906. Estimated deaths from cancer in the United States for 1907 was 63,508.

"The crude death rates from cancer continue to increase, and slightly higher rates are recorded for each main subdivision of the registration area. For the year 1908, 33,465 deaths from this disease were returned, and the death rate was 74.3 per 100,000 of population, as compared with 30,514 deaths and a death rate of 73.1 for 1907."[1]

Schuster,[2] in his statistical study of carcinoma, shows the death rate from cancer between 1863 and 1867 to have been 7.14 per 10,000; from 1873 to 1877, 10.39; from 1893 to 1897, 12.21; from 1903 to 1907, 14.76.

According to K. Sato,[3] of 64,030 patients treated in Japanese hospitals, 1372, or 2.14 per cent., suffered from cancer. The proportions in which the various organs were affected are as follows: Uterus, 33.53; stomach, 32; intestines, 6.2; breast, 5.69; skin, 2.17; esophagus, 1.53 per cent.

Various attempts have been made from time to time, particularly by Newsholme and his followers, to question the reality of the increase of cancer. Some have declared it

---

[1] Department of Commerce and Labor, Bureau of the Census, 1908, Bulletin, No. 104.

[2] Zur Carcinom Frage, Bamberg, 1909.

[3] Gann, Results of Cancer Research in Japan, 1907.

due simply to the increase of population, but, as Williams has pointed out, while the population of Great Britain doubled between 1850 to 1905, the cancer mortality increased six times.

Another explanation of the increase of cancer which has been more widely accepted is, that during recent years, due to improved hygienic conditions, a larger number of people have reached mature life, or the cancer age, and for this reason a larger number would be affected by cancer. Williams' reply to this is that the saving of life in modern times has been almost entirely confined to the precancerous period, the death rates of males over thirty-five years and of females over forty-five years having remained almost stationary, while the proportion attaining old age has decreased.

The objection so strongly urged by Newsholme is that the increase of the cancer death rate is due chiefly to improved methods in diagnosis.

This objection was answered many years ago by Mitchell Banks, one of the most careful students of cancer in Great Britain, and a man of wide experience. Banks stated that while the diagnosis of cancer in its early stages is probably made much more frequently now than in former times, it required little skill to make the diagnosis at the time of the death of the patient. The diagnosis at such a time was by no means beyond the ability of even the rural practitioner of fifty years ago.

Williams further points out that the increase has been far too uniform and steadily progressive during this long succession of years to leave any basis for such an argument, and, taking the increase over the entire period, he believes it to be so enormous as to make the explanation seem far-fetched. While it is possible that improved methods in diagnosis may add slightly to the total cancer death rate, Williams points out that these very improvements in diagnosis may also cause subtractions from it, and he shows that in the report of the Registrar-General as late as 1880 such diseases as fibroid tumor, polypus, and lupus were usually classed as cancer. Since then these diseases, as well as a a number of other conditions at one time regarded as malignant, have been assigned to other causes.

A careful study of the whole subject shows the increase to be a general one and not limited to a few parts of the body. In other words, intra-abdominal or inacessible cancer, which would be the type most likely to be affected by improved methods of diagnosis, shows even less relative increase than external cancer. In 1868 the death rate for cancer of the stomach per 1,000,000 living, thirty-five years and upward, was 283.65 for males and 193.45 for females. In 1888 the rate had increased to 346.15 for males and 277.75 for females, making an increase of 22 per cent. for males and 44 per cent. for females; but in this particular period the death rate of cancer in general had increased 50 per cent.

The greater death rate of malignant disease in women is due to the large number of cases which occur in the breast and the uterus. In all other localities the liability in the male is much greater than in the female.

Cancer has already increased to such an extent that at the present date it causes more deaths among women than tuberculosis, in 1905 the rate being 100 cancer deaths to 94 from tuberculosis. Even taking men and women together, and at all ages, the death rate from cancer is rapidly approaching that of tuberculosis. From 1851 to 1860 the death rate per 1,000,000 living was 317 for cancer, 2676 for phthisis, and 807 for other tuberculous disease; while from 1891 to 1900 the rate was 754 for cancer, 1391 for phthisis, and 619 for other tuberculous diseases.

That the death rate of cancer is often much higher among the rich and well-to-do is shown by some of the Irish statistics. In prosperous Armagh the rate was 104, while in poverty-stricken Kerry it was as low as 26.

In Switzerland we have a low tuberculosis mortality, but an exceedingly high cancer death rate; and even here the rate is steadily increasing, having risen from 114 in 1889 to 132 per 100,000 living in 1898. Here two-thirds of the people are engaged in industrial and commercial work and only one third in agriculture.

Williams states there are no millionaires in Switzerland and no paupers; prosperity is more widely diffused than even in France.

In Denmark the mortality from cancer is 130 per 100,000 living, with a phthisis rate of 150.

In studying the statistics of France we have to consider that they are based entirely upon urban population, excluding the rural populace, thus covering only 12,000,000 out of a total of 39,000,000. The population of France has remained relatively more stationary than in most other countries of which statistics exist, and yet the death rate of cancer shows the same constant increase as elsewhere. In Paris the death rate of cancer in 1865 was 84; 1870, 91; 1880, 94; 1890, 108; 1900, 120.

The towns above 10,000 show, in 1887, 76; 1890, 91; 1895, 100; 1900, 106.

In Australia the death rate per 100,000 living has been as follows: In 1851, 14; 1861, 19; 1871, 25; 1881, 32; 1891, 45; 1901, 57.

The Australian statistics show a remarkable difference between the Australian-born and British and foreign population. Of the former, 58 in 100,000 living died of cancer, as against 137 of the British and foreign-born.

There is much difference of opinion as to the frequency of cancer in China, but there is no question that the Chinese in other parts of the world suffer severely from the disease. In 1900 the rate among Chinese in Australia was 72 in 100,000. On the other hand, among the Australian natives, i. e., the aborigines, which in 1891 numbered 60,000, cancer is very rare.

Medical men who have lived among the Pacific Islanders for many years state they have never seen a case of cancer.

In Ceylon and Java the cancer mortality is very low. This, however, may be partly explained by the fact that the death statistics are very incomplete, the causes of death in the large majority of cases not having been medically certified.

In nearly all the countries from which reliable returns have been obtained the cancer mortality has shown a general tendency to increase in recent years. On the other hand the statistics of tuberculosis show 56,841 deaths, or 6041 less than the average for ten years.

The cancer statistics of last year show 31,668 to have died of cancer in England and Wales, being 2882 more than the average for ten years, the male increase over the decennial average being 16 per cent., the female increase 6 per cent., making 794 deaths from cancer per 1,000,000 living males and 732 for females, both being the highest rates on record.

A careful analysis of the statistics of cancer that are obtainable at the present time forces one to the conclusion that there is a constant and considerable increase in the number of people afflicted with cancer in all civilized countries. How can we best explain this increase?

The pathologists together with the clinicians who accept Cohnheim's theory as the true explanation of the cause of cancer try to explain this increase of the cancer mortality by changes in the mode of living as compared with previous years. Many, like Roger Williams, believe that the increased consumption of nitrogenous food has much to do with the increase of cancer. Attempts have been made to show that it is more prevalent among the rich and well-to-do than among the poor and ill-fed. A careful study of the cancer statistics, however, does not fully bear out this assumption. Some of the districts in which the cancer mortality is the highest are rural districts, in which the people live in a very simple manner. Some writers attribute a high cancer mortality to luxurious living, especially to large consumption of meat and alcohol. This is hardly true, as the mortality of

Copenhagen, 138 per 100,000, is nearly double that of London, Paris, or New York.

My own feeling is that the most rational explanation is to assume that cancer is of extrinsic or microbic origin.

New evidence in favor of the endemic and, possibly, infectious nature of cancer, is found in a paper on "Cancer in New Zealand," by Hyslop and Fenwick.[1]

They state that although New Zealand has the lowest death rate for the world, there is, nevertheless, a persistent increase in the percentage of deaths from cancer. In the year 1898 the rate per 100,000 living was 64; in 1907 it was 73. The alimentary tract was the seat of invasion in the great majority of cases of both males and females. In males the stomach was the seat of the cancer in 32.5 per cent. of the total number; intestine and rectum, 10.8 per cent.; liver, 11.8 per cent. In the females: stomach, 21.9 per cent.; intestine and rectum, 12 per cent; liver, 16 per cent.

One of the writers collected 31 cases of cancer which had come under his personal observation in his own district, and found that of 16 male cases, 11 occurred in the bowel.

Dr. Hyslop describes at length the topography of the district in which his cases were observed—a flat tract, lying between a snow-fed river and a smaller stream. A large portion of the district is seasonally flooded by these streams, and the high mortality from cancer is in harmony with the conclusions of Haviland, based on a careful study of the geographical distribution of cancer.

It is of further interest to note that 6 of the 31 patients all lived in the same house. These 6 persons were all shepherds, agricultural laborers, or farmers, and they were not related by blood, thus entirely excluding the element of heredity.

As regards the habits of the patients, all drank tea with

[1] British Medical Journal, October 23, 1909.

their meals three times a day, and nearly all of them had meat three times a day.

The great variation in the death rate from cancer in the different parts of New Zealand is also interesting:

Dr. Britton who, at one time practised at Ross, on the West Coast, found from his note-books and death certificates that during a practice of three years he had 35 deaths. Of these, 20 were under nine years of age; the remaining 15 between ten and seventy-eight years; in 5 of these, or 33.3 per cent., death was due to cancer. While in his ten years' practice on the East Coast his records showed 71 deaths, only 1 of which was due to cancer.

CONCLUSIONS. A great mass of evidence, based upon vital statistics, shows a well-marked and steady increase in cancer in practically every civilized country.

Attempts to explain away this increase as an apparent and not a real increase are far from convincing.

Without any further increase the present death rate from cancer is appalling.

Furthermore, the actual death rate from cancer is much higher than the known rate, by reason of the fact that in many cases of patients dying from internal metastases the strong prejudice of the relatives against the name of cancer is respected by the family physician, and some secondary cause of death appears in the certificate, instead of the primary cause, cancer.

The object in pointing out the ravages of this disease is to awaken a more profound interest on the part of the laity as well as the profession in cancer problems. Physicians can help toward the solution of this problem by making a careful study of every case of cancer that comes under their observation, recording every fact. When collected in sufficient numbers, such facts may throw some light upon the etiology of the disease and help to settle the vexed questions of heredity and contagion.

The pathologists are already deeply interested in the

study of cancer, but the laboratory studies alone of cancerous tumors can never solve this great problem of the cause of cancer. The problem must be attacked from all sides— the clinical as well as the laboratory.

Once aroused to the importance of this problem the laity will lend its support by way of greatly increased endowments for cancer research work, and better and more efficient coöperation of State and National Boards of Health will follow.

BIBLIOGRAPHY.

Williams, Roger. Natural History of Cancer, 1909.

United States Census Reports, 1900 to 1908.

Reports of Registrar-General of Great Britain, 1900 to 1906.

Edwards, R. F. Medical Record, December 18, 1909.

Sato, K. Gann, Results of Cancer Research in Japan, 1907.

Bashford, E. T. Reports of Imperial Cancer Research Fund, 1908.

Lewin. Deutsch. med. Wochenschrift, April 22, 1909.

Hislop and Fenwick. Cancer in New Zealand, British Medical Journal, October 23, 1909, 1222.

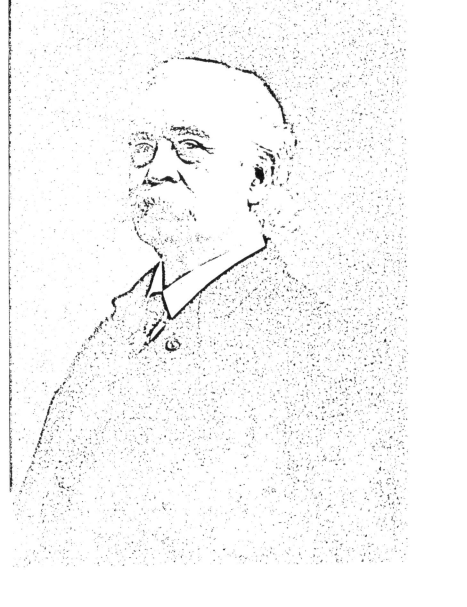

Faithfully,
Thad. H. Re

IN MEMORIAM.

THADDEUS A. REAMY.

By Robert Carothers, M.D.

On March 11, 1909, Dr. Thaddeus Asbury Reamy, of Cincinnati, an Honorary Member of the Southern Surgical and Gynecological Association, died, in his eightieth year, at the home of his niece, who is the wife of Dr. William Gillespie, of Cincinnati. He had been a sufferer for several years from arterial sclerosis and chronic interstitial nephritis, the diseases which ultimately caused his death.

He was born in Warren County, Virginia, about five miles from Fort Royal, April 28, 1829, his family being of French extraction. From a people of rough and rugged habits, of the agricultural class, living close to the soil, he acquired in his early childhood habits of industry and toil. His early education was what the little red schoolhouse, and afterward the nearby village, offered, which, when backed by vim and determination, wrested success from unpromising beginnings.

He graduated in medicine from Starling Medical College, Columbus, Ohio, in 1854. His first location was Chickenville, Licking County, Ohio, where he practised his profession, and also acted as striker for the village blacksmith as part payment for his board. He remained here only a short time, and then removed to Mt. Sterling, a village in Muskingum County, Ohio, where he did an active practice for some nine years, and then removed to Zanesville, Ohio, where he was actively engaged in medicine and surgery until he settled in Cincinnati, in 1871, where he remained until the time of his death.

In 1853, at Mt. Sterling, he married Miss Sarah Catallier, and during his residence there his only daughter and child was born. She married Dr. Giles Mitchell, of Cincinnati, but lived only a few years afterward. Though childless after the death of his only daughter, many of his nieces and nephews have received many benefits from him.

He served as a professor of materia medica and therapeutics for two sessions—1859 to 1861—in the Cincinnati College of Medicine and Surgery, at Cincinnati. He travelled each week from home to Cincinnati to deliver his lectures, and also attended to a large practice as well.

From 1863 to 1870 he was professor of puerperal diseases of women and diseases of infants in Starling Medical College, Columbus, Ohio. His attainments as a teacher and reputation as a practitioner seem to have travelled ahead, that he should have been called from a village and afterward a small city to these medical centres to assist in the training of future doctors.

In 1871, after taking up his residence in Cincinnati, he became professor of obstetrics and diseases of children in the Medical College of Ohio. He held this position until 1887, when he became professor of clinical gynecology in the same school (afterward the Medical Department of the University of Cincinnati), and remained in that position until he resigned in 1905.

During his career he held many hospital positions. He was obstetrician and gynecologist to the Good Samaritan Hospital of Cincinnati, 1871 to 1905; obstetrical and gynecological staff physician of the Cincinnati Hospital, 1882 to 1892; surgeon-in-charge of Reamy's Private Hospital for Women, Cincinnati, 1877 to 1898; consulting abdominal surgeon to Christ Hospital, Cincinnati, 1887 to 1905; consulting gynecologist to the Presbyterian Hospital, Cincinnati, 1893 to 1898.

Dr. Reamy was an enthusiastic and energetic medical society man. He was a member of the American Medical Association since 1858, and was chairman of the Section on Obstetrics and Diseases of Women in 1880. He joined the Ohio State Medical Society in 1855, and was president in 1871. In 1871 he became a member of the Cincinnati Academy of Medicine, and served as its president in 1877. In 1877 he founded the Cincinnati Obstetrical Society, which is still a prosperous organization, and was its president in 1884. He became a member of the American Gynecological Society in 1877; vice-president in 1881; a member of the council in 1883; and president in 1885. In 1890 he joined the Southern Surgical and Gynecological Society, and in 1902 was made, by request, an Honorary Member. He was also a member of the Medico-Chirurgical Society of Philadelphia, corresponding member of Boston Gynecological Society and Detroit Academy of Medicine.

In 1870 the Ohio Wesleyan University conferred upon him the honorary degree of Master of Arts, and in 1890 Cornell College, Iowa, conferred upon him the degree of LL.D

In summing up the goodness and greatness of Dr. Reamy, one hardly would know where to begin or end. Dr. Reamy was, above all things, a man, with all the virile and worthy attributes with which we imbue the highest type. He was a good citizen, a devoted husband, and a stanch and never-failing friend. He did love his friends, and would have hated his enemies if any there had been. He was a Christian man, a devout member of the Methodist Church, the pulpits of which he not infrequently occupied as a public speaker, with both pleasure and profit to his audiences, for his fund of information was great and his ability to impart it was supreme. He also was an orator. In the classroom, in the clinical amphitheatre, on the floor of the Society, in the pulpit, his words were from the silver-tongued orator. Stories were circulated among his acquaintances that once he was a minister and again a political speaker. I never heard that he was an actor, although he was.

Dr. Reamy also was a good surgeon. Although of a past generation, it was surprising with what ability he was able to adopt the innovations in the surgical field. His best work was done in obstetrics, in which department he was a master, and in his prime had no equal. As a teacher of obstetrics he made a profound impression, and during the sixteen years he held this chair in the old Medical College of Ohio the student body felt his enthusiasm, wisdom, and strength.

Dr. Reamy was an indefatigable worker, arising early and working late; a voluminous writer, a good teacher, a true, friend, a loving husband, a good citizen, and, above all, a great big, strong, handsome, manly man.

One time, after he had retired to his farm, near Cincinnati, some friends, who were driving in that neighborhood, wished to pay him a visit. In order to locate his farm, a passerby on the road was asked the way, and the answer was, "A mile ahead between a schoolhouse and a church, a road to the left will lead directly to Dr. Reamy's house." What a beautiful inscription on a tombstone for the man—"Between the schoolhouse and the church."

In Muskingum County, Ohio, they buried him with his fathers.

INDEX.

Lightning Source UK Ltd.
Milton Keynes UK
UKHW011838140219
337137UK00005BA/518/P